AF683785

FREE Study Skills DVD Offer

Dear Customer,

Thank you for your purchase from Mometrix! We consider it an honor and a privilege that you have purchased our product and we want to ensure your satisfaction.

As a way of showing our appreciation and to help us better serve you, we have developed a Study Skills DVD that we would like to give you for FREE. This DVD covers our *best practices* for getting ready for your exam, from how to use our study materials to how to best prepare for the day of the test.

All that we ask is that you email us with feedback that would describe your experience so far with our product. Good, bad, or indifferent, we want to know what you think!

To get your FREE Study Skills DVD, email freedvd@mometrix.com with *FREE STUDY SKILLS DVD* in the subject line and the following information in the body of the email:

- The name of the product you purchased.
- Your product rating on a scale of 1-5, with 5 being the highest rating.
- Your feedback. It can be long, short, or anything in between. We just want to know your impressions and experience so far with our product. (Good feedback might include how our study material met your needs and ways we might be able to make it even better. You could highlight features that you found helpful or features that you think we should add.)
- Your full name and shipping address where you would like us to send your free DVD.

If you have any questions or concerns, please don't hesitate to contact me directly.

Thanks again!

Sincerely,

Jay Willis
Vice President
jay.willis@mometrix.com
1-800-673-8175

Mometrix
TEST PREPARATION
The World's #1 Test Preparation Company

Maternal Newborn Nursing Exam SECRETS

Study Guide

Your Key to Exam Success

Mometrix TEST PREPARATION

Written and edited by the Mometrix Nursing Certification Test Team

Printed in the United States of America

This paper meets the requirements of ANSI/NISO Z39.48-1992 (Permanence of Paper).

Paperback
ISBN 13: 978-1-62120-168-7
ISBN 10: 1-62120-168-6

Ebook
ISBN 13: 978-1-62733-507-2
ISBN 10: 1-62733-507-2

Dear Future Exam Success Story

First of all, **THANK YOU** for purchasing Mometrix study materials!

Second, congratulations! You are one of the few determined test-takers who are committed to doing whatever it takes to excel on your exam. **You have come to the right place.** We developed these study materials with one goal in mind: to deliver you the information you need in a format that's concise and easy to use.

In addition to optimizing your guide for the content of the test, we've outlined our recommended steps for breaking down the preparation process into small, attainable goals so you can make sure you stay on track.

We've also analyzed the entire test-taking process, identifying the most common pitfalls and showing how you can overcome them and be ready for any curveball the test throws you.

Standardized testing is one of the biggest obstacles on your road to success, which only increases the importance of doing well in the high-pressure, high-stakes environment of test day. Your results on this test could have a significant impact on your future, and this guide provides the information and practical advice to help you achieve your full potential on test day.

Your success is our success

We would love to hear from you! If you would like to share the story of your exam success or if you have any questions or comments in regard to our products, please contact us at **800-673-8175** or **support@mometrix.com**.

Thanks again for your business and we wish you continued success!

Sincerely,
The Mometrix Test Preparation Team

Need more help? Check out our flashcards at:
http://mometrixflashcards.com/MaternalNewborn

TABLE OF CONTENTS

Introduction

Thank you for purchasing this resource! You have made the choice to prepare yourself for a test that could have a huge impact on your future, and this guide is designed to help you be fully ready for test day. Obviously, it's important to have a solid understanding of the test material, but you also need to be prepared for the unique environment and stressors of the test, so that you can perform to the best of your abilities.

For this purpose, the first section that appears in this guide is the **Secret Keys**. We've devoted countless hours to meticulously researching what works and what doesn't, and we've boiled down our findings to the five most impactful steps you can take to improve your performance on the test. We start at the beginning with study planning and move through the preparation process, all the way to the testing strategies that will help you get the most out of what you know when you're finally sitting in front of the test.

We recommend that you start preparing for your test as far in advance as possible. However, if you've bought this guide as a last-minute study resource and only have a few days before your test, we recommend that you skip over the first two Secret Keys since they address a long-term study plan.

If you struggle with **test anxiety**, we strongly encourage you to check out our recommendations for how you can overcome it. Test anxiety is a formidable foe, but it can be beaten, and we want to make sure you have the tools you need to defeat it.

Secret Key #1 – Plan Big, Study Small

There's a lot riding on your performance. If you want to ace this test, you're going to need to keep your skills sharp and the material fresh in your mind. You need a plan that lets you review everything you need to know while still fitting in your schedule. We'll break this strategy down into three categories.

Information Organization

Start with the information you already have: the official test outline. From this, you can make a complete list of all the concepts you need to cover before the test. Organize these concepts into groups that can be studied together, and create a list of any related vocabulary you need to learn so you can brush up on any difficult terms. You'll want to keep this vocabulary list handy once you actually start studying since you may need to add to it along the way.

Time Management

Once you have your set of study concepts, decide how to spread them out over the time you have left before the test. Break your study plan into small, clear goals so you have a manageable task for each day and know exactly what you're doing. Then just focus on one small step at a time. When you manage your time this way, you don't need to spend hours at a time studying. Studying a small block of content for a short period each day helps you retain information better and avoid stressing over how much you have left to do. You can relax knowing that you have a plan to cover everything in time. In order for this strategy to be effective though, you have to start studying early and stick to your schedule. Avoid the exhaustion and futility that comes from last-minute cramming!

Study Environment

The environment you study in has a big impact on your learning. Studying in a coffee shop, while probably more enjoyable, is not likely to be as fruitful as studying in a quiet room. It's important to keep distractions to a minimum. You're only planning to study for a short block of time, so make the most of it. Don't pause to check your phone or get up to find a snack. It's also important to **avoid multitasking**. Research has consistently shown that multitasking will make your studying dramatically less effective. Your study area should also be comfortable and well-lit so you don't have the distraction of straining your eyes or sitting on an uncomfortable chair.

The time of day you study is also important. You want to be rested and alert. Don't wait until just before bedtime. Study when you'll be most likely to comprehend and remember. Even better, if you know what time of day your test will be, set that time aside for study. That way your brain will be used to working on that subject at that specific time and you'll have a better chance of recalling information.

Finally, it can be helpful to team up with others who are studying for the same test. Your actual studying should be done in as isolated an environment as possible, but the work of organizing the information and setting up the study plan can be divided up. In between study sessions, you can discuss with your teammates the concepts that you're all studying and quiz each other on the details. Just be sure that your teammates are as serious about the test as you are. If you find that your study time is being replaced with social time, you might need to find a new team.

Secret Key #2 – Make Your Studying Count

You're devoting a lot of time and effort to preparing for this test, so you want to be absolutely certain it will pay off. This means doing more than just reading the content and hoping you can remember it on test day. It's important to make every minute of study count. There are two main areas you can focus on to make your studying count:

Retention

It doesn't matter how much time you study if you can't remember the material. You need to make sure you are retaining the concepts. To check your retention of the information you're learning, try recalling it at later times with minimal prompting. Try carrying around flashcards and glance at one or two from time to time or ask a friend who's also studying for the test to quiz you.

To enhance your retention, look for ways to put the information into practice so that you can apply it rather than simply recalling it. If you're using the information in practical ways, it will be much easier to remember. Similarly, it helps to solidify a concept in your mind if you're not only reading it to yourself but also explaining it to someone else. Ask a friend to let you teach them about a concept you're a little shaky on (or speak aloud to an imaginary audience if necessary). As you try to summarize, define, give examples, and answer your friend's questions, you'll understand the concepts better and they will stay with you longer. Finally, step back for a big picture view and ask yourself how each piece of information fits with the whole subject. When you link the different concepts together and see them working together as a whole, it's easier to remember the individual components.

Finally, practice showing your work on any multi-step problems, even if you're just studying. Writing out each step you take to solve a problem will help solidify the process in your mind, and you'll be more likely to remember it during the test.

Modality

Modality simply refers to the means or method by which you study. Choosing a study modality that fits your own individual learning style is crucial. No two people learn best in exactly the same way, so it's important to know your strengths and use them to your advantage.

For example, if you learn best by visualization, focus on visualizing a concept in your mind and draw an image or a diagram. Try color-coding your notes, illustrating them, or creating symbols that will trigger your mind to recall a learned concept. If you learn best by hearing or discussing information, find a study partner who learns the same way or read aloud to yourself. Think about how to put the information in your own words. Imagine that you are giving a lecture on the topic and record yourself so you can listen to it later.

For any learning style, flashcards can be helpful. Organize the information so you can take advantage of spare moments to review. Underline key words or phrases. Use different colors for different categories. Mnemonic devices (such as creating a short list in which every item starts with the same letter) can also help with retention. Find what works best for you and use it to store the information in your mind most effectively and easily.

Secret Key #3 – Practice the Right Way

Your success on test day depends not only on how many hours you put into preparing, but also on whether you prepared the right way. It's good to check along the way to see if your studying is paying off. One of the most effective ways to do this is by taking practice tests to evaluate your progress. Practice tests are useful because they show exactly where you need to improve. Every time you take a practice test, pay special attention to these three groups of questions:

- The questions you got wrong
- The questions you had to guess on, even if you guessed right
- The questions you found difficult or slow to work through

This will show you exactly what your weak areas are, and where you need to devote more study time. Ask yourself why each of these questions gave you trouble. Was it because you didn't understand the material? Was it because you didn't remember the vocabulary? Do you need more repetitions on this type of question to build speed and confidence? Dig into those questions and figure out how you can strengthen your weak areas as you go back to review the material.

Additionally, many practice tests have a section explaining the answer choices. It can be tempting to read the explanation and think that you now have a good understanding of the concept. However, an explanation likely only covers part of the question's broader context. Even if the explanation makes sense, **go back and investigate** every concept related to the question until you're positive you have a thorough understanding.

As you go along, keep in mind that the practice test is just that: practice. Memorizing these questions and answers will not be very helpful on the actual test because it is unlikely to have any of the same exact questions. If you only know the right answers to the sample questions, you won't be prepared for the real thing. **Study the concepts** until you understand them fully, and then you'll be able to answer any question that shows up on the test.

It's important to wait on the practice tests until you're ready. If you take a test on your first day of study, you may be overwhelmed by the amount of material covered and how much you need to learn. Work up to it gradually.

On test day, you'll need to be prepared for answering questions, managing your time, and using the test-taking strategies you've learned. It's a lot to balance, like a mental marathon that will have a big impact on your future. Like training for a marathon, you'll need to start slowly and work your way up. When test day arrives, you'll be ready.

Start with the strategies you've read in the first two Secret Keys—plan your course and study in the way that works best for you. If you have time, consider using multiple study resources to get different approaches to the same concepts. It can be helpful to see difficult concepts from more than one angle. Then find a good source for practice tests. Many times, the test website will suggest potential study resources or provide sample tests.

Practice Test Strategy

When you're ready to start taking practice tests, follow this strategy:

Untimed and Open-Book Practice

Take the first test with no time constraints and with your notes and study guide handy. Take your time and focus on applying the strategies you've learned.

Timed and Open-Book Practice

Take the second practice test open-book as well, but set a timer and practice pacing yourself to finish in time.

Timed and Closed-Book Practice

Take any other practice tests as if it were test day. Set a timer and put away your study materials. Sit at a table or desk in a quiet room, imagine yourself at the testing center, and answer questions as quickly and accurately as possible.

Keep repeating timed and closed-book tests on a regular basis until you run out of practice tests or it's time for the actual test. Your mind will be ready for the schedule and stress of test day, and you'll be able to focus on recalling the material you've learned.

Secret Key #4 – Pace Yourself

Once you're fully prepared for the material on the test, your biggest challenge on test day will be managing your time. Just knowing that the clock is ticking can make you panic even if you have plenty of time left. Work on pacing yourself so you can build confidence against the time constraints of the exam. Pacing is a difficult skill to master, especially in a high-pressure environment, so **practice is vital**.

Set time expectations for your pace based on how much time is available. For example, if a section has 60 questions and the time limit is 30 minutes, you know you have to average 30 seconds or less per question in order to answer them all. Although 30 seconds is the hard limit, set 25 seconds per question as your goal, so you reserve extra time to spend on harder questions. When you budget extra time for the harder questions, you no longer have any reason to stress when those questions take longer to answer.

Don't let this time expectation distract you from working through the test at a calm, steady pace, but keep it in mind so you don't spend too much time on any one question. Recognize that taking extra time on one question you don't understand may keep you from answering two that you do understand later in the test. If your time limit for a question is up and you're still not sure of the answer, mark it and move on, and come back to it later if the time and the test format allow. If the testing format doesn't allow you to return to earlier questions, just make an educated guess; then put it out of your mind and move on.

On the easier questions, be careful not to rush. It may seem wise to hurry through them so you have more time for the challenging ones, but it's not worth missing one if you know the concept and just didn't take the time to read the question fully. Work efficiently but make sure you understand the question and have looked at all of the answer choices, since more than one may seem right at first.

Even if you're paying attention to the time, you may find yourself a little behind at some point. You should speed up to get back on track, but do so wisely. Don't panic; just take a few seconds less on each question until you're caught up. Don't guess without thinking, but do look through the answer choices and eliminate any you know are wrong. If you can get down to two choices, it is often worthwhile to guess from those. Once you've chosen an answer, move on and don't dwell on any that you skipped or had to hurry through. If a question was taking too long, chances are it was one of the harder ones, so you weren't as likely to get it right anyway.

On the other hand, if you find yourself getting ahead of schedule, it may be beneficial to slow down a little. The more quickly you work, the more likely you are to make a careless mistake that will affect your score. You've budgeted time for each question, so don't be afraid to spend that time. Practice an efficient but careful pace to get the most out of the time you have.

Secret Key #5 – Have a Plan for Guessing

When you're taking the test, you may find yourself stuck on a question. Some of the answer choices seem better than others, but you don't see the one answer choice that is obviously correct. What do you do?

The scenario described above is very common, yet most test takers have not effectively prepared for it. Developing and practicing a plan for guessing may be one of the single most effective uses of your time as you get ready for the exam.

In developing your plan for guessing, there are three questions to address:

- When should you start the guessing process?
- How should you narrow down the choices?
- Which answer should you choose?

When to Start the Guessing Process

Unless your plan for guessing is to select C every time (which, despite its merits, is not what we recommend), you need to leave yourself enough time to apply your answer elimination strategies. Since you have a limited amount of time for each question, that means that if you're going to give yourself the best shot at guessing correctly, you have to decide quickly whether or not you will guess.

Of course, the best-case scenario is that you don't have to guess at all, so first, see if you can answer the question based on your knowledge of the subject and basic reasoning skills. Focus on the key words in the question and try to jog your memory of related topics. Give yourself a chance to bring the knowledge to mind, but once you realize that you don't have (or you can't access) the knowledge you need to answer the question, it's time to start the guessing process.

It's almost always better to start the guessing process too early than too late. It only takes a few seconds to remember something and answer the question from knowledge. Carefully eliminating wrong answer choices takes longer. Plus, going through the process of eliminating answer choices can actually help jog your memory.

Summary: Start the guessing process as soon as you decide that you can't answer the question based on your knowledge.

How to Narrow Down the Choices

The next chapter in this book (**Test-Taking Strategies**) includes a wide range of strategies for how to approach questions and how to look for answer choices to eliminate. You will definitely want to read those carefully, practice them, and figure out which ones work best for you. Here though, we're going to address a mindset rather than a particular strategy.

Your chances of guessing an answer correctly depend on how many options you are choosing from.

How many choices you have	How likely you are to guess correctly
5	20%
4	25%
3	33%
2	50%
1	100%

You can see from this chart just how valuable it is to be able to eliminate incorrect answers and make an educated guess, but there are two things that many test takers do that cause them to miss out on the benefits of guessing:

- Accidentally eliminating the correct answer
- Selecting an answer based on an impression

We'll look at the first one here, and the second one in the next section.

To avoid accidentally eliminating the correct answer, we recommend a thought exercise called **the $5 challenge**. In this challenge, you only eliminate an answer choice from contention if you are willing to bet $5 on it being wrong. Why $5? Five dollars is a small but not insignificant amount of money. It's an amount you could afford to lose but wouldn't want to throw away. And while losing $5 once might not hurt too much, doing it twenty times will set you back $100. In the same way, each small decision you make—eliminating a choice here, guessing on a question there—won't by itself impact your score very much, but when you put them all together, they can make a big difference. By holding each answer choice elimination decision to a higher standard, you can reduce the risk of accidentally eliminating the correct answer.

The $5 challenge can also be applied in a positive sense: If you are willing to bet $5 that an answer choice *is* correct, go ahead and mark it as correct.

Summary: Only eliminate an answer choice if you are willing to bet $5 that it is wrong.

Which Answer to Choose

You're taking the test. You've run into a hard question and decided you'll have to guess. You've eliminated all the answer choices you're willing to bet $5 on. Now you have to pick an answer. Why do we even need to talk about this? Why can't you just pick whichever one you feel like when the time comes?

The answer to these questions is that if you don't come into the test with a plan, you'll rely on your impression to select an answer choice, and if you do that, you risk falling into a trap. The test writers know that everyone who takes their test will be guessing on some of the questions, so they intentionally write wrong answer choices to seem plausible. You still have to pick an answer though, and if the wrong answer choices are designed to look right, how can you ever be sure that you're not falling for their trap? The best solution we've found to this dilemma is to take the decision out of your hands entirely. Here is the process we recommend:

Once you've eliminated any choices that you are confident (willing to bet $5) are wrong, select the first remaining choice as your answer.

Whether you choose to select the first remaining choice, the second, or the last, the important thing is that you use some preselected standard. Using this approach guarantees that you will not be enticed into selecting an answer choice that looks right, because you are not basing your decision on how the answer choices look.

This is not meant to make you question your knowledge. Instead, it is to help you recognize the difference between your knowledge and your impressions. There's a huge difference between thinking an answer is right because of what you know, and thinking an answer is right because it looks or sounds like it should be right.

Summary: To ensure that your selection is appropriately random, make a predetermined selection from among all answer choices you have not eliminated.

Test-Taking Strategies

This section contains a list of test-taking strategies that you may find helpful as you work through the test. By taking what you know and applying logical thought, you can maximize your chances of answering any question correctly!

It is very important to realize that every question is different and every person is different: no single strategy will work on every question, and no single strategy will work for every person. That's why we've included all of them here, so you can try them out and determine which ones work best for different types of questions and which ones work best for you.

Question Strategies

Read Carefully

Read the question and answer choices carefully. Don't miss the question because you misread the terms. You have plenty of time to read each question thoroughly and make sure you understand what is being asked. Yet a happy medium must be attained, so don't waste too much time. You must read carefully, but efficiently.

Contextual Clues

Look for contextual clues. If the question includes a word you are not familiar with, look at the immediate context for some indication of what the word might mean. Contextual clues can often give you all the information you need to decipher the meaning of an unfamiliar word. Even if you can't determine the meaning, you may be able to narrow down the possibilities enough to make a solid guess at the answer to the question.

Prefixes

If you're having trouble with a word in the question or answer choices, try dissecting it. Take advantage of every clue that the word might include. Prefixes and suffixes can be a huge help. Usually they allow you to determine a basic meaning. Pre- means before, post- means after, pro - is positive, de- is negative. From prefixes and suffixes, you can get an idea of the general meaning of the word and try to put it into context.

Hedge Words

Watch out for critical hedge words, such as *likely*, *may*, *can*, *sometimes*, *often*, *almost*, *mostly*, *usually*, *generally*, *rarely*, and *sometimes*. Question writers insert these hedge phrases to cover every possibility. Often an answer choice will be wrong simply because it leaves no room for exception. Be on guard for answer choices that have definitive words such as *exactly* and *always*.

Switchback Words

Stay alert for *switchbacks*. These are the words and phrases frequently used to alert you to shifts in thought. The most common switchback words are *but*, *although*, and *however*. Others include *nevertheless, on the other hand, even though, while, in spite of, despite, regardless of.* Switchback words are important to catch because they can change the direction of the question or an answer choice.

Face Value

When in doubt, use common sense. Accept the situation in the problem at face value. Don't read too much into it. These problems will not require you to make wild assumptions. If you have to go beyond creativity and warp time or space in order to have an answer choice fit the question, then you should move on and consider the other answer choices. These are normal problems rooted in reality. The applicable relationship or explanation may not be readily apparent, but it is there for you to figure out. Use your common sense to interpret anything that isn't clear.

Answer Choice Strategies

Answer Selection

The most thorough way to pick an answer choice is to identify and eliminate wrong answers until only one is left, then confirm it is the correct answer. Sometimes an answer choice may immediately seem right, but be careful. The test writers will usually put more than one reasonable answer choice on each question, so take a second to read all of them and make sure that the other choices are not equally obvious. As long as you have time left, it is better to read every answer choice than to pick the first one that looks right without checking the others.

Answer Choice Families

An answer choice family consists of two (in rare cases, three) answer choices that are very similar in construction and cannot all be true at the same time. If you see two answer choices that are direct opposites or parallels, one of them is usually the correct answer. For instance, if one answer choice says that quantity *x* increases and another either says that quantity *x* decreases (opposite) or says that quantity *y* increases (parallel), then those answer choices would fall into the same family. An answer choice that doesn't match the construction of the answer choice family is more likely to be incorrect. Most questions will not have answer choice families, but when they do appear, you should be prepared to recognize them.

Eliminate Answers

Eliminate answer choices as soon as you realize they are wrong, but make sure you consider all possibilities. If you are eliminating answer choices and realize that the last one you are left with is also wrong, don't panic. Start over and consider each choice again. There may be something you missed the first time that you will realize on the second pass.

Avoid Fact Traps

Don't be distracted by an answer choice that is factually true but doesn't answer the question. You are looking for the choice that answers the question. Stay focused on what the question is asking for so you don't accidentally pick an answer that is true but incorrect. Always go back to the question and make sure the answer choice you've selected actually answers the question and is not merely a true statement.

Extreme Statements

In general, you should avoid answers that put forth extreme actions as standard practice or proclaim controversial ideas as established fact. An answer choice that states the "process should be used in certain situations, if..." is much more likely to be correct than one that states the "process should be discontinued completely." The first is a calm rational statement and doesn't even make a definitive, uncompromising stance, using a hedge word *if* to provide wiggle room, whereas the second choice is a radical idea and far more extreme.

BENCHMARK

As you read through the answer choices and you come across one that seems to answer the question well, mentally select that answer choice. This is not your final answer, but it's the one that will help you evaluate the other answer choices. The one that you selected is your benchmark or standard for judging each of the other answer choices. Every other answer choice must be compared to your benchmark. That choice is correct until proven otherwise by another answer choice beating it. If you find a better answer, then that one becomes your new benchmark. Once you've decided that no other choice answers the question as well as your benchmark, you have your final answer.

PREDICT THE ANSWER

Before you even start looking at the answer choices, it is often best to try to predict the answer. When you come up with the answer on your own, it is easier to avoid distractions and traps because you will know exactly what to look for. The right answer choice is unlikely to be word-for-word what you came up with, but it should be a close match. Even if you are confident that you have the right answer, you should still take the time to read each option before moving on.

General Strategies

TOUGH QUESTIONS

If you are stumped on a problem or it appears too hard or too difficult, don't waste time. Move on! Remember though, if you can quickly check for obviously incorrect answer choices, your chances of guessing correctly are greatly improved. Before you completely give up, at least try to knock out a couple of possible answers. Eliminate what you can and then guess at the remaining answer choices before moving on.

CHECK YOUR WORK

Since you will probably not know every term listed and the answer to every question, it is important that you get credit for the ones that you do know. Don't miss any questions through careless mistakes. If at all possible, try to take a second to look back over your answer selection and make sure you've selected the correct answer choice and haven't made a costly careless mistake (such as marking an answer choice that you didn't mean to mark). This quick double check should more than pay for itself in caught mistakes for the time it costs.

PACE YOURSELF

It's easy to be overwhelmed when you're looking at a page full of questions; your mind is confused and full of random thoughts, and the clock is ticking down faster than you would like. Calm down and maintain the pace that you have set for yourself. Especially as you get down to the last few minutes of the test, don't let the small numbers on the clock make you panic. As long as you are on track by monitoring your pace, you are guaranteed to have time for each question.

DON'T RUSH

It is very easy to make errors when you are in a hurry. Maintaining a fast pace in answering questions is pointless if it makes you miss questions that you would have gotten right otherwise. Test writers like to include distracting information and wrong answers that seem right. Taking a little extra time to avoid careless mistakes can make all the difference in your test score. Find a pace that allows you to be confident in the answers that you select.

Keep Moving

Panicking will not help you pass the test, so do your best to stay calm and keep moving. Taking deep breaths and going through the answer elimination steps you practiced can help to break through a stress barrier and keep your pace.

Final Notes

The combination of a solid foundation of content knowledge and the confidence that comes from practicing your plan for applying that knowledge is the key to maximizing your performance on test day. As your foundation of content knowledge is built up and strengthened, you'll find that the strategies included in this chapter become more and more effective in helping you quickly sift through the distractions and traps of the test to isolate the correct answer.

Now it's time to move on to the test content chapters of this book, but be sure to keep your goal in mind. As you read, think about how you will be able to apply this information on the test. If you've already seen sample questions for the test and you have an idea of the question format and style, try to come up with questions of your own that you can answer based on what you're reading. This will give you valuable practice applying your knowledge in the same ways you can expect to on test day.

Good luck and good studying!

Pregnancy, Birth Risk Factors and Complications

Antenatal Factors

Maternal Health Status

General maternal health status is discussed below:

- **Dental**
  - **Gingival disease** increases and gums bleed easily.
- **Gastrointestinal**
  - Appetite increases, reflux occurs, motility and intestinal transit decrease, and gall bladder dilates. Constipation and hemorrhoids are common.
- **Respiratory**
  - Oxygen requirement, oxygen pressure, tidal volume, inspiratory and vital capacity, minute volume, and PO_2 **increase**, while carbon dioxide pressure, expiratory reserve volume, residual volume, total lung capacity, HCO_3, and PcO_2 **decrease**.
- **Cardiovascular**
  - Cardiac output, stroke volume, heart rate, and blood flow to uterus, kidneys, breasts, skin, and brain **increase**. Systemic vascular resistance and pulmonary vascular resistance **decrease**.
- **Hematologic**
  - Plasma volume, total erythrocyte volume, mean cell volume, total iron-binding capacity, E-sed rate, and alkaline phosphatase **increase**. Hemoglobin, hematocrit, serum iron, total protein, albumin, and osmolality **decrease**.
- **Renal**
  - Kidneys enlarge and bladder tone **decreases**. Residual volume, renal plasma flow, and GFR **increase**. Renin, angiotensin I and II, and renin substrate **increase**.
- **Ophthalmic**
  - Blurred vision is common.
- **Integumentary**
  - Vascular spiders, palmar erythema, striae gravidarum, and hyperpigmentation occur. Significant hair loss occurs 2 to 4 months after pregnancy.

Maternal Age

Adolescent

Adolescent mothers >15 are not at higher risk than those >20 if they have **adequate prenatal care** and follow **guidelines and recommendations**, but this is often not the case. Teenage mothers are more likely to smoke and to gain inadequate weight, increasing the likelihood of premature delivery, low-birth weight infants, iron deficiency anemia, and preeclampsia/eclampsia. Additionally, there is increased risk of cephalopelvic disproportion, because the mother may not be fully mature physically. Teenagers 15 to 19 also have increased risk of sexually transmitted diseases, such as gonorrhea, herpes, chlamydia, and syphilis. Many also drink alcohol and take illicit drugs, increasing the incidence of fetal abnormalities. In many cases, the male partner has little education, lacks employment, and may not be able to provide emotional or financial support. Adolescent partners are often of similar social and educational background to the mothers, may not have completed development, and may not be prepared for fatherhood. The nurse should remain non-judgmental and supportive, educating the adolescent and encouraging good prenatal care.

Mature, Over 35

Many women have chosen to delay pregnancy, resulting in a marked increase in pregnant women >35. These mothers tend to be better educated and more financially secure than younger mothers. If the mother is in good health, pregnancy poses little increased risk; however, the risk of **death associated with pregnancy** does increase with age. Those >40 have about 5 times the risk of those ≤24. Additionally, those >35 are more likely to have **preexisting health problems**, such as diabetes or hypertension, which increases risk. They are more likely to have a C-section, placenta previa, abruptio placentae, and spontaneous abortion. There may also be increased risk to the fetus. The incidence of Down syndrome increases with mothers >35, and more markedly in those >40, so these mothers are more likely to want genetic testing. Macrosomia and congenital malformations are also more common. Older mothers with unplanned pregnancies may be concerned about their age, long-term care of the child, retirement plans, and lifestyle changes.

Maternal Nutrition

The **nutrition** of the mother has a profound effect on the developing embryo/fetus. Caloric needs vary widely depending on the mother's age, size, weight, metabolism, and general health. Energy needs of the mother usually remain stable during the first trimester, but an additional **300 kilocalories** a day are needed during the second and third trimesters for a singleton, and **600 kilocalories** a day for twins. Recommended nutrient intake for pregnant women is shown below:

Vit. A (μg/d)	Vit. C (mg/d)	Vit. D (μg/d)	Vit. E (mg/d)	Vit. K (μg/d)	Ca (mg/d)	Phos. (mg/d)
750- 770	80-85	≥5	15	75-90	1000-1300	700-1250

Generally, a pregnant woman requires about 71 g of **protein** daily (3 meat servings or equivalent) and 4 to 5 cups of milk (or equivalent). Diet should include 2 to 4 servings of fruit and 3 to 5 servings of vegetables. **Simple carbohydrates** (sugar, flour) should be limited and replaced by whole grains, which are high in B vitamins. **Fat** should constitute about 30% of total caloric intake. Iron intake should be about 27mg per day.

Malnutrition

Maternal malnutrition can have a profound effect on the developing fetus. If malnutrition occurs during the stages of cell division, then cells may not divide properly, causing permanent damage. If malnutrition occurs when cells are enlarging, then correcting the nutritional deficit can reverse damage. Maternal weight gain must be adequate:

- Underweight: 28-40 lb.
- Normal weight: 25-35 lb.
- Overweight: 15-25 lb.
- Obese: 15 lb.

Mothers who are malnourished or underweight have increased perinatal losses and preterm births. Neonates often have lower Apgar score and low birth weight (<2500 g). Women with eating disorders are more likely to have infants that are small for gestational age. Vitamin and mineral deficiencies can result in a number of problems for the developing fetus:

- Thiamine: Congestive heart failure, stillbirths.
- Folic acid: Megaloblastic anemia, neural tube defects.
- Vitamin D and calcium: Skeletal defects.

Infants of obese and morbidly obese women are often macrosomic (large) and may suffer fetal distress, early neonatal death, meconium aspiration, shoulder dystocia, and/or complications from Caesarean birth.

Grand Multiparity

Grand multiparity is ≥5 deliveries of live or stillborn infants at ≥20 weeks, although some studies suggest risks increase after 4 deliveries. **Great grand multiparity** is usually considered ≥10 deliveries.

Risks associated with multiparity include increased incidence of placenta previa, abruptio placentae, preeclampsia, and hemorrhage. Rates of C-sections are increased significantly. Grand multiparas often have **poor prenatal care** and tend to have increased rates of disease, such as diabetes mellitus and hypertension, but studies show that with proper prenatal care, those without health problems have risks comparable to those with lower parity. Younger multiparous women have fewer complications than older multiparous women, so some of the increased risks may be primarily age-related. Fetal complications include macrosomia, SGA, and malpresentation (breech).

Psychosocial Issues

Almost all mothers have feelings of **ambivalence** about the challenges of parenthood. These feelings are normal and healthy, representing a transitional stage leading to acceptance. Areas of concern include:

- **Changing body image/sexuality**: Weight gain, varicose veins, growing abdomen, stretch marks, and breast changes may cause the mother to fear she is no longer attractive.
- **Labile moods**: Hormonal and body changes can lead to rapid mood swings and emotional outbursts that may affect relationships, especially if the partner is unprepared.
- **Personality changes**: Pregnancy often results in a tendency toward introversion, with the mother requiring more rest and personal time, and this can lead to conflicts.

If the pregnancy was **unintended**, the mother may resent the pregnancy and consider abortion, leading to feelings of guilt. Many mothers are able to work through these issues and reach acceptance, especially by the third trimester when pregnancy is obvious and people are often more solicitous and supportive.

Cultural Influences During Pregnancy

Family Structure

Families may range from nuclear families to extended families in which grandparents or godparents are important and may be consulted regarding decisions. Some immigrants or religious groups may practice polygamy.

Family Size

While having 2 to 3 children is the norm in the United States, some religious groups and cultures do not practice birth control and believe they should have large families, regardless of financial or health circumstances. Some cultures attach shame to pregnancy out of wedlock, and women may face ostracism, injury, or even death.

Pregnancy Beliefs

Beliefs vary widely. Some people believe pregnancy is a natural occurrence, so they may not seek help unless a problem arises. Other people believe women are more vulnerable during pregnancy and need protection to some degree. People may exercise caution and avoid taboos, depending on cultural beliefs and superstitions.

Health Practices

While most women in the United States depend on obstetricians during pregnancy, some cultures may prefer lay midwives, indigenous healers, or spiritualists.

Female Infertility

Cause	Discussion	Tests
Non-patent fallopian tubes	Fallopian tubes may be scarred by PID, endometriosis, or adhesions.	Hysterosalpingography Laparoscopy
Ovulation failure	Hormone levels may be inadequate to promote ovulation. Ovarian cysts may interfere with ovulation.	Ultrasound (transvaginal)
Cervical obstruction or uterine abnormality	Excess production of mucus or narrowing of the cervical os may prevent sperm from entering the uterus. Thickening, abnormalities, or growths (fibroids, cysts) of the uterus may prevent implantation.	Hysteroscopy Endometrial biopsy Postcoital test Ultrasound (hysterosonogram)

Male Fertility Tests

In up to 30% of infertility cases, the male is responsible, so **male fertility testing** should be done as part of fertility assessment:

Urogenital History and Examination

A history should review drug abuse, smoking, exercise, STDs, and sexual behaviors. The male is examined for physical abnormalities, such as varicocele, and the testes are evaluated for size.

Semen Analysis

Usually, two different semen samples, from different times, are examined. Two normal tests, taken at different times, usually indicate the male is fertile. The sperm count is calculated, and the sperm examined for size, shape, and motility.

Hormone Levels

Testosterone and other hormone levels may be evaluated, but abnormal hormone levels are associated with only about 3% of male infertility cases.

Genetic Testing

Testing may identify Klinefelter's syndrome (male with an extra X chromosome) or Y microdeletion (cause of aspermia).

Assisted Reproduction Methods

The following are methods of assisted reproduction:

- **Assisted reproduction therapy (ART) with egg and/or sperm donation** - Donor eggs or sperm are combined with the partner's eggs or sperm before intrauterine insemination.
- **Gamete intrafallopian transfer (GIFT)** - Sperm and ovum (gametes) are harvested, collected and inserted next to each other in the fallopian tube, where normal fertilization takes place.
- **Intracytoplasmic sperm injection (ICSI)** - Individual harvested ovum is injected directly with individual sperm before intrauterine insemination (May be part of ART).
- **Intrauterine insemination (IUI)** - Sperm are inserted directly into the uterus through a catheter. This procedure may follow hormone treatments to stimulate ovulation.
- **In vitro fertilization (IVF)** - Harvested and fertilized ova are inserted into the uterus, often after the woman takes drugs to stimulate ova production. Ova, sperm, or both, may be donated.
- **Zygote intrafallopian transfer (ZIFT)** - Sperm and ova are combined, and fertilization occurs outside the body. The zygotes are inserted into the fallopian tube. From there, they travel to the uterus to implant.

Gonadotropins Treatment for Infertility

Gonadotropin treatment requires administration of natural or recombinant hormones: **follicle stimulating hormone (FSH)** and **luteinizing hormone (LH)**. Drugs include human chorionic gonadotropin (hCG), human menopausal gonadotropin (hMG), and recombinant human FSH (rFSH).

- **Females** who are not ovulating usually receive injections of hCG or hMG for 12 days to stimulate maturity of follicles and then one dose of hCG to trigger ovulation. About 50% become pregnant, but over half of the pregnancies result in miscarriage. There is increased risk of multiple gestations, and ovarian enlargement or ovarian hyperstimulation syndrome may occur. Gonadotropins may also be used prior to harvesting of ova. Frequent ultrasounds and hormone level measurements are required to monitor the development of follicles.
- **Males** with low testosterone levels usually receive injections of hCG 3 times weekly for 4 to 6 months until testosterone levels increase. They then continue to receive injections of hCG or hMG 2 times weekly until sperm count is adequate. Gynecomastia may occur.

Fertility Drugs

Bromocriptine and Cabergoline

Bromocriptine reduces prolactin levels. Increased prolactin levels can interfere with ovulation in females and decrease testosterone levels and sperm production in males, resulting in impotence or erectile dysfunction. This drug is taken vaginally or orally 1 to 4 times daily, increasing the dose slowly to minimize side effects, which include headaches, dizziness, and GI disturbances.

The actions of **cabergoline** are the same as bromocriptine, but cabergoline is only taken 1 to 2 times a week. Side effects, usually only headache, are milder than with bromocriptine.

Clomiphene and GnRH

Clomiphene stimulates hormone production and ovulation in women whose estrogen levels and pituitary function are normal. Clomiphene is taken orally for 5 days during menstruation for 3 to 6 months with dosage adjusted according to results of clomiphene challenge test (FSH levels). Males may take clomiphene to increase sperm counts. Clomiphene is often used to stimulate production of multiple ova prior to harvesting.

Gonadotropin-releasing hormone (GnRH) is administered prior to gonadotropin treatment to prevent the pituitary from stimulating production of FSH and LH, so production can be controlled.

Physiological Changes Related to Pregnancy

Amenorrhea

Amenorrhea, absence of menstruation, is one of the first signs of pregnancy. Most women menstruate on a 28-day cycle, with ovulation occurring at about day 14 of the cycle. The ovum remains fertile for 12 to 24 hours. For conception to occur, intercourse must take place on, or five to six days before, the day of **ovulation**. Sperm are most fertile during the first 24 hours in female reproductive tract. Fertilization (conception) usually takes place in the **fallopian tube**, and during the first 14 days (pre-embryonic stage), cell division and cell multiplication occur, forming an inner layer (blastocyst) and outer layer (trophoblast). If fertilization of the egg does not occur, the uterine lining begins to shed, and **menstruation** occurs on about day 23 of the cycle. However, if the trophoblast attaches to the endometrium of the uterus (**implantation**), usually 7 to10 days after fertilization, the uterine lining thickens and the trophoblast cells grow into the lining. The placenta forms, and hormonal changes associated with pregnancy prevent menstruation.

Breast Changes

Breast changes—growth, engorgement, tenderness, prominent veins, stretch marks, and itching—often begin to occur even before the first missed period. Hormone changes promote growth of the **ductal system** to prepare the breasts for milk production. Breasts usually grow about a cup size. At six to eight weeks, the nipples begin to enlarge, and **Montgomery's tubercles**—bumps around the areola—become more obvious. Discomfort usually recedes after the first trimester. A support bra may help relieve discomfort.

Quickening

Movement of the fetus is usually detected at 18 to 20 weeks after the LMP in a primigravida or 16 weeks in a multigravida. Quickening is often described as a "fluttering" within the abdomen.

Abdominal Enlargement

Progressive abdominal enlargement associated with amenorrhea is characteristic of pregnancy. Little change is evident during the first trimester, as the fundal height remains within the pelvis, but the abdomen enlarges as the **uterus** grows and **fundal height** moves upward.

Nausea and Vomiting

In the **first trimester**, HCG secretion of the blastocyst and changes in carbohydrate metabolism cause nausea. In the **second and third trimesters**, pressure of growing uterus displaces the stomach upward and the intestines laterally and downward. Gastric emptying and peristalsis slow, causing bloating and constipation. Smooth muscles relax (from elevated progesterone), resulting in gastric reflux and heartburn, which further aggravate nausea and can lead to vomiting.

Preventive measures are as follows:

- Eat small frequent meals
- Avoid fatty, spicy foods
- Eat simple carbohydrate foods, such as saltine crackers
- Drink herbal tea with sugar or ginger ale

Medical treatments include the following:

- Antacids: calcium carbonate, magnesium hydroxide, or magnesium oxide
- Antihistamine/anticholinergic: meclizine
- Antiemetics: ondansetron, prochlorperazine, promethazine, metoclopramide, or trimethobenzamide

HEARTBURN

Heartburn results when increased progesterone combined with decreased GI motility, relaxation of the cardiac sphincter, and upward displacement of stomach from pressure of the growing uterus increase esophageal reflux.

Management:

- Eat 4-5 small meals rather than 3 large meals daily.
- Take low sodium antacids (NOT sodium bicarbonate).
- Avoid lying down within two hours of eating.
- Avoid fried or spicy foods that trigger symptoms.

URINARY FREQUENCY

Pressure of growing uterus on the bladder during the first and third trimesters increases frequency of urination.

Management:

- Increase fluids in the daytime and decrease in the evening ONLY if nocturia is present.
- Urinate when the urge is felt.

ANKLE/FOOT EDEMA

Edema is caused by increased sodium retention from hormonal changes, circulatory impairment to lower extremities from pressure of uterus during second and third trimesters, prolonged sitting/standing, and increased permeability of capillaries.

Management:

- Elevate feet and legs when sitting.
- Avoid restrictive clothing, socks, or other bands around legs.
- Exercise feet frequently while sitting.
- Walk to promote increased circulation.

PTYALISM

The cause of bitter saliva during the first trimester is unclear.

Management:

- Use astringent mouthwashes.
- Chew gum or suck on hard candy.

Leg Cramps

Leg cramps are caused by calcium/phosphorus imbalance, increased pressure on nerves, or impaired lower peripheral circulation from the growing uterus. General fatigue, pointing toes, and shortening muscles may also cause cramps.

Management:

- Dorsiflex feet to stretch muscles.
- Modify diet to improve
- calcium/phosphorus balance.
- Apply heat to cramping muscles.
- Change position slowly.

Constipation

Increased progesterone levels slow intestinal motility. Pressure on intestines from enlarging uterus, inadequate diet/fluid intake, lack of exercise, and iron supplements all slow motility.

Management:

- Increase fluids and fiber in diet.
- Use stool softeners, such as DSS.
- Avoid laxatives, which may increase constipation over time.

Hemorrhoids

Constipation and pressure on hemorrhoidal veins from the growing uterus cause veins to dilate.

Management:

- Treat constipation.
- Apply ice packs.
- Take sitz baths.
- Apply topical ointments, such as Preparation H® or cortisone ointment.
- Apply topical anesthetic agent.

Varicose Veins

Venous congestion from pressure of uterus causes impaired circulation. Increased weight, age, and hereditary factors contribute to varicosities.

Management:

- Elevate feet and legs frequently.
- Avoid prolonged standing, crossing legs, and wearing constrictive hosiery or clothing.
- Wear support hose.

Backache

Increased hormone levels cause softening of cartilage and increased lumbosacral curvature. Muscle strain, fatigue, poor body mechanics, and carrying twins contribute to backache.

Management:

- Do the pelvic-tilt exercise.
- Utilize correct body mechanics. Avoid heavy lifting, reaching for things on high surfaces, and wearing high heeled shoes.
- Adjust height of work surfaces. Apply heat to lower back. Use back support in chair/bed. Begin modified exercise program, such as swimming, beginning with stretching. Stand straight and avoid slumping.

Nasal Stuffiness/Bleeding

Increased production of estrogen during first trimester causes swelling and irritation of mucus membranes.

Management:

- Use cool-air vaporizer.
- DO NOT use nasal sprays or decongestants.

Vaginal Discharge/Monilial Infection

Increased estrogen promotes hyperplasia of vaginal mucosa and increased production of mucus. Warm moist environment promotes *Candida* monilial infection.

Management:

- Bathe daily.
- Wear cotton panties (NOT nylon or pantyhose).
- Avoid douching, panty liners, and tight clothing.
- Topical treatments include miconazole, butoconazole, clotrimazole, ticconazole, nystatin, or terconazole.

Pregnancy Tests

Pregnancy should be verified by a positive **pregnancy test:**

- **Urine tests:** All tests measure human chorionic gonadotropin (hCG). Laboratory tests, such as the hemagglutination-inhibition test and the latex agglutination test, are 95 to 98% accurate at about two weeks after the first missed period. Home urine tests may detect pregnancy within a day of a missed period, and most are more accurate at one to two weeks after a missed period. False negatives are more common than false positives.
- **Serum tests:** These tests are more accurate than urine tests as they detect a sub-unit of hCG, so they may detect pregnancy even before a missed period. Additionally, monitoring of progesterone levels may help to determine if a pregnancy is viable. Levels >25 ng/mL suggest viability, and levels <5 ng/mL are inconsistent with viability.
- **Ultrasound:** The gestational sac can be seen transabdominally five to six weeks after the beginning of the LMP and transvaginally at three to four weeks.

Laboratory Changes Associated with Pregnancy

Test	Normal value	Pregnancy value
Hemoglobin	11.7 to 15.5 gm/dl	11.5 to 15 gm/dl
Hematocrit	38 to 44%	32 to 36.5%
Red blood cell count	4.20 to 4.87	Unchanged
White blood cell count	4500 to 11,000	6000 to 20,000 (increase often related to neutrophils)
Serum creatinine	0.5 to 1.1 mg/dL	0.53 to 0.9 mg/dL
Serum BUN	8 to 21 mg/dL	8 to 10 mg/dL
Serum uric acid	3.5 to 7.3 mg/dL	2 to 5.8 mg/dL
Creatinine clearance (urine)	75 to 115 mL/min	150 to 200 mL/min
Alkaline phosphatase (ALP)	25 to 125 U/L	Increase 2 to 4 times

Antepartum Risk Factors

Pregnancy and Diabetes Mellitus

About 2% of women have or develop **diabetes mellitus** during pregnancy. Factors that affect maternal health include change in **dietary habits** (such as inadequate intake because of nausea and diarrhea), changes in **hormones** that affect glucose metabolism, and increased **renal blood flow** that interferes with tubular reabsorption and results in increased glucosuria. All of these factors make control of diabetes more difficult. Mothers are at increased risk of diabetic ketoacidosis, pregnancy-induced hypertension (preeclampsia), and diabetic retinopathy. Polyhydramnios (>2000 mL amniotic fluid) occurs in about 10% of diabetic pregnancies, increasing the risk of abruptio placentae, premature labor, and postpartal uterine atony. The risk of spontaneous abortion increases markedly if glucose levels are poorly controlled. Urinary tract infections, including pyelonephritis, may occur. Patient education is important to help the mother maintain adequate control of glucose, with fasting AM plasma glucose at 90 to 100mg/100 mL and <120 to 140 mg/100 mL during the day. Dietary recommendations include 35 kilocalories per kg of ideal body weight. Induction at week 38 or 39 is common.

Review Video: Diabetes Type I
Visit mometrix.com/academy and enter code: 501396

Hypertensive Disorders of Pregnancy

Hypertensive disorders of pregnancy comprise a continuum ranging from mild to severe.

- **Hypertension:** BP >140/90 or 20 mm Hg increase in systolic or 10 mm diastolic. May be chronic or transient without signs of preeclampsia or eclampsia.
- **Preeclampsia:** New onset hypertension with or without proteinuria (300mg/24h) and edema (peripheral or generalized) or increase of ≥5 pounds of weight in one week after the twentieth week of gestation. Preeclampsia with severe features is BP ≥160/110. Symptoms include headache, abdominal pain, and visual disturbances.
- **Eclampsia:** Preeclampsia with seizures occurring at the twentieth week of gestation to 1 month after delivery.
- **HELLP syndrome** (hemolysis, elevated liver enzymes (AST and ALT), and low platelets (<100,000): Usually accompanied by epigastric or right upper quadrant pain.

These conditions are treated as follows:

- **Chronic hypertension**: Methyldopa beginning with 250mg every 6 hours.
- **Preeclampsia, eclampsia, HELLP:**
    - Delivery of fetus (may be delayed with mild preeclampsia if <37 weeks).
    - Magnesium sulfate IV 4 to 6 g over 15 minutes initially and then 1 to 2 g per hour.
    - Antihypertensive drugs.

Review Video: Hypertension
Visit mometrix.com/academy and enter code: 999599

CHEAP TORCHES

CHEAP TORCHES is the acronym used to recall common causes of congenital and neonatal infections. Many congenital infections are present for at least a month prior to birth and remain present at birth:

C	Chickenpox (varicella)
H	Hepatitis (B, C, & E)
E	Enterovirus (RNA viruses, including coxsackievirus, echovirus, and poliovirus)
A	AIDS (HIV)
P	Parvovirus (B 19)
T	Toxoplasmosis
O	Other (Group B streptococcus, *Candida, Listeria*, TB, lymphocytic choriomeningitis)
R	Rubella (measles)
C	Cytomegalovirus
H	Herpes simplex virus
E	Every other STD (*Chlamydia,* gonorrhea, *Ureaplasma,* papillomavirus
S	Syphilis

Exposure to these pathogens *in utero* may cause a miscarriage or congenital defect, especially if the exposure was during the first trimester.

HIV/AIDS IN PREGNANCY

Women with **HIV/AIDS** taking **anti-retroviral drugs** before conception should continue with the medications, although efavirenz is contraindicated because of teratogenic effects. If HIV is diagnosed during the first trimester, treatment should begin at that point or at the beginning of the second trimester. With treatment during pregnancy, the transmission rate from mother to fetus is about 2%. Usual treatment is 500 to 600 mg **zidovudine** (ZDV) in 2 to 5 doses daily from week 14. Cesarean delivery poses less chance of HIV transmission for the neonate, but increases the risk of maternal infection. **C- section** is recommended if mother lacked adequate prenatal care, viral load is unclear, or >1000 copies per mL were measured at 36 weeks, or if the mother has not received antiretroviral drugs or has taken only ZDV or azidothymidine (AZT) during her pregnancy. IV ZDV is started 3 hours prior to C-section and used continuously through labor and delivery for vaginal delivery. HIV increases risk of maternal and fetal infections.

Anemia

Clinical indications of anemia are as follows:

- **Mild – Hemoglobin 10 to14 g/dL**
    - Usually asymptomatic, but patient may experience palpitations, especially on exertion.
- **Moderate – Hemoglobin 6 to 10 g/dL**
    - Palpitations increase, even at rest.
    - Patient may experience dyspnea and general fatigue.
- **Severe – Hemoglobin <6 g/dL**
    - Pallor is evident, and hemolysis of RBCs may cause increased bilirubin, resulting in jaundice and itching.
    - Increased cardiovascular abnormalities may include tachycardia, systolic murmur, angina, and intermittent claudication leading to congestive heart failure and MI.
    - Dyspnea, tachypnea, and orthopnea are evident at rest.
    - CNS involvement causes headache, vertigo, cognitive impairment, depression, and irritability.
    - Mouth becomes sore, with glossitis and smooth tongue, difficulty swallowing, anorexia, weight loss, and dysphagia.
    - Bone pain and sensitivity to cold may occur.

Pregnancy and Iron-Deficiency Anemia

Iron is necessary for the development of red blood cells. During pregnancy, the mother's plasma volume increases by about 50% but red cell mass increases less, so the **hematocrit** drops from a normal of 38 to 47% to as low as 34% (physiologic/iron deficiency anemia of pregnancy). Because the fetus takes iron from the mother, the mother's iron intake must compensate for this loss. Recommended daily iron supplements include

- If the hematocrit is within normal range: 30 mg elemental iron daily.
- If the mother has iron deficiency anemia: 60 to 120 mg/daily until hematocrit normalizes, at which point the dose should decrease to 30 mg daily

When **hemoglobin** falls <11 g/dL, the mother is at increased risk of infection, preeclampsia, and postpartal hemorrhage, with associated dangers to the fetus. If hemoglobin falls <6 g/dL, the mother may suffer cardiac failure, and the fetus is at high risk, with increased rates of miscarriage and stillbirths, low birth rate, and neonatal death. Initial *symptoms* of iron deficiency include pallor, glossitis, headache, and pica, progressing to weakness, lethargy, confusion, ataxia, and cardiovascular abnormalities.

Pregnancy and Folate/Folic Acid Deficiency Anemia

Folate/folic acid deficiency can result in **megaloblastic anemia**. Folic acid is necessary for DNA synthesis and for the formation and maturation of red blood cells. Causes of folic acid deficiency include inadequate diet, malabsorption syndromes (especially of the small intestine), medications that interfere with absorption (oral contraceptives, methotrexate, phenobarbital, and diphenylhydantoin), anorexia, alcoholism, and dialysis. Diagnostic findings include decreased hemoglobin, hematocrit, and folate (normal value—3 to 25 mg/mL), as well as increased MCV and MCHV. Cobalamin level is normal and gastric analysis is positive for hydrochloric acid. Other blood studies are usually within normal range. RBCs are macrocytic and normochromic. Folic acid deficiency is associated with **neural tube defects**, such as myelomeningocele, spina bifida, and anencephaly in the fetus.

Signs and symptoms include:

- Asymptomatic (initially)
- GI disturbances, such as indigestion, anorexia, and weight loss
- Red beefy-appearing tongue
- Pallor
- Weakness, fatigue
- Forgetfulness, impaired concentration

Treatment is as follows:

- Diet high in folic acid: green leafy vegetables, liver, citrus fruits, legumes, nuts, and grains
- Oral supplementation: folic acid 1 mg to 5 mg per day, with duration varying according to cause of deficiency

Classes I to IV Cardiac Disease in Pregnancy

The New York Heart Association classifies **heart disease** by the functional capacity:

I. No cardiac insufficiency or activity limitations.
II. Slight activity limitations: symptoms present with ordinary physical activity.
III. Marked activity limitations: mild activity causes symptoms.
IV. Inability to carry out physical activities without severe symptoms.

The **maternal classification** affects the fetus. There is minimal danger to the fetus for mothers in Class I or Class II, but increased risk to both the mother and the fetus for Classes III and IV. Most medications cross the placenta, and the degree of safety during pregnancy has not been established for all of these. The most common drugs—heparin, digitalis glycosides, antiarrhythmics, thiazide, and loop diuretics—are not **teratogenic**. For Classes III and IV, delivery may be facilitated by low forceps or vacuum assistance, and caesarian may be done if mother or fetus is in danger. Labor and delivery are particularly dangerous to the fetus because of inadequate oxygen and blood supply, so continuous fetal monitoring is essential.

Pregnancy and Congenital Heart Defects

With improved surgical repair techniques for **congenital heart defects,** many women survive to childbearing age. These are common **maternal defects**:

- Tetralogy of Fallot
- Ventricular and atrial septal defects
- Patent ductus arteriosus
- Coarctation of the aorta

If surgical correction was successful, there is no added **fetal risk**, but if the condition has not been completely repaired or involves cyanosis, pregnancy can put the fetus at risk because of inadequate oxygen supply. There is a 2 to 4% risk that the child will inherit the condition.

Marfan syndrome poses severe risks to the mother, with mortality rates of 25 to 50% because of possible rupture of the aorta, which also puts the fetus at risk. Additionally, because this is an autosomal dominant disorder, there is a 50% chance that an infant will inherit the syndrome.

Mitral valve prolapse usually does not pose a risk to the fetus. Severe maternal cardiopulmonary disorders can result in death of the mother and/or fetus. However, the most common fetal complications are premature labor/birth and a fetus that is small for gestational age.

Fetal Exposure to Amphetamines

Amphetamines are a class of drugs that cause CNS stimulation. The most commonly abused amphetamine is methamphetamine. Maternal use of these substances causes hypertension and tachycardia, which can cause miscarriage, abruptio placentae, and premature delivery. Vasoconstriction affects placental vessels, decreasing circulation, nutrition, and oxygen to the fetus. Methamphetamines can cross the placental barrier and cause fetal hypertension and prenatal strokes and damage to the heart and other organs. The neonate is commonly small for gestational age, often ≤5 pounds, full term but ≤10 percentile for weight, with shortened length and smaller head circumference. The neonate in withdrawal from maternal amphetamine use will suffer abnormal sleep patterns, often characterized by lethargy and excessive sleeping during the first few weeks, poor feeding, tremors, diaphoresis, miosis, frantic fist sucking, high-pitched crying, fever, excessive yawning, and hyperreflexia.

Fetal Exposure to Cocaine

Cocaine/crack (freebase cocaine) is a nonopioid substance that readily crosses the placenta through simple diffusion. One of the most potent properties of cocaine is the ability of it to act as a vasoconstrictor. When a mother uses cocaine, the blood supply to the placenta is severely compromised when the vessels constrict, compromising blood flow and resulting in growth restriction and hypoxia. Cocaine also causes a programmed cell death (known as apoptosis) in the heart muscle cells of the fetus, resulting in cardiac dysfunction for the fetus. Maternal cocaine use increases the risk of premature birth and causes serious consequences for the neonate after birth. Maternal cocaine use can cause cerebral infarctions, nonduodenal intestinal atresia, anal atresia, NEC, defects of the limbs, and genitourinary defects. Cocaine stimulates the central nervous system by limiting the uptake of certain neurotransmitters norepinephrine, serotonin, and dopamine. Cocaine has a direct toxic effect on the nervous system, so the infant will exhibit extreme irritability and tremors followed by sluggish, lethargic behavior.

Fetal Exposure to Methadone

Methadone is commonly used to treat women who are addicted to opioids, such as heroin or prescriptive narcotics, as it blocks withdrawal symptoms and drug craving. An associated risk is that methadone crosses the placental barrier and exposes the fetus to the drug. Many female heroin users are of reproductive age and methadone is often administered to pregnant women to decrease dangers associated with heroin, such as fluctuating levels of drug and exposure to hepatitis and HIV from sharing of needles. Exposure to methadone may result in miscarriage, stillbirth, intrauterine growth restriction, fetal distress, and low birth rate although symptoms are usually less severe than with heroin. However, if the mother takes methadone and other drugs, this can compound the adverse effects. Additionally, sudden withdrawal from methadone may cause preterm labor or death of the fetus, so methadone should be monitored carefully.

Fetal Exposure to Tobacco/Nicotine

Tobacco smoke contains many substances known to be detrimental to a person's health. When a pregnant woman smokes, her fetus is exposed to carbon monoxide, nicotine, and hydrogen cyanide that all cross the placenta. Carbon monoxide displaces oxygen from hemoglobin, resulting in decreased oxygen delivery to the fetus. Exposure increases risk of miscarriage and perinatal death. Infants exposed *in utero* to tobacco may have the following problems:

- Decreased length, weight, and head circumference.
- Increased rates of congenital birth defects, such as cleft palate or lip, limb reduction defects, and urinary tract anomalies.
- Increased incidence of placenta previa, placental abruption, and preterm birth.

If smoking continues after delivery, these further detrimental effects may occur:

- Sudden infant death syndrome.
- Increased infant respiratory tract infections and childhood asthma.
- Behavioral problems in later childhood.

Substance Abuse During Pregnancy

Heroin

Heroin, an illegal opioid narcotic, is highly addictive. Users are at increased risk of HIV/AIDS from sharing needles, as well as cellulitis, endocarditis, and abscesses. Pregnant users may experience poor nutrition, iron deficiency anemia, and preeclampsia to eclampsia, all negatively affecting the fetus. Premature birth, early placental separation, and breech presentation are common. If the mother tries to stop using heroin, she may go into withdrawal, which can trigger premature labor, spontaneous abortion, or stillbirth. Symptoms of **withdrawal** usually start within 12 hours and include agitation, insomnia, increased sweating, and runny nose, progressing to gastrointestinal effects that include cramping, diarrhea, nausea, and vomiting. Pregnant women may be placed on a program of **methadone maintenance** under careful medical supervision. Methadone, while posing less danger to the fetus, is also addictive. However, methadone may delay withdrawal symptoms and reduce cravings. Additionally, while neonates may exhibit jitteriness, fever, poor feeding, and vomiting after birth, the symptoms are usually transient.

Alcohol

No safe limit for **alcohol** use during pregnancy has been established, and pregnant women should be advised to have **no alcoholic beverages**. Long-term exposure to alcohol may cause more damage to the fetus than a single use at a higher dose. Women who drink alcohol may not seek prenatal care or eat an adequate diet. Women who drink alcoholic beverages more than twice weekly have double the rate of spontaneous abortion as those who do not drink. Those who drink ≥5 alcoholic beverages weekly have a 70% increased risk of stillbirth. Alcohol use is also associated with **intrauterine growth restriction (IUGR)** and **fetal alcohol syndrome (FAS)**. More than 10% of pregnant women continue to drink and 3% engage in binge drinking, so it is essential to assess the mother for drinking, to educate about the effects of drinking alcohol, and to provide access to rehabilitation programs. Alcohol can also be passed in the human milk to the infant.

Preterm/Premature Labor

Preterm or premature labor occurs within weeks 20 to 37. Premature rupture of membrane (PROM) occurs when the membranes rupture before the onset of labor and may lead to premature labor. There are numerous causes for PROM, including infections and digital pelvic exams. When a woman presents in labor, the estimated date of delivery should be obtained by determining the date of the last menstrual period (LMP) and using a gestation calculator wheel or estimating with Naegele's rule: First day LMP minus 3 months plus 7 days equals estimated date of delivery.

Fetal viability is very low before 23 weeks of gestation; by 25 weeks, delaying delivery for 2 days can increase survival rates by 10%. Tocolytic drugs, which have many negative side effects, may be used to delay delivery in order to administer glucocorticoids, such as betamethasone or dexamethasone, to improve fetal lung maturity between weeks 24 and 36.

Post-Term Pregnancy

Post-term pregnancy (>294 days or 42 weeks past 1st day of last menstrual period) occurs in 3-7% of pregnancies, and is often the result of errors in calculating due date, but true post-term pregnancies, while posing little risk to the mother, can increase risk to the fetus, and vaginal birth may be facilitated by forceps or vacuum extractor. Increased fetal risks include:

- **Large for gestational age** (LGA), >4500g (about 10 pounds), which may result in prolonged labor, birth trauma with fractures or neurological injury, or Caesarean section.
- **Aspiration of meconium** occurs more frequently because a large fetus is more likely to expel meconium.
- **Post-maturity syndrome** related to restriction of growth in the uterus, often because of restricted blood flow, putting the fetus at risk for respiratory and neurological disorders.

Multiple Gestations

In vitro fertilization and ovulation-inducing drugs have increased the incidence of high order **multiple gestations** over the past 30 years. The trend of delayed childbearing has led to an increase in twin/multiple gestations. Infants born from multiple gestations are more likely to be born prematurely and with low birth weights. The incidence of premature birth and low birth weight is proportional to the number of fetuses. There may be growth restriction/growth discordance, oligohydramnios, and restriction of movement of one or more of the fetuses. Approximately 50% of twins and 90% of triplets are born premature, compared to 10% of singletons. With this increase in prematurity and the proportion of infants born with low birth weight, there are increased morbidities, such as cerebral palsy and intellectual disability. The risk for genetic disorders, such as neural tube defects, gastrointestinal defects, and cardiac abnormalities is twice that of single gestations.

Intrauterine Growth Restriction

When a fetus does not fulfill his or her growth potential for any reason, the diagnosis is **intrauterine growth restriction (IUGR)**. Prenatal ultrasound is used to diagnose IUGR, which is associated with oligohydramnios (decreased amniotic fluid) and preeclampsia (pregnancy-induced hypertension and proteinuria). IUGR is classified as symmetric or asymmetric, based on the size of the newborn's head:

- **Symmetric IUGR**
  - Both head and body are small (growth-restricted).
  - The restriction occurs early in pregnancy.
  - Common causes are chromosomal abnormalities and infections.
- **Asymmetric IUGR**
  - The head is large in proportion to the body; the head is spared.
  - The head is normal in size for gestational age, while the body is growth-restricted.
  - Restriction occurs late in pregnancy.
  - Common causes include placental insufficiency and preeclampsia.

Oligohydramnios

Oligohydramnios is decreased amounts of amniotic fluid (<500mL). Amniotic fluid cushions the fetus during development and is also necessary for normal development of the lungs. After 20 weeks of gestation, amniotic fluid is mainly produced by the fetus' excretion of urine. Fluids secreted by the respiratory tract and the oral/nasal cavity also contribute to the production of amniotic fluid. Oligohydramnios signals significant congenital pathology in the fetus and is associated with an elevated perinatal mortality rate. Some conditions associated with oligohydramnios include:

- Urinary tract anomalies:
  - Obstructive uropathy.
  - Renal agenesis.
  - Polycystic kidneys.
- Pulmonary hypoplasia.
- Pressure deformities, such as clubbed feet.
- Compression of the umbilical cord, leading to fetal hypoxia.
- Meconium staining.
- Post term gestation.
- Leaking of amniotic fluid, prolonged or premature rupture of membranes, which are risk factors for neonatal infections.

Polyhydramnios

Polyhydramnios is increased amounts of amniotic fluid (>500 mL) present during fetal development and is associated with an elevated perinatal mortality rate. Approximately 25% of pregnant women with polyhydramnios experience preterm labor and delivery of a premature infant. Approximately 20% of infants born to mothers with polyhydramnios have an associated anomaly. Some conditions associated with polyhydramnios include:

- Obstructional lesions in the GI tract, such as duodenal atresia or tracheoesophageal fistula with esophageal atresia.
- Anencephaly.
- Central nervous system anomalies that impair the swallowing reflex.
- Cardiovascular rhythm anomalies associated with hydrops.
- Twin-twin transfusion syndrome in multiple pregnancies.
- Macrosomia.
- Fetal or neonatal hydrops.
- Chromosomal abnormalities such as trisomy 21, 18, or 13.
- Skeletal malformations such as congenital hip dislocation, clubfoot, or limb reduction.
- Increased risk for prolapsed umbilical cord and placental abruption.

Impact of Maternal Obesity and Age on Pregnancy

The numbers of mothers who are **obese** or **older than 35 years of age** are increasing. Both conditions increase the risk of **morbidity and mortality** for mother and fetus. Complications of pregnancy are more numerous in these two groups and include a higher risk of ischemic events, preeclampsia, gestational diabetes, stillbirth, and premature births. Labor and delivery can be complicated by macrosomia, failure to progress, cesarean section deliveries, problems with anesthetics, and postpartum hemorrhages. Infection and wound dehiscence are more common. Fetal anomalies such as spina bifida and ventral wall defects, distress during labor and delivery, and postnatal neonatal problems occur at a higher rate because of the complications rather than the obesity and age.

Effects of Obesity on Labor, Fetus, and Newborn

A pregnant woman is considered **obese** with weight 50% greater than ideal weight, weight greater than 200 lb. (91 kg), or BMI greater than 29. The woman is at increased risk of developing gestational diabetes mellitus and hypertension. The second stage of labor is often prolonged because the myometrium is overstretched. Additionally, labor is difficult and associated with macrosomia and shoulder dystocia, which can cause permanent brachial plexus injury in the newborn. Because of excessive fatty tissue in the abdomen, monitoring of fetal heart rate and contractions may be difficult. During labor and delivery, the woman is at increased risk of uterine rupture and lacerations. The obese pregnant woman is more likely to require Caesarean but is at risk for excessive blood loss during surgery (>1000 mL), difficulty with intubation, and prolonged operative time as well as the need for hysterectomy. Postoperatively, the woman is at greater risk of complications (DVT and infection).

Issues of Pregnancy Post-Bariatric Surgery

Patients are usually advised to avoid pregnancy for at least 12 months to as long as 24 months **post-bariatric surgery** to give the patient time to stabilize weight loss. Pregnancy soon after surgery may result in small-for-gestational age neonates. The primary concern with pregnancy post-bariatric surgery is the **maternal nutritional status** because many patients have deficiencies of protein, iron, and calcium as well as vitamin deficiencies (especially vitamins B12 and D), and their caloric intake may be 500 to 1000 kcal/day, which is not sufficient to support pregnancy. Thus, patient's nutritional status should be monitored at least every trimester. The patient may need to eat several small nutritious meals daily. Additionally, absorption of medications may be impaired, and symptoms of pregnancy (nausea, vomiting, discomfort) may mimic those of post-bariatric complications, so careful evaluation is necessary. Patients still overweight are at increased risk of hypertension and gestational diabetes. Labor and delivery should progress normally in post-bariatric patients. Bariatric surgery is not an indication for cesarean although rates tend to be high.

Fetal Assessment

Biophysical Profile

The **fetal biophysical profile** includes 5 measurements that are taken to assess the health of the fetus.

Measure	Discussion	Normal (2)	Abnormal (0)
Fetal heart rate	Measures fetal heart rate and acceleration with movement as measured by the NST.	≥2 FHR accelerations of 15 bmp above baseline for ≥15 seconds in a 20-40-minute period. (Reactive)	0-1 FHR accelerations in 40 minutes. (Nonreactive)
Fetal respirations	Assessed by ultrasound.	≥1 episode of rhythmic breathing for ≥30 seconds in a 30-minute period.	≤30 seconds of rhythmic breathing in 30 minutes.
Fetal movement	Assessed by ultrasound and tocodynamometer	≥3 separate movements in 30 minutes.	≤2 movements in 30 minutes.
Fetal tone	Assessed by ultrasound	≥2 episodes of extension and flexion of arm/leg (or opening/ closing of a hand)	No extension/ flexion.
Amniotic fluid volume	Assessed by ultrasound and amniotic fluid index.	At least one single vertical pocket >2 cm.	Largest single vertical pocket is ≤2 cm.

Scoring: 10 normal, 8 little risk, 8 with abnormal amniotic fluid volume suspected chronic asphyxia, 6 possible asphyxia, 4 probable asphyxia, 2 almost certain asphyxia, 0 asphyxia.

Scoring

The 5 different measurements for the **biophysical profile** are completed, and scores (2 for normal and 0 for abnormal) are compiled and interpreted according to risk for asphyxia. Max score is 10:

Score	Risk of fetal asphyxia	Discussion
10	Normal fetus with no risk	No intervention is indicated.
8	Little/rare risk to fetus	No intervention is indicated.
8 (with abnormal amniotic fluid)	Suspected chronic asphyxia	Induce birth because of increased risk of perinatal mortality ≤1 week (89:1000).
6	Possible asphyxia	Induce birth if amniotic fluid volume is abnormal or if fluid level is normal at >36 weeks with cervix favorable and repeat test is ≤6. Observe and repeat tests according to protocol if the repeat test is >6.
4	Probable asphyxia	Repeat the test the same day to verify scores; induce birth if the score ≤6.
2	Asphyxia virtually certain	Marked increase in risk of perinatal mortality (125:1000), so birth should be induced.
0	Certain asphyxia	Risk of perinatal mortality is extremely high (600:1000), so birth should be induced.

Fetal Ultrasound

Ultrasound is an imaging technique using high-frequency sound waves to create computer images of vessels, tissues, and organs. Newer scans include two-dimensional Doppler readings. Fetal ultrasound can be done at about the fifth week of gestation and is commonly done at 20 weeks for all pregnant women. Ultrasound may be done **transvaginally** or, more commonly, **transabdominally**, to evaluate the gestational sac and embryo/fetus, providing the most accurate measurement of gestational age.

Trimester	Purpose
First	Estimate gestational age (accuracy ±5-7 days) Assess vaginal bleeding Determine if multiple fetuses Examine for indications of birth defects of the brain/spine
Second	Estimate gestational age (accuracy ±7-10 days) Determine size and position of placenta, fetus, and umbilical cord Examine for indications of major birth defects (cardiovascular/neural tube)
Third	Estimate gestational age (accuracy ±21-30 days) Assess fetal viability Determine size and position of placenta, fetus, and umbilical cord Estimate volume of amniotic fluid

Tests for Fetal Lung Maturity

Tests for fetal lung maturity are important for monitoring fetuses if there is an indication for early termination of pregnancy. Pulmonary maturity is often an important factor in neonatal survival, as immaturity can result in respiratory distress syndrome (RDS). Commonly, two tests are used to confirm lung maturity. Tests of amniotic fluid include:

- **Lecithin/sphingomyelin (L/S) ratio:** The ratio of the phospholipid's lecithin and sphingomyelin (two components of surfactant) changes during pregnancy, with L/S ratio at 0.5:1 early in pregnancy, 1:1 at 30-32 weeks, and 2:1 at 35 weeks. At 2:1, RDS is unlikely, although this finding is not always accurate for infants of diabetic mothers (IDM), as they may show adequate ratio but still develop RDS. These neonates must be monitored carefully. This test is not accurate if the amniotic fluid contains blood or meconium.
- **Phosphatidylglycerol (PG):** This phospholipid first appears in surfactant at about week 35 in IDM with complications and week 36 in other pregnancies. Its presence is a sign of lung maturity.

Amniocentesis

Amniocentesis is done at 15 to 20 weeks for **genetic diagnoses** and at 30 to 35 weeks to determine **fetal lung maturity**. Ultrasound locates the placenta and fetus and identifies an area with adequate amniotic fluid. The needle is inserted carefully to avoid major structures, the fetus, and arteries. A local anesthetic may be administered before insertion of a 22-gauge spinal needle into the uterine cavity. The first drops of fluid are discarded and a syringe attached. About 15 to 20 mL of amniotic fluid are withdrawn and placed in tubes, brown-tinted to shield the fluid from light that might break down bilirubin or other pigments. Ultrasound is again used to monitor removal of the needle, and the insertion point is checked for streaming (leakage of fluid). If the mother is Rh-negative, she is given Rh immune globulin immediately, unless already sensitized. The fetal heart rate is monitored. Miscarriage occurs in about 1 in 1600 amniocenteses. If the procedure is performed at 11 to 14 weeks, there is increased risk to the fetus. Infection of the placenta (chorioamnionitis) is a rare complication.

Quad Screen

The **Quad Screen** is done between weeks 16 and 20 gestation to assess for risk of genetic abnormalities and is usually offered to all pregnant women but is especially important for those with risk factors: history of birth defects in family, age ≥35, use of teratogenic medications during pregnancy, diabetes mellitus with insulin use, exposure to high-dose radiation, and history of viral infection during pregnancy. The Quad Screen includes: (1) Alpha-fetoprotein (AFP), (2) Human chorionic gonadotropin (hCG), (3) Estriol (uE^3), and (4) Inhibin A (INH-A).

Disorder	AFP	hCG	uE^3	INH-A
Neural tube defects	High	Normal	Normal	Normal
Trisomy 21	Low	High	Low	High
Trisomy 18	Low	Low	Low	Low
Multiple gestation	High	High	Normal	Normal

The fourth marker, inhibin A, improves the accuracy of screening for trisomy 21, especially in patients <35 years of age. With abnormal findings, an ultrasound may be used to verify weeks of gestation and an amniocentesis to confirm trisomy 21 or neural tube defects because of possible false positives.

Cell-Free Fetal DNA Testing

Cell-free fetal DNA (cffDNA) testing is done during or after week 10 of gestation and after genetic counseling to screen for chromosomal disorders, such as trisomy 21, 18, and 13. CffDNA is fetal DNA that has entered the maternal blood. CffDNA is usually detectable by about week 7 and continues to increase through pregnancy. Testing is especially recommended for those at **high risk** including those ≥35, with a positive first or second trimester screening test, with family history of chromosomal abnormalities, and/or with abnormal ultrasound findings. While cell-free DNA is more accurate than the Quad Screen, especially for trisomy 21, false positives can occur (most commonly with trisomy 18), so a positive finding must still be confirmed with CVS (10-12 weeks gestation) or amniocentesis (15 to 20 weeks gestation). CffDNA testing can also be used for prenatal paternity testing and fetal gender identification (especially important with X-linked disorders).

Intrapartum Factors

Fetal Heart Rate

Continuous Fetal Heart Rate Monitoring

Fetal heart rate (FHR) monitoring is usually done by **electronic fetal monitoring (EFM)**, as it provides a continuous tracing. FHR can be assessed by auscultation or ultrasound with an abdominal transducer, but tracings can be poor with an active fetus, with maternal movement, and with hydramnios. Intermittent monitoring is usually every 15 minutes in the first stage of labor and every 5 minutes in the second. Internal monitoring requires cervical dilation of ≥2cm so an electrode can be applied to the fetal presenting part (head or buttocks). Internal scalp electrodes should not be used if the mother has a communicable disease, such as HIV, or with preterm infants. Telemetry with ultrasound or fetal ECG transducers and external uterine pressure transducers can also be used to monitor FHR. This type of battery-operated monitoring can be used while the mother ambulates, as it is less invasive. FHR patterns are evaluated against a baseline rate (rate for 10 minutes between contractions), usually 110 to 160 bpm.

Fetal Heart Rate Abnormalities

Fetal heart rate usually varies with accelerations and decelerations. Fetal reactivity (accelerated fetal heart rate with fetal activity) begins at about 32 weeks. Heart rate often increases for periods of 20 to 40 minutes. These are causes for accelerated or decelerated fetal heart rate.

- **Tachycardia:** >160 for ≥10 minutes, severe >180. Transient tachycardia occurs <10 minutes and is usually not significant. Tachycardia may result from early fetal hypoxia, prematurity, medications (such as terbutaline), fetal infection, maternal fever or anxiety.
- **Bradycardia:** <120 for ≥10 minutes, severe <80. Bradycardia at 100 to 119 is usually not significant, but bradycardia may indicate heart block or placentae abruptio. Uterine contractions slow the fetal heart rate because of compression of the head affecting cerebral blood flow, compression of the myometrial vessels of the uterus, and/or occlusion of the umbilical cord causing fetal hypertension or hypoxemia. Epidural anesthesia and medications such as narcotics and oxytocin can also cause decreased heart rate.

Review Video: Fetal Heart Rate
Visit mometrix.com/academy and enter code: 980576

Fetal Heart Rate Variability and Accelerations

Fetal heart rate variability shows sensitivity to oxygenation and acid-base status. Good variability indicates adequate oxygenation of the fetus's central nervous system (CNS). Decreased variability corresponds to fetal hypoxia and acidemia. Fetal heart rate variability is fluctuation in the fetal heart rate of two cycles or more, graded according to the range of amplitude:

- Absent: range not detectable
- Minimal: ≤5 bpm
- Moderate: 6 to 25 bpm
- Marked: >25 bpm

Short-term variability is a variation in amplitude of 3 to 8 bpm on a beat-to-beat basis. Long-term variability is an irregular pattern of variability of 3 to 5 cycles per minute with amplitude of 5 to 15 bpm.

FHR accelerations are transient increases in fetal heart rate. Non-periodic accelerations relate to fetal movement. Periodic accelerations accompany contractions and/or compression of the umbilical cord and may indicate low amniotic fluid or dangerous cord compression.

Fetal Heart Rate Decelerations

Decelerations are transient decreases in FHR. They are categorized according to contraction cycle and waveform.

- **Early**: Caused by head compression as it descends the birth canal. Waveform is uniform, with onset just before or at the onset of contraction and the lowest level at the midpoint of contraction, inversely mirroring contraction. Range is usually 120 to 160 bpm. Deceleration may occur once or may repeat.
- **Late**: Caused by compression of vessels and uteroplacental insufficiency. Waveform is uniform, with shape reflecting contraction. Onset is late in the contraction and the lowest point is after the midpoint of the contraction. Range is 120 to130 bpm. Deceleration may be occasional, consistent, or repetitive.
- **Variable**: Caused by umbilical cord compression. Waveform is variable with sharp drops and increases. Onset may be abrupt with fetal insult and not related to contraction. The lowest point is around the midpoint. The range is usually outside normal. Deceleration may be variable and occur once or repetitively. Repetitive deceleration may indicate fetal distress.

Fetal Scalp Sampling and Stimulation

Fetal scalp sampling involves making a small cut in the fetal scalp and collecting a blood sample to monitor **blood gas and pH**. Fetal scalp sampling is used to determine if the fetus is receiving enough oxygen during labor, to measure fetal platelets, and to rule out acidosis. The results of the sampling are normal if the pH is greater than 7.25, prepathological if between 7.20 to 7.25, and pathological if less than 7.20. The test must be repeated every 20 to 30 minutes because the results are time-limited. This technique has several limiting factors, such as inadequate cervical dilation, fetal head too high, membranes still intact, or sampling errors due to hematoma of the fetus's scalp. The procedure requires specific technical skills, equipment, trained staff, and is costly. For the reason, it is not common practice in United States hospitals anymore.

Fetal scalp stimulation is done during the vaginal examination by gently massaging the scalp for 15 seconds. The result of scalp stimulation should be an **increase in the fetal heart rate** of 10 to 15 beats over baseline for 10 to 15 seconds. Failure of the heartbeat to accelerate is an indication of acidosis.

CORD BLOOD GAS TESTING

Umbilical cord blood gas testing, preferably arterial, should be done within ≤60 minutes of birth for infants who are at risk or depressed, to determine pH and **acid-base balance**. Testing is most applicable to infants with low Apgar scores (0 to 3) persisting for ≥5 minutes. A pH of <7 may indicate birth asphyxia/hypoxia severe enough to cause neurological deficits. Infants with normal Apgar scores may also have pH <7 but without pathology, so results must be evaluated in relation to the Apgar scores and the child's general condition. Preterm infants often have low Apgar scores and may be suspected of having birth asphyxia, but if they have suffered no birth asphyxia or hypoxia, the pH level is usually normal.

Normal cord blood values			**Abnormal cord blood values**	
	Venous	**Arterial**	**Respiratory acidosis**	**Metabolic acidosis**
pH	7.25 to 7.35	7.28	<7.25	<7.25
pO_2	28 to 32 mm Hg.	16 to 20 mm Hg.	Varies	<20 mm Hg.
PCO_2	40 to 50 mmHg.	40 to 50 mm Hg.	>50 mm Hg.	44 to 55 mm Hg.
Base excess	0 to 5 mEq/L	0 to 10 mEq/L	<10 mEq/L	>10mEq/L

Medications Used in Labor

Tocolytics

Tocolysis suppresses preterm labor and premature birth, sometimes allowing time to administer betamethasone to accelerate maturity of fetal lungs. Tocolytics (some off-label) include these.

- **Indomethacin,** an NSAID that inhibits prostaglandin production, can be used up to 32 weeks of gestation. It crosses the placenta and can cause reduction in amniotic fluid, leading to fetal distress, especially >32 weeks. Indomethacin can also cause premature closure of the ductus arteriosus. This medication is the first-line therapy for women 24-32 weeks gestation.
- **Nifedipine,** a calcium channel blocker that reduces muscle contractility, is most commonly used, as it is more effective and safer than many other drugs. It may increase fetal heart rate (FHR). This is second-line therapy for women 24-32 weeks gestation, and first-line therapy for women 32-34 weeks gestation.
- **Terbutaline** is a beta-adrenergic asthma drug that also relaxes the uterine muscle. It may increase FHR. It can be used as second-line therapy at 32-34 weeks gestation when nifedipine is used in the 24-32 weeks gestational period.
- **Magnesium sulfate** is similar in action to terbutaline, but it requires close monitoring for maternal adverse effects. It crosses the placenta, and the neonate may suffer respiratory and motor depression.
- **Ritodrine** is a beta-2 agonist that relaxes smooth muscles and can delay delivery for 24 to 48 hours but may increase fetal heart rate.

Concurrent use of tocolytics is discouraged.

Use of Opioids and Sedatives During Labor

Opioids and sedatives are usually given only in the **early stages of labor**, sometimes with PAC, because they readily cross the placental barrier and can cause **central nervous system depression** in the fetus. This depression can persist after delivery, especially in premature infants, affecting Apgar scores. Some drugs, such as morphine and benzodiazepines, are avoided because they can cause excessive fetal depression.

- **Meperidine** (1 to 25 mg IV or 25 to 50 mg IM to a maximum of 100 mg) is the most common. IV onset is 1 to 20 minutes and IM is 1 to 3 hours. Its use is limited to >4 hours before delivery.
- **Fentanyl** (25 to100 µg/hr IV) has shorter onset (3 to10 minutes) with one-hour duration and causes less fetal depression.
- **Butorphanol** (1 to 2 mg) and **nalbuphine** (10 to 20 mg IV or IM) cause little respiratory effect and provide adequate relief of pain, but may result in excessive sedation if given repeatedly.
- **Promethazine** (25 to 50 mg IM) and **hydroxyzine** may be used in combination with meperidine or alone to provide relief of anxiety and to reduce the dose of opioids.

Anesthesia Used During Labor

Pudendal Nerve Block

Visceral pain occurs in the first stage of labor from contractions and cervical dilation with afferent impulses entering the spinal cord at T10 and T11. However, during the second stage of labor, the stretching of the vagina and perineum caused by the descent of the fetus causes **somatic pain** with impulses carried by the pudendal nerves to the spinal cord at S2 to S4. **Pudendal nerve block** is used during the second stage (sometimes along with perineal infiltration) to reduce **somatic pain** when neuraxial blocks are contraindicated and for episiotomy and relaxation of the pelvic floor for forceps delivery. With the patient in lithotomy position, a transvaginal or transperineal approach is used to block the nerve. For the transvaginal approach (the most common), a Kobak needle or special guide (Iowa trumpet) is used to prevent inadvertent injection into the fetal head. Anesthetic agents include 10 mL of 1% lidocaine or 2% chloroprocaine. The transperineal approach may be used if the head is engaged.

Lumbar Epidural

The most common form of regional anesthesia/analgesia for labor and delivery is the **lumbar epidural**. Dilute mixtures of local anesthetic and opioids are combined. The catheter is usually placed early so that it is available when pain relief is needed. At one time, epidurals were delayed until labor was well established, but current trend is to administer it earlier if the fetus is in no distress, contractions are 3 to 4 minutes apart and persisting at least 60 seconds, and the fetal head is engaged with 3 to 4 cm of cervical dilation. The catheter is usually placed with the mother in a sitting position to ensure sacral spread. Placement is usually at L3 to L4 or L4 to L5. If inadvertent spinal placement occurs, spinal anesthesia/analgesia may be given or the catheter removed and replaced at a higher level. Most commonly, bupivacaine or ropivacaine (0.0625 to 0.125%) is given in combination with fentanyl (2 to 3 µg/ mL) or sufentanil (0.3 to 0.5 µg/mL). If dilute anesthetic agents are used, the mother may be able to ambulate while receiving the epidural.

Intrathecal Analgesia with Opioids

Intrathecal (spinal) analgesia, injected into the subarachnoid space with only **opioids,** is sometimes used during the **first stage of labor**. Commonly used agents include morphine (0.25 to 0.5 mg), meperidine (10 to 15 mg), fentanyl, 12.5 to 15 µg, and sufentanil 92 to10 µg). Meperidine is the only agent that has local anesthetic characteristics. Higher doses are needed if spinal opioids are used alone, administered as a single dose, or given intermittently per catheter. This can result in higher risk of complications, maternal respiratory depression, and fetal depression. However, if given alone, opioids (except for meperidine) do not provide motor blockade or maternal hypotension, so the mother is able to push. However, the analgesic effect may not be adequate, and side effects (pruritis, nausea, and vomiting) related to the agent may occur. Morphine alone has a slow onset (45 to 60 minutes), although it provides 4 to 6 hours of analgesia with spinal administration. However, low doses may not provide adequate relief, and high doses increase side effects. Morphine is frequently combined with fentanyl for more rapid onset. Commonly, opioids are combined with local anesthetics.

Spinal Anesthesia (Saddle Block)

A **saddle block**, or **spinal anesthesia**, is usually given just before vaginal delivery to provide rapid **perineal anesthesia**. Spinal blocks are avoided during labor because they interfere with motor function. Because of this, other agents may be used during labor. Prior to receiving the spinal anesthesia, the patient is given a bolus of 500 to 1000 mL fluid. With the patient in sitting position, a very small spinal needle (to prevent CSF leakage and post-spinal headache) is inserted into the subarachnoid space. Local anesthetics used include hyperbaric tetracaine, bupivacaine, or lidocaine, often with the addition of fentanyl or sufentanil to potentiate the effect. The agents are administered between contractions over about 30 seconds. The patient remains sitting for 3 minutes and then is placed in lithotomy position with left uterine displacement to prepare for delivery.

Induction of Labor

Induction of labor stimulates uterine contractions to speed birth and may be done for many conditions, including diabetes mellitus, pre-eclampsia, post-term gestation, mild *abruptio placentae*, oligohydramnios, and poor biophysical profile. Induction is contraindicated with abnormal fetal heart rate patters, breech or uncertain presentation, multiple gestation, maternal heart disease or hypertension, and polyhydramnios. Common induction methods include:

- **Stripping/sweeping amniotic membrane***:* A gloved finger is inserted through the cervical os and rotated (360°) two times to separate the amniotic membrane from the lower part of the uterus in order to release prostaglandins and stimulate contractions. Although not always effective, labor usually begins in 24-48 hours.
- **Oxytocin infusion***:* Oxytocin (Pitocin®) is used to stimulate contractions of the uterus for induction of labor, but risks include over-stimulating the uterus, causing too frequent/intense contractions as well as uterine rupture, and water intoxication.
- **Complementary methods**: These methods include sexual intercourse, nipple stimulation, and herbal/homeopathic preparations. These methods have few negative effects.

Complications of Labor

Fetal Macrosomia

Fetal macrosomia, an **exceptionally large fetus**, poses problems for vaginal delivery because of the size of the infant. Fetal macrosomia is defined variably as >90th percentile for weight according to gestational age or >4500 g. Fundal height >4 cm above expected for gestational age may be an indication. Fetal macrosomia is common with infants of diabetic mothers, obese mothers, or those who gain an excessive amount of weight during pregnancy. Complications include prolonged second stage of labor because of over-stretching of the myometrium. If the fetus is too large to descend, uterine rupture may occur. Vaginal birth often results in lacerations or extensive episiotomy. The mother has an increased risk of post-partum hemorrhage. The most common complication is **shoulder dystocia**, sometimes resulting in permanent brachial plexus injury to the neonate. Identifying fetal macrosomia prior to labor helps to prevent complications, but ultrasound and palpation are not always reliable when estimating fetal size/weight.

Cephalopelvic/Fetopelvic Disproportion

Cephalopelvic/fetopelvic disproportion is usually diagnosed when labor does not progress, although in rare cases it may be diagnosed prior to labor. It may relate to pelvic diameters that are too small (most common with android and platypelloid pelvic types) or due to contractures of the pelvic inlet (<10 cm anteroposterior diameter or <12 cm transverse diameter), contracted midpelvis, or contracted outlet (<8 cm interischial tuberous diameter). Rarely is this disproportion caused by excessive fetal size as most fetuses are within normal size and weight limits. Usually labor is extended and premature rupture of the membranes occurs, increasing danger of cord prolapse. The fetal head is often markedly molded and continued pressure can cause neurological injury or even death of the fetus if the labor continues and the fetus cannot be delivered, but when labor fails to progress, the mother is usually given a Caesarean section (within 2 hours of labor onset) to prevent further injury to the fetus.

Fetal Malpresentation

Military

The head is erect and neck not flexed. This poses little problem because flexion often occurs as the head descends.

Brow

The neck is extended so that the brow presents first. This presentation may relate to SGA, LGA, hydramnios, and uterine or fetal anomalies. Brow presentation, with the largest diameter (about 13.5cm), increases fetal mortality because of birth trauma, which can include compression of the neck and cerebrum, and tracheal and laryngeal damage. Vaginal delivery with episiotomy, or caesarian, is usually required.

Face

The neck is severely extended so that the face presents first (about 9.5 cm diameter). This often prolongs labor and may result in increased edema of the fetus and trauma to the neck and internal structures. The neonate usually has bruising in the facial skin.

Breech

This occurs in 4% of births and is frequently related to early labor and delivery (25% are at 25 to 26 weeks). Frank breech (buttocks presentation with legs extended upward) is most common, but single or double footling breech or complete breech (buttocks presentation with legs flexed) can occur. Breech presentation is most common with placenta previa, hydramnios, fetal anomalies, and multiple gestations. Cord prolapse is more likely. Head trauma may occur because molding does not occur, and the head can become entrapped. Mortality and morbidity are reduced with caesarian section, especially with low or high fetal weight, hyperextension of neck (>90°), fetal anomalies, and pelvic disproportion.

Shoulder

This transverse lie poses extreme risk of uterine rupture. The fetus cannot be delivered, and caesarian section is required.

Compound

This is when there are two presenting parts, such as the head and a hand, increasing the chance of laceration. With fetal distress or uterine dysfunction, a caesarian section is required.

Meconium in Amniotic Fluid

When **meconium is present in the amniotic fluid**, the following steps should be taken immediately following birth to avoid meconium aspiration syndrome:

- If the infant is crying and showing no signs of distress, the mouth, nose and throat should be suctioned with a suction catheter and the usual steps of drying and stimulation completed.
- If the infant shows signs of respiratory distress in the presence of meconium stained fluid, the infant should be immediately intubated with an endotracheal tube for the purpose of suctioning the trachea. Once intubated, the trachea can be suctioned with a large catheter attached to wall suction.
- Once the airway has been adequately suctioned and cleared, the stomach may need to be suctioned as well in order to prevent the regurgitation of the swallowed meconium. Meconium that is swallowed and then regurgitated can be aspirated into the lungs.

Shoulder Dystocia

Shoulder dystocia occurs when the head has been delivered but the infant's shoulder is wedged behind the mother's **symphysis pubis**. Shoulder dystocia is sometimes associated with macrosomia, postterm pregnancies, gestational diabetes, protracted labor, or assisted vaginal delivery. Special precautions are indicated during delivery. If meconium is noted, the infant's nose and mouth should be suctioned before the shoulders are delivered.

- Get help immediately.
- Consider episiotomy.
- Do McRoberts maneuver: The thighs are lifted and hyperflexed to elevate the pubic bone.
- Apply suprapubic pressure externally over the wedged shoulder while traction is continued.
- Manually rotate the infant's head and upper body while continuing suprapubic pressure.
- Pull the posterior arm out of the birth canal, flex the elbow, and deliver the forearm over the chest wall.

PROM, SROM, PPROM, and Prolonged PROM

Premature rupture of membranes (PROM): The chorioamniotic membrane breaks, ideally at term (40 weeks), prior to onset of labor. Rupture of membranes is premature if labor fails to begin within an hour. About 80% of women go into labor within 24 hours. If labor doesn't begin in 12 to 24 hours, the patient must be frequently monitored to ensure that adequate amniotic fluid remains, or labor may be induced/augmented to prevent infection, if the child is at term.

Spontaneous rupture (SROM) usually occurs in the early stage of labor during an intense contraction, causing the fluid to gush out of the vagina.

Preterm premature rupture of membranes (PPROM) occurs in a woman <37 weeks of gestation and prior to the onset of labor. The patient is monitored, as with premature rupture. It is one of the leading causes of premature birth.

Prolonged rupture of membranes: Prolonged PROM persists for greater than 18 to 24 hours prior to the onset of labor. It is associated with increased risk of infection in the neonate.

Chorioamnionitis

Chorioamnionitis is an intraamniotic infection caused by bacterial infection of the membranes before delivery. Chorioamnionitis occurs in 3 to 15% of cases of PROM and up to 25% of cases of PPROM. Chorioamnionitis poses a risk of sepsis to both the mother and fetus. The mother usually exhibits fever ≥100.5, tachycardia (>120 bpm), hypotension, and uterine tenderness. The fetus exhibits tachycardia (160 to180 bpm). The mother's white blood cell count may be elevated >15,000 cell/μL, and purulent cervical discharge (usually a late sign) may occur. Chorioamnionitis may cause spontaneous onset of labor. Infants are at increased risk of cerebral palsy and early-onset sepsis. The most common pathogenic agents are Gram-negative organisms, particularly *Escherichia coli.* Treatment includes intravenous antibiotics and prompt delivery through induction, labor augmentation, or caesarian. The infant must be evaluated at birth and may require treatment for infection.

Prolonged Labor

Prolonged labor results from dysfunctional uterine contractions, accounting for 50% of caesarians in nulliparous women, but only 5% of caesarians in multiparous women. Dysfunctional contractions are often irregular, exhibiting low amplitude, and result in <1cm cervical dilation/hr. In some cases, contractions continue but cervical dilation is arrested. The labor patterns below are associated with prolonged labor:

- **Hypertonic:** Ineffectual contractions in the latent phase of labor become more frequent but do not result in dilation or effacement. The resting tone of the myometrium increases. The contractions may interfere with uteroplacental exchange, resulting in fetal distress. The pressure on the fetal head may result in cephalhematoma, caput succedaneum, or excessive molding. Oxytocin infusion or amniotomy may be used after assessment for cephalopelvic disproportion (CPD).
- **Hypotonic**: Fewer than 3 contractions occur in 10 minutes during active phase, with less than 1 cm dilatation per hour or arrest of dilatation. Treatment is the same as for hypertonic patterns.

Placenta Previa and Abruptio Placentae

Placenta previa: Implantation of the placenta is over or near the internal cervical os. Women with placenta previa have increased incidences of hemorrhage in the third trimester. In infants, placenta previa is associated with poor growth, anemia, and increased risk of congenital anomalies in their central nervous systems, heart, respiratory and gastrointestinal tracts. Placenta previa may also cause premature birth with associated neonatal complications of prematurity.

Abruptio placentae: The placenta prematurely detaches, partially or completely, from the uterine. Abruptio placentae is related to maternal hypertension and incidence increases with cocaine abuse. Partial detachment interferes with the functioning of the placenta, causing intrauterine growth restriction. Severe bleeding occurs with total detachment. Common fetal complications are preterm labor, hypoxia, and anemia. Fetal mortality is about 25% with partial detachment and 100% with complete. Irreversible brain damage may occur with fetal hypoxia, and neurological deficits occur in about 14% of survivors.

Prolapsed Umbilical Cord

A **prolapse of the umbilical cord** occurs when the umbilical cord precedes the fetus in the birth canal and becomes entrapped by the descending fetus. An **occult cord prolapse** occurs when the umbilical cord is beside or just ahead of the fetal head. About half of prolapses occur in the second stage of labor and relate to premature delivery, multiple gestation, polyhydramnios, breech delivery, and an excessively long umbilical cord. Some cases are precipitated by obstetric interventions, such as amniotomy, external eversion, and application of scalp electrode for monitoring. As contractions occur and the head descends, this applies pressure to the umbilical cord, occluding blood flow and causing hypoxia and bradycardia. The decrease in blood flow through the umbilical vessels can cause impaired gas exchange, and if pressure on the cord is not relieved, the fetus can suffer severe neurological damage or death. *Management* includes elevating the presenting part off the cord, having the mother elevate her knees to the chest, and preparing for C-section.

Precipitous Labor/Birth

Precipitous labor and birth occurs when onset of labor to birth takes 3 hours or less, often because of strong uterine contractions and low muscle resistance in maternal tissue that promotes rapid dilation of the cervix (or lacerations) and descent of the fetus. A primigravida may dilate 5 cm per hour; and a multigravida, 10 cm per hour. The neonate may have a low Apgar score and is at increased risk for aspiration of meconium and intracranial injury, such as subdural/dural tears. The strong uterine contractions may interfere with uterine blood flow and oxygenation of the fetus. Precipitous birth alone, by contrast, is usually an unexpected and sudden birth that takes place outside of the hospital or is unattended by a physician because there is no time to travel or get help. In these cases, the neonate is sometimes expelled into a toilet or onto the floor, causing injury.

Fetal/Neonatal and Maternal Complications Related to Multiple Births

Multiple births, such as twins, triplets, and quadruplets, are increasing in incidence because of fertility treatments and increased maternal age. Multiple gestations are always considered **high risk** for both the fetuses and mother. Mothers may require bed rest during the last trimester, especially with ≥3 fetuses, and may require hospitalization for close monitoring during last month prior to delivery. Complications include:

Fetal/neonatal	Increased incidence of spontaneous abortion and neonatal death. Risk of cerebral palsy correlating with decreased gestational age Increased risk of IUGR. Increased disabilities related to premature status. Increased incidence of respiratory distress syndrome, necrotizing enterocolitis, intraventricular hemorrhage, ROP, and PDA
Maternal	Severe hypertension/preeclampsia (risk increases 2 to 3 times). Anemia (usually hemoglobin about 10 g/dL) from 20 weeks. Iron deficiency anemia is common if serum ferritin concentration is low. Preterm delivery (61%) with average gestational age in weeks of 28 (quadruplets), 33 (triplets), and 37 (twins). Increased PROM, incompetent cervix, uterine dysfunction, and malpresentation. Increased incidence of instrumental and cesarean births

Methods of Delivery

VAGINAL DELIVERY

EXPULSIVE PERIOD

During the **expulsive period of delivery**, the mother will need to be coached to achieve effective pushing effort. Two types of pushing are effective—open glottis physiologic pushing and closed glottis (Valsalva) pushing. The mother should be coached on the method most effective for her. During crowning, the mother should be instructed to "pant like a puppy." The integrity of the perineum needs to be taken into consideration. Most mothers would like to avoid an episiotomy if at all possible; however, there are several factors that may make an episiotomy necessary:

- Fetal malposition
- Anticipation of the delivery of a large baby
- Possibility of shoulder dystocia, where the anterior shoulder cannot pass below the symphysis pubis
- Poor elasticity of the perineal tissue
- Difficulty in maintaining adequate control of the patient's expulsive efforts

PLACENTA

The **placenta** will generally deliver 5 to 30 minutes after delivery of the fetus. The mechanism of **placental separation** starts with the change in the size of the uterus and then proceeds with the formation of a hematoma between the placenta and uterine wall, the separation of the placenta, the descent of the placenta through the lower uterine segment and vagina, and then expulsion. *Signs and symptoms* of placental separation include a sudden increase in vaginal bleeding, lengthening of the umbilical cord, and the rising of the uterus in the abdomen. *Management* of placental delivery includes obtaining cord blood samples after the cord is clamped, inspecting the cord for the number of vessels, and avoiding uterine massage and cord traction until the placenta is separated. Pushing by the mother may assist in expulsion of the placenta. If membranes follow the placenta, hold the placenta and roll it over and over until the membranes are delivered.

OPERATIVE DELIVERY

FORCEPS-ASSISTED BIRTH

Forceps-assisted birth utilizes a variety of specialized tools to assist with the birth of the fetus by providing traction and a method of rotating the fetal head into proper occiput-anterior position. Most forceps are used with the fetus in the head-down position and the forceps positioned on the sides of the head.

- **Outlet forceps application** can be used when the perineum is bulging, the scalp is visible between contractions, or the sagittal suture is not >45 degrees from midline. The fetal skull must be at station +2 or below.
- **Midforceps application** requires that the head be engaged with the leading edge above +2 station.
- **High forceps** are no longer used.

Indications for forceps-assisted birth include conditions that pose a risk to the mother or fetus and are relieved by birth. Maternal risks of forceps-assisted birth include infection, cervical and birth canal lacerations, extension of episiotomy, anal sphincter injury, and weakening of pelvic floor muscles. Neonatal risks include bruising and edema of face, caput succedaneum, cephalhematoma, transient low Apgar score, retinal hemorrhage, ocular trauma, Erb's palsy, and elevated bilirubin.

Vacuum-Assisted Birth

Vacuum-assisted birth utilizes a soft suction cup attached to a suction pump that creates negative pressure of 50 to 60 mm Hg. The suction cup is applied to the **occiput** of the fetus, and traction is applied with contractions. Suction use should be limited to 20 to 30 minutes, with scalp trauma more likely after 10 minutes of use. If the suction cup dislodges more than 3 times, its use should be discontinued. Indications include prolonged second stage of labor or nonreassuring heart pattern. Vacuum-assisted birth may also be used if the mother is too fatigued to push. Neonatal risks include scalp lacerations, subdural hematoma, cephalhematoma, intracranial hemorrhage, subconjunctival hemorrhage, Erb's palsy, sixth and ninth cranial nerve trauma, retinal hemorrhage, and death. A caput forms on the neonate's head, but this should subside in 2 to 3 days. Maternal risks include perineal trauma, lacerations, pain, and infection.

Caesarian Section

Caesarean sections are done if there is increased risk of uterine rupture, maternal hemorrhage, dystocia, fetal-pelvic disproportion, breech presentation, active herpes infection, and emergent situations such as fetal distress or impending maternal death. Regional anesthesia (spinal, epidural) is associated with lower mortality than general anesthesia, so it is the preferred anesthetic approach. Additionally, there is less fetal depression, reduced risk of maternal pulmonary aspiration, and an opportunity to provide neuraxial analgesia for postoperative pain relief. Regional anesthesia must provide a T4 sensory level, which causes a high sympathetic blockade. In some cases, general anesthesia may be administered for caesarian section, although the risks to the mother are intensified, so general anesthesia is usually limited to emergent situations in which the mother or fetus is at risk. Reasons for caesareans are:

- Fetal distress during the second stage of labor.
- Tetanic uterine contractions.
- Patient confused, uncontrollable, and unable to cooperate (such as psychiatric patients).
- Inverted uterus.
- Retained placenta.
- Breech extraction or other position requiring version and extraction.

VBAC

There has been decreasing interest in **vaginal birth after caesarean section (VBAC)** with only 10% attempting it in recent years, but many mothers are able to undergo vaginal delivery without complications. Risks include hemorrhage and uterine rupture (1%). Women who attempt vaginal birth have a 60 to 80% success rate. Below are the guidelines for vaginal delivery after caesarean.

- A woman with one previous caesarean section and a low transverse uterine incision should be advised to try vaginal birth. A woman with 2 or more previous caesarean sections may attempt vaginal birth.
- In all cases, a physician, an anesthesiologist, and adequate staff must be present and available throughout labor to provide a caesarean section if necessary.

Contraindications to attempting a VBAC are:

- T or classic incision.
- History of myomectomy.
- Contracted pelvis.
- Obstetrical complications precluding vaginal birth.
- Inadequate facilities or staff to provide emergency Caesarean section if it is needed.

Delayed Cord Clamping

Practice since the 1950s has been to clamp the umbilical cord within about 15 seconds of birth, but recent research indicates benefits to **delayed cord clamping** to 30-60 seconds with some recommending 2 to 5 minutes to allow **increased blood** to flow to the newborn (approximately 80 mL within the first minute and 100 mL in the first three) as well as **fetal stem cells** and **immunoglobulins**. Benefits to the term infant include increased hemoglobin and improves iron status for the first few months of life. Benefits to preterm infants include lower rates of intraventricular hemorrhage and necrotizing enterocolitis. Delayed cord clamping is contraindicated in infants that require positive pressure ventilation or if mothers are hemodynamically unstable. While there are some concerns that the infant may develop polycythemia, studies have not supported this; however, there is some increase in jaundice and the need for phototherapy. Delayed cord cutting does not appear to increase risk of maternal hemorrhage.

ABO Incompatibility

Rhesus and ABO Incompatibility

Both **Rhesus** and **ABO incompatibility** involve a mother and fetus with **different blood types**. If fetal blood escapes into maternal circulation and the mother is D- or has blood type O, she will make antibodies if the fetal blood is D+, or type A or B. These antibodies can then threaten subsequent pregnancies if the fetus has D+ or type A or B blood. The antibodies cause **hemolysis** of the fetal red blood cells, which results in **anemia**. If the anemia is severe, erythroblastosis fetalis can occur and the fetus may die without an intrauterine blood transfusion. As a neonate, hyperbilirubinemia can occur with the threat of kernicterus, and cause CNS damage and cerebral palsy if bilirubin levels are high. Infant deaths occur much less frequently in the United States since the advent of the use of D-immunoglobulin.

Maternal Rh Alloimmunization

Rh incompatibility occurs if the mother is Rh- and the father is Rh+, putting their infant is at risk for hemolytic disease of the newborn (HDN) or Rh disease, (erythroblastosis fetalis). **Rh alloimmunization** (formation of antibodies against foreign antigens) can occur during abortion, abruptio placenta, amniocentesis, cesarean section, chorionic villus sampling, cordocentesis, delivery, ectopic pregnancy, and toxemia. To prevent erythroblastosis fetalis, a woman who is Rh- with an Rh+ mate receives the serum **RhoGAM®**, containing anti Rh+ antibodies. The purpose of the antibodies is to agglutinate any fetal red blood cells that pass over into the mother's circulatory system and thus prevent the mother from forming antibodies against them that will attack the infant and sensitize her for future pregnancies:

- Mother receives 300 mcg RhoGAM (Rhlg, Rh immunoglobulin) intramuscularly at 26 to 28 weeks of pregnancy and again within 72 hours after her delivery.
- Miscarriage, ectopic, abortion: At ≤12 weeks, the mother receives 50 mcg of MICRhoGAM®. At ≥13 weeks, the mother receives RhoGAM® as for pregnancy.

ABO incompatibility is similar but usually less severe although some infants require phototherapy for jaundice and/or exchange transfusion.

ABO Incompatibility

About 20-25% of pregnancies involve **ABO incompatibility**, usually with the mother type O and the fetus A or B. **Anti-A and anti-B antibodies** occur naturally when a woman is exposed to A and B antigens in foods or bacteria, so these antibodies can cross the placenta and result in **hemolysis of fetal RBC**; however, the antibodies are relatively large and do not enter the fetal circulation easily. If fetal blood leaks into maternal blood (a common occurrence), then smaller antibodies form and these can cross the placenta more easily. There is no difference in affect between the first pregnancy and subsequent pregnancies. There are rarely serious complications for the fetus although the neonate may develop hyperbilirubinemia, so the infant should be observed carefully. Only in severe cases of hemolysis (rare), does the child require exchange transfusions. Anemia may develop in the weeks after delivery because of increased rate of RBC breakdown, so the neonate should be monitored with blood counts.

Pregnancy Terms

Gravida—Any pregnancy (including present), regardless of duration/outcome.

Nulligravida—A woman who has never been pregnant.

Primigravida—A woman with her first pregnancy.

Multigravida—A woman in her second (or more) pregnancy.

Para—Delivery of live or stillborn fetus/neonate >20 weeks.

Nullipara—Woman who has not given birth >20 weeks.

Primipara—A woman who has given birth, live or stillborn, one time >20 weeks.

Multipara—A woman who has given birth, live or stillborn, ≥2 times >20 weeks.

Grand multipara—A woman who has given birth, live or stillborn, ≥5 times >20 weeks.

Term—38 to 48 weeks, i.e., duration of pregnancy.

Gestation—Number of weeks since the first day of last menstrual period (LMP).

Abortion—Death of fetus <20 weeks' gestation.

Stillbirth—Death of fetus >20 weeks' gestation.

Maternal Postpartal Assessment, Management, and Education

Physiologic Changes and Physical Assessment

Postpartal Uterine Involution

The normal uterus weighs about 70 to 100 g and has a capacity of 5 mL. During pregnancy, the uterus increases in weight to 1000 g with a capacity of 5000 mL. After delivery, the weight of the uterus decreases to 500 g by the end of the first week, 300 by the second, and 100 by the third. **Uterine involution** (the process of the uterus returning to the pre-pregnant state) begins immediately after the placenta separates. The changes occur over the first 3 weeks, except for the placental site, which takes 6 to 7 weeks to heal over.

- **Estrogen and progesterone levels** drop markedly, causing cells to atrophy, reversing hyperplasia.
- **Autolysis** occurs as proteolytic enzymes are released and macrophages migrate to the uterus.
- The **spongy layer of decidua** sloughs off as lochia.
- The **basal layer of decidua** separates into two layers within 48 to 72 hours with the outer layer becoming necrotic and sloughing off as lochia with the inner layer providing the base for the new endometrium.

Postpartal Fundus Evaluation

The uterus contracts after the placenta is expelled to about grapefruit size, with the **fundus** about midway to two-thirds the distance between the symphysis pubis and the umbilicus. The contraction of the uterus brings the uterine walls together and compresses the vessels to prevent bleeding.

- Over the 6 to12 hours after delivery, blood and clots pool in the uterus, and the fundus rises midline to the level of the **umbilicus**, where it stays for about 12 hours. A **boggy fundus** above the umbilicus indicates excessive bleeding. A **high fundus** that deviates from midline often indicates a distended bladder.
- By first postpartum day, the fundus is about 1 cm (one finger-width) below the umbilicus.
- The fundus continues to descend about 1 cm per day until it is no longer palpable (usually within 2 weeks).

If a boggy uterus is felt on fundal examination, it should be massaged until the uterus contracts, expels clots and debris, and firms. If it fails to firm, the physician should be notified.

Postpartal Assessment of Lochia

Lochia, vaginal discharge after delivery, rids the uterus of remaining debris. The total volume of discharge is about 240 to 480 mL, with discharge decreasing over time. Discharge is usually increased in the morning because of pooling. Lochia should be examined to assess both hemorrhage and uterine involution.

Rubra (days 1 to 3 or 4) - Dark red discharge, containing epithelial cells, red and white blood cells, bacteria, decidua shreds, lanugo, vernix caseosa, and sometimes meconium. Clots should not exceed nickel size, as large clots may indicate hemorrhage—although this should be differentiated from bleeding from vaginal lacerations.

Serosa (days 4 to10) - Pinkish to brownish discharge, containing serous exudate, decidua shreds, red and white blood cells, cervical mucus, and various microorganisms. Gradually lightens as the number of red blood cells decreases.

Alba (the following 2 to 85 days [average 24]) - Yellowish discharge contains primarily white blood cells, epithelial cells, decidual cells, fat, mucus, and bacteria. The cervix is closed when lochia alba flow stops, so the danger of infection ceases.

POSTPARTAL PHYSIOLOGICAL CHANGES

CARDIOVASCULAR AND RESPIRATORY SYSTEMS

The **cardiovascular system** remains fairly stable after delivery. Blood pressure readings are usually within normal limits for the mother. Decreased BP may indicate physiological adaptation to decreased intrapelvic pressure, but can also indicate hemorrhage. Orthostatic hypotension is common for the first few hours postpartum. Elevated BP may indicate preeclampsia. A slow heart rate (puerperal bradycardia) of 50 to70 bpm is common from days 6 to 10 because of decreased strain on the heart, decreased blood volume, and increased stroke volume. Tachycardia may result from excessive blood loss or prolonged labor.

The **respiratory system** adapts to pregnancy by increased minute ventilation, tidal volume, and respiratory rate. By the time of delivery, **functional residual capacity (FRC)** and residual volume have decreased because of the pressure of the uterus against the diaphragm. The FRC returns to normal within about 1 to 2 weeks, while other respiratory changes usually return to baseline within 6 to 12 weeks.

URINARY AND GASTROINTESTINAL SYSTEMS

Urinary system changes in the postpartal period include

- Increased bladder capacity
- Edema and bruising about urethra
- Decreased sensitivity to bladder filling and fluid pressure
- Increased urinary output (puerperal diuresis) for 12 to 24 hours

Combined, these put the woman at risk for **excessive bladder distention** and **residual urine**. Anesthetic blocks may inhibit neural function and cause difficulty voiding, as well as bladder distention. If the mother received oxytocin as a uterotonic, this causes an antidiuretic effect, and the bladder tends to fill rapidly. Because the ureters and renal pelvis dilate during pregnancy, the mother is at increased risk of infection for about 6 weeks postpartum. Hematuria, which may be an indication of infection, may be overlooked because of lochia.

Gastrointestinal concerns include a lack of **muscle tone** and slow **motility** from lasting effects of progesterone, which can lead to constipation. The mother is usually hungry and thirsty after birth. Concerns about opening an episiotomy may cause mothers to delay elimination, but bowel movements are usually not painful.

Hematological System

Most women lose approximately 200 to 500 mL of **blood** during vaginal delivery and 700 to 1000 mL with cesarean, with a 2 point drop in hematocrit corresponding to about 500 mL of blood loss, so both **hemoglobin** and **hematocrit** fall after delivery, resulting in **anemia** in up to 50% of new mothers, usually related to low iron levels. Hemoglobin and hematocrit usually return to prelabor levels within 2 to 6 weeks. Coagulation factors are activated during pregnancy, putting mothers at increased risk of thromboembolism, although early ambulation and activity reduces incidence. The sedimentation rate is elevated for about a week after delivery because of increased plasma fibrinogen levels. The white blood cell count elevates and may increase to 30,000 in the days after delivery without indicating infection. However, a WBC increase of >30% in a 6-hour period may indicate infection. Vasomotor changes may cause women to have chills immediately after delivery, but this does not indicate infection.

Hypothyroidism

Symptoms of **hypothyroidism** may include chronic fatigue, menstrual disturbances, hoarseness, subnormal temperature, low pulse rate, weight gain, thinning hair, thickening skin. Some dementia may occur with advanced conditions. *Treatment* involves hormone replacement with synthetic levothyroxine (Synthroid®) based on TSH level. The same dosage is usually adequate during pregnancy. Weekly nonstress tests should be done >35 weeks. Without treatment, fetal loss is 50%. Newborns should be screened for T4 level.

Hyperthyroidism

Hyperthyroidism is caused by excess production of T3 and T4 thyroid hormones and suppression of TSH may be present in neonates born to thyrotoxic mothers or those with genetic disorders, such as McCune-Albright syndrome. Hyperthyroidism may develop during the fetal stage, resulting in IUGR, fetal hydrops (non-immune), and fetal death. *Symptoms* of neonates include:

- Hyperkinesis.
- Diarrhea.
- Vomiting.
- Failure to thrive or gain weight.
- Tachycardia with ↑ pulse pressure.
- Hypertension (systemic and pulmonary).
- Hepatosplenomegaly.
- Thrombocytopenia.
- Hyperviscosity syndrome.
- Ophthalmic abnormalities.
- Craniosynostosis.

Treatment includes the use of antithyroid medications, such as Propacil® or Tapazole®, β-adrenergic blockers, and iodine. Digoxin may be necessary as well as glucocorticoids. Remission usually occurs in 20-48 weeks. In rare cases, thyroid ablation (thyroidectomy) may be necessary.

TYPES OF INSULIN

There are a number of different types of **insulin,** with varying action times. Insulin is used to metabolize glucose for those whose pancreases do not produce insulin. People may need to take a combination of insulins (short and long-acting) to maintain glucose control. Duration of action may vary according to the individual's metabolism, intake, and level of activity.

- **Humalog (Lispro H)** is a fast-acting, short duration insulin that acts within 5 to15 minutes, peaking between 45 to 90 minutes and lasting 3 to 4 hours.
- **Regular (R)** is a relatively fast-acting (within 30 minutes) insulin that peaks in 2 to 5 hours and lasts 5 to 8 hours.
- **NPH (N)** or **Lente (L)** insulin is intermediate acting with onset in 1 to 3 hours, peaking at 6 to 12 hours and lasting 16 to 24 hours.
- **Ultralente (U)** is long-acting insulin with onset in 4 to 6 hours, peaking at 8 to 20 hours and lasting 24 to 28 hours.
- **Combined NPH/Regular** (70/30 or 50/50) has an onset of 30 minutes, peaks at 7 to 12 hours, and lasts 16 to 24 hours.

Comprehensive Postpartum Assessment and Postoperative Care

Postpartum Assessment

- **Vital signs**
  - VS should be checked every 15 minutes and evaluated in relation to baseline VS and VS prior to delivery.
  - Normal BP varies from 90/60 to 140/90.
  - Falling BP and increased pulse may indicate uterine bleeding.
  - Pulse (60 to 90) is usually slightly decreased from that found during labor.
  - Respirations should be relaxed and not labored, usually ranging 12 to 20/min.
- **Temperature**
  - Slight elevation immediately after delivery (≤100.4), but this should return to normal within 24 hours.
- **Alertness**
  - The mother should be awake, alert, responsive, and able to hold the infant.
- **Fundus**
  - Fundus is palpated to determine if it is firm, midline, and in the expected position (at the umbilicus).
  - A boggy fundus may indicate uterine bleeding.
  - Bladder distention may cause the fundus to deviate from midline.
- **Lochia**
  - Lochia should be checked every 15 minutes for signs of excess bleeding, such as copious discharge or large clots.
  - Lochia must be observed while fundus is massaged to determine if there is free flow of blood or expulsion of clots, which may indicate hemorrhage.
  - Lochia rubra should be present with moderate amount of discharge, <1 perineal pad/hr.
- **Perineum**
  - The perineal area should be examined and amount of swelling and bruising noted, along with the condition of episiotomy (if present) and sutures.
  - Severe perineal/rectal pain requires further examination.
- **Bladder**
  - The bladder should be palpated to determine if it is distended.
  - The mother should be given the opportunity to urinate within the first hour after delivery before catheterization is considered.
  - Mother should spontaneously urinate >100 mL clear urine with no distention noted after urination.
- **Rectum**
  - Rectum should be examined for presence of tearing or hemorrhoids.
  - No severe rectal pain should be present.
  - If hemorrhoids are present, engorgement must be reported to physician, especially if ≥2 cm in size.

- **Pain**
  - Mother should have only mild pain, <3 on 1 to10 scale.
  - Severe pain requires further examination to determine cause.
  - Analgesia should be provided to control pain.
- **Legs/feet**
  - Feet and legs should be warm and pulses palpable.
  - Edema, which may have been present before delivery, should remain stable or decrease.
- **Anesthesia**
  - If the mother had an anesthetic, such as epidural or spinal, the level of anesthesia should be assessed every 15 minutes.

Cesarean

The initial assessments of the mother who has had a **cesarean** and of the neonate are similar to those for vaginal birth, but the mother also must recover from a surgical procedure and anesthesia. These assessments constitute standard **postoperative care** during the first hour postpartum:

- **VS** checked every 5 minutes until stable, then every 15 minutes for one hour, and finally every 30 minutes until mother released from the recovery area
- **Abdominal dressing and perineal pad** checked every 15 minutes for bleeding for the first hour; fundus gently palpated with a hand supporting the area of the incision
- **IV oxytocin** administered to promote contraction of the uterine muscles
- If general anesthesia, patient positioned on side and **turned** every 2 hours for 24 hours
- If epidural or spinal anesthesia, level of **anesthesia** checked every 15 minutes
- **Intake and output** monitored, and urine checked for signs of blood (indicating bladder trauma)
- **Analgesia** as needed to control pain

Postoperative Care After Cesarean Birth

The mother who has had a **cesarean** birth has both routine postpartal and surgical needs. The mother should deep-breathe and cough (while supporting the abdomen with a pillow) and use an **incentive spirometer** every 2 to 4 hours during the daytime for the first few days. The mother should sit on the side of the bed within 12 hours of surgery and ambulate within 24 hours. **Pain management** with PCA, oral, and parenteral medications and/or relaxation techniques helps the mother to ambulate and care for her infant. Epidural analgesia may continue for 24 hours after delivery and must be monitored carefully. Flatus and abdominal distention are common complaints, so the mother should avoid carbonated beverages and drinking through straws. Taking an antiflatulent (Mylicon®), turning frequently, rocking, or lying on the left side may help to expel gas. The mother should be encouraged to breastfeed but may be more comfortable sitting with the baby supported by a pillow or lying on her side to prevent pressure on the incision.

Common Medications

NSAIDs

Non-steroidal anti-inflammatory drugs (NSAIDs) include cyclooxygenase (COX) inhibitors that block COX enzymes that develop with inflammation and with precancerous/cancerous tissues. COX enzymes form these prostanoids:

- **Prostaglandins**—cell growth, inflammatory reactions, sensitivity to pain, platelet aggregation/disaggregation, hormone and calcium regulation
- **Prostacyclin**—platelet aggregation and vasodilation
- **Thromboxane**—platelet aggregation and vasoconstriction

COX inhibitors are used as anti-inflammatory, analgesic, and antiplatelet drugs. Some drugs, such as ibuprofen and aspirin, block both COX-1 and COX-2 enzymes (non-selective inhibitors). Aspirin should be used with caution in the postpartal period because of increased risk of bleeding. Non-selective NSAIDs are associated with irritation of gastric mucosa because of inhibition of COX-1, which has a protective effect on gastrointestinal mucosa. Other drugs, such as celecoxib, block only COX-2 enzymes (selective inhibitors). These tend to have fewer adverse gastrointestinal effects, but they have been implicated in increased risk for cardiovascular disease and thrombus formation. COX-2 NSAIDs specifically target inflammation.

Acetaminophen

Acetaminophen is an antipyretic and non-opioid analgesic suitable for **mild to moderate pain**. Acetaminophen reduces fever by acting on the hypothalamic heat-regulating center to cause vasodilation and increased perspiration to dissipate heat. Acetaminophen is especially indicated for those who are sensitive to aspirin or at increased risk of bleeding. Acetaminophen may relieve musculoskeletal pain, but it lacks the anti-inflammatory action of NSAIDs.

- Oral adult dose: 1000 mg TID to QID, not to exceed 4 g/day.
- Pediatric dose (0 to 3 months): 40 mg 4 to 5 times daily.

Acetaminophen should be used cautiously with impaired hepatic function, alcoholism, and pregnancy as well as during lactation. While side effects are uncommon if recommended doses are adhered to, adverse effects may include headache, chest pain, dyspnea, hepatic toxicity, jaundice, acute renal failure, methemoglobinemia, hemolytic anemia, rash, and fever. Women should be cautioned not to exceed recommended dose and to avoid multiple analgesic preparations as some others may contain acetaminophen.

Antibiotic Medications

Antibiotics may be classified according to their chemical nature, origin, action, or range of effectiveness. There are hundreds of antibiotics. **Broad-spectrum antibiotics** are useful against both gram-positive and gram-negative bacteria. **Medium-spectrum antibiotics** are usually effective against gram-positive bacteria, although some may be effective against gram-negative as well. **Narrow-spectrum antibiotics** are effective against a small range of bacteria. Antibiotics are bacteriocidal, meaning they function by killing the bacteria by interfering with its biological functions, or bacteriostatic, meaning they prevent reproduction of bacteria. The main classes of antibiotics are described here:

- **Macrolides**: Medium-spectrum antibiotics that prevent protein production by bacteria and are primarily bacteriostatic, but may be bactericidal at high doses. They may be irritating to the gastric mucosa, but are less likely to cause allergic responses than penicillins or cephalosporins. Macrolides include erythromycin (E-Mycin®), clarithromycin (Biaxin®), and azithromycin (Zithromax®)
- **Penicillins:** Medium-spectrum antibiotics, which may be combined with beta-lactamase inhibitors. They are bacteriocidal, causing breakdown of the bacterial cell wall. Penicillins may cause severe allergic reactions in sensitive individuals. Penicillins include penicillin, ampicillin, and amoxicillin.
- **Cephalosporins:** Medium-spectrum antibiotics effective against gram-negative organisms. They are bacteriocidal and inhibit cell wall synthesis. They are divided into different "generations" according to antimicrobial properties, with succeeding generations having more a powerful effect against resistant strains. First generation includes cephazolin (Kefzol®), cephalexin (Keflex®), and cephradine (Velosef®). Second generation includes cefaclor (Ceclor®), cefuroxime (Zinacef®), and loracarbef (Lorabid®). Third generation includes cefotaxime (Claforan®), cefixime (Suprax®), cefpodoxime (Vantin®), ceftazidime (Fortaz®), and cefdinir (Omnicef®). Fourth generation includes cefixime (Maxipime®).
- **Polymyxins:** Narrow-spectrum antibiotics effective against gram-negative organisms. They interfere with the cell membrane of bacteria and are bacteriocidal. Polymyxins have both neurotoxic and nephrotoxic properties and are not used unless other antibiotics are ineffective. They must be given intravenously. Polymyxins include Polymyxin B Sulfate®.
- **Fluoroquinolones:** Broad-spectrum antibiotics that inhibit bacterial reproduction and repair of genetic material in the bacterial DNA. Drugs include ciprofloxacin (Cipro®), levofloxacin (Levaquin®), and ofloxacin (Floxin®).
- **Sulfonamides**: Medium-spectrum with action against gram-positive and many gram-negative organisms, as well as plasmodium and toxoplasma. Some people are sensitive and may develop an allergic response. Resistance to sulfa drugs is widespread. Sulfa drugs interfere with folate synthesis and prevent cell division, so they are bacteriostatic. Sulfonamides include cotrimoxazole (Bactrim®) and trimethoprim (Proloprim®).
- **Tetracyclines**: Broad-spectrum antibiotics, which are also used for rickettsias and psittacosis- producing agents. Tetracyclines include tetracycline, doxycycline (Vibramycin®), and minocycline.
- **Aminoglycosides:** Effective against gram-negative bacteria. They interfere with protein production in the bacteria and are bacteriocidal. Aminoglycosides cannot be taken orally. They are often given in conjunction with other classes of antibiotics, such as penicillin. Aminoglycosides include gentamicin (Garamycin®), tobramycin (Tobrex®), neomycin, and streptomycin.

Vasodilators and Antihypertensives Medications

Calcium Channel Blockers

Primarily arterial vasodilators that may affect the peripheral and/or coronary arteries. Side effects include lethargy, flushing, abdominal and peripheral edema, and indigestion. Examples:

- **Dihydropyridines**, such as nifedipine (Procardia®), which should be avoided in older adults, and nicardipine (Cardene®) are primarily arterial vasodilators that affect both coronary and peripheral arteries and are used to treat acute hypertension.
- **Benzothiazepines**, such as diltiazem (Cardizem®) and phenylalkylamines, such as verapamil (Calan®, Isoptin®), dilate primarily coronary arteries and are used for angina and supraventricular tachycardias.

Angiotensin Converting Enzyme (ACE) Inhibitors

Limit production of the peripheral vasoconstricting angiotensin, resulting in vasodilation, which can cause a precipitous fall in blood pressure, so use must be carefully monitored. They are often the first line of drugs to be used for acute hyper-tension and heart failure, and are also used to prevent diabetic nephropathy. The most common ACE inhibitors, captopril (Capoten®) and enalapril (Vasotec®), decrease afterload and preload for heart failure.

Angiotensin receptor blockers (ARBs)

Examples: Losartan (Cozaar®) and valsartan (Diovan®)

Decrease afterload and preload and reverse ventricular remodeling, causing vasodilation and reducing blood pressure. They are used for those who cannot tolerate ACE inhibitors. Side effects include cough (less common than with ACE inhibitors), hyperkalemia, hypotension, headache, dizziness, metallic taste, and rash.

Beta-blockers

Examples: Metoprolol (Lopressor®), carvedilol (Coreg®) and esmolol (Brevibloc®)

Slow the heart rate, reduce hypertension, prevent dysrhythmias, and reverse ventricular remodeling, but should not be used during decompensation and should be monitored carefully for those with airway disease, uncontrolled diabetes, slow or irregular pulse, or heart block.

Aldosterone agonists

Example: Spironolactone (Aldactone®)

Decreases preload and myocardial hypertrophy and reduces edema and sodium retention, but may increase serum potassium.

Loop Diuretics

Diuretics increase **renal perfusion and filtration**, thereby reducing preload and decreasing peripheral and pulmonary edema, hypertension, CHF, diabetes insipidus, and osteoporosis. There are different types of diuretics: loop, thiazide, and potassium sparing. Diuretics are rarely used during pregnancy.

Loop diuretics inhibit the reabsorption of sodium and chloride (primarily) in the ascending loop of Henle. They also cause increased secretion of other electrolytes, such as calcium, magnesium, and potassium, and this can result in imbalances that cause dysrhythmias. Other side effects include frequent urination, postural hypotension, and increased blood sugar and uric acid levels. They are short acting and so are less effective than other diuretics for control of hypertension.

- **Bumetanide** (Bumex®) should be avoided while breastfeeding. High doses may suppress lactation.
- **Ethacrynic acid** (Edecrin®) should be avoided while breastfeeding.
- **Furosemide** (Lasix®) is used for the control of congestive heart failure as well as renal insufficiency. It may suppress lactation.

THIAZIDE DIURETIC MEDICATIONS

Thiazide diuretics inhibit the reabsorption of **sodium and chloride**, primarily in the early distal tubules, forcing more sodium and water to be excreted. Thiazide diuretics increase secretion of **potassium and bicarbonate**, so they are often given with supplementary potassium or in combination with potassium- sparing diuretics. Thiazide diuretics are the first line of drugs for treatment of hypertension. They have a long duration of action, 12 to 72 hours, depending on the drug, so they are able to maintain control of hypertension better than short-acting drugs. They may be given daily or 3 to 5 days per week. There are numerous thiazide diuretics.

- **Chlorothiazide** (Diuril®): Low doses do not interfere with lactation.
- **Bendroflumethiazide** (Naturetin®): Shorter acting diuretics are usually preferred, but low doses should not interfere with lactation.
- **Chlorthalidone** (Hygroton): This drug may suppress lactation and may accumulate in the infant.
- **Trichlormethiazide** (Naqua®): Large doses may suppress lactation.

Side effects include dizziness, lightheadedness, postural hypotension, headache, blurred vision, and itching, especially during initial treatment. Thiazide diuretics cause sensitivity to sun exposure, so patients should be counseled to use sunscreen.

POTASSIUM-SPARING DIURETIC MEDICATIONS

Potassium-sparing diuretics inhibit the reabsorption of sodium in the **late distal tubule and collecting duct**. They are weaker than thiazide or loop diuretics, but do not cause a reduction in potassium level; however, if used alone, they may cause an increase in potassium, which can cause weakness, irregular pulse, and cardiac arrest. Because potassium-sparing diuretics are less effective alone, they are often given in a combined form with a thiazide diuretic (usually chlorothiazide), which mitigates the potassium imbalance. Typical side effects include dehydration, blurred vision, nausea, insomnia, and nasal congestion, especially in the first few days of treatment.

- **Spironolactone** (Aldactone®) is a synthetic steroidal diuretic that increases the secretion of both water and sodium and is used to treat congestive heart failure. It may be given orally or intravenously. By itself, it does not usually affect lactation and has minimal effects on the infant.
- **Eplerenone** is similar to spironolactone but has fewer side effects, so it may be used with patients who can't tolerate the other drug.

Review Video: Diuretics
Visit mometrix.com/academy and enter code: 373276

Uterotonic Medications

Uterotonics are drugs used to prevent and treat post-partum hemorrhage, most often related to uterine atony:

- **Oxytocin (Pitocin)** - Used to stimulate contractions of the uterus for induction of labor, but also used in the postpartum period to stimulate uterine contractions and prevent atony through rhythmic contractions. Onset is immediate with IV administration. Adverse effects include uterine hyperstimulation, transient hypertension, and water intoxication (rare).
- **Methyl-ergonovine maleate (Methergine)** - A semisynthetic ergot alkaloid used routinely after placental delivery to prevent uterine atony and hemorrhage. Administration may begin after the anterior shoulder is delivered, during the second stage of labor, and causes sustained uterine contractions. Numerous adverse effects include hypertension, dizziness, flushing, tinnitus, nausea, vomiting, palpitations, and chest pain. Overdose or sensitivity reaction may result in vasoconstriction with distal peripheral numbness and tingling, and seizures. It is contraindicated in women with high blood pressure.
- **Ergonovine maleate (Ergotrate Maleate®)** - An ergot alkaloid that is used to prevent and control hemorrhage after delivery or abortion. It provides sustained contractions of the uterus. Adverse effects are similar to those of methylergonovine maleate and include hypertension, dizziness, flushing, tinnitus, nausea, vomiting, palpitations, and chest pain. It is contraindicated in women with high blood pressure.
- **Prostaglandins** - Include carboprost tromethamine (Hemabate®) and dinoprostone (Prostin®). Used for control of refractory post-partum hemorrhage related to uterine atony after other agents have failed to control hemorrhage. Adverse effects include gastrointestinal disorders, headache, flushing, bradycardia, respiratory distress (wheezing, cough, and bronchospasm), chills, and fever. It is contraindicated in women with cardiovascular, kidney, or liver disease or asthma. Women receiving prostaglandins must be monitored carefully for signs of fever or respiratory distress. Antipyretic medications may be needed to control fever/chills.

GI Motility (Laxative) Drug Categories

Bulk Formers

Have high fiber content and both soften stool and create more formed stools. These include products such as Metamucil®, Citrucel®, and FiberCon®, which are usually added to liquids, because without adequate fluids they can increase constipation. These can be safely used while breastfeeding.

Lubricants

Include both oral mineral oil and glycerin suppositories. They coat the stool, preventing fluid absorption and keeping the stool soft. Mineral oil absorbs fat-soluble vitamins and should be avoided, but glycerin suppositories pose no risk.

Saline

Includes Milk of Magnesia® and Epsom salt, which contain ions (such as magnesium phosphate, magnesium hydroxide, and citrate) that are not absorbed through the intestines and draw more fluid into the stool. The magnesium in the preparations also stimulates the bowel. People with impaired kidney function should avoid magnesium products, and saline laxatives should be used infrequently to avoid dependence. Epsom salt often has a purging effect and is rarely used. Milk of Magnesia in small doses may be used during breastfeeding.

Stimulants

Increase intestinal motility, moving the stool through the bowel faster and reducing the absorption of fluids so the stool remains softer. Common ingredients include cascara in Castor Oil®, senna in Senokot® and sennosides in Ex-lax®. Stimulants work quickly and are effective, but can result in electrolyte imbalance, abdominal distention, and cramping. Chronic use may cause a cycle of constipation and diarrhea. Stimulant suppositories, such as Dulcolax®, are also available. Large doses of stimulant laxatives may be excreted in the milk and can cause diarrhea in the infant.

Metoclopramide (Reglan®)

Used to reduce nausea and vomiting from a wide range of causes. It is also a prokinetic drug that increases gastrointestinal contractions and promotes faster gastric emptying, so it is used for heartburn, GERD, and diabetic gastroparesis. Infants receive <10% of the dose through breastfeeding with little effect. Metoclopramide may increase milk supply by increasing serum prolactin. It may cause depression, so care must be used with postpartum women.

Stool softeners

Include emollients, such as Colace®, and Phillip's Liqui-Gels®. They use wetting agents such as docusate sodium to increase liquid in the stool, thereby softening it. They should not be used with mineral oil because of increased absorption of the oil through the intestines. Stool softeners are safe to use while breastfeeding.

Hyperosmotics

Contain materials that are not digestible and serve to retain fluid in the stool. Products such as Kristalose® and MiraLax® soften the stool. May result in increased abdominal distention and flatus, especially initially. There are 3 types of hyperosmolar laxatives: lactulose, polymer, and saline. Lactulose types use a form of sugar and work similarly to saline laxatives, but more slowly, and may be used for long-term treatment. Salines empty the bowels quickly and are used short-term. Polymers contain polyethylene glycol, which retains fluid in the stool and is used short-term.

Combination

Use two or more types together, such as stool softener with stimulant. Short-term only.

Vaccines

Influenza

A different **influenza ("flu") vaccine** is formulated each year, and administration begins in September prior to flu season. There are two types of flu vaccine:

- **Trivalent inactivated influenza vaccine (TIV)** (injectable) is available for use in those over 6 months old, including older people who are healthy or have chronic medical conditions.
- **Live attenuated influenza vaccine (LAIV)** is a nasal spray for use in those 2 to 49 years of age. It is not for use in pregnant women and is not used for older adults.

Antibodies against the viruses used to formulate the vaccines develop in about 2 weeks. Vaccination is **recommended** for all people over six months of age.

The flu vaccine is **contraindicated** in individuals with an allergy to eggs, a history of reaction to flu vaccine, and a history of Guillain-Barré. The vaccine should not be administered 6 weeks or less after a previous flu vaccine. *Adverse effects* include infection with local inflammation, fever, and aching.

HPV

Human papillomavirus (HPV) comprises >40 viruses. It is sexually transmitted and invade mucosal tissue, causing genital warts, which are low risk for cancer or changes in the mucosa, which can lead to cervical cancer. Most HPVs cause few or no symptoms, but they are very common, especially in those 15 to 25. Over 99% of cervical cancers are caused by HPV, and 70% are related to HPVs 16 and 18. The HPV vaccine Gardasil®, protects against HPVs 6 and 11, which cause genital warts, against 16, and 18, which can cause cancer. Protection is only conveyed if the female has not yet been infected with these strains. The vaccine is currently recommended for females ≤26 years of age. Studies are determining the benefit for males and women over 18. A series of **3 injections** is required over a 6-month period:

- Initial dose 11 to12 years (but may be given as young as 9 or ≥18)
- 2 months after first dose
- 6 months after first dose

Diphtheria, Tetanus, and Pertussis Vaccine

Diphtheria and pertussis (whooping cough) are highly contagious bacterial diseases of the upper respiratory tract. Cases of diphtheria are now rare; however, recent outbreaks of pertussis have occurred in the United States. Tetanus is a bacterial infection contracted through cuts, wounds, and scratches. The **diphtheria, tetanus, and pertussis (DTaP) vaccine** is recommended for all children. DTaP requires 5 doses:

- 2 months
- 4 months
- 6 months
- 5-18 months
- 4-6 years (or at 11-12 years if booster missed between 4-6)

Rotavirus Vaccine

Rotavirus is a cause of significant morbidity and mortality in children, especially in developing countries, but most children, without vaccination, will suffer from severe diarrhea caused by rotavirus within the first 5 years of life. The new rotavirus vaccine is advised for all infants but should not be initiated after 12 weeks or administered after 32 weeks, so there is a narrow window of opportunity. Three doses are required:

- 2 months (between 6-12 weeks)
- 4 months
- 6 months

Nicotine Patches and Antiretroviral Drugs

Nicotine patches are sometimes used for pregnant women who smoke, but there is little consensus about the use during pregnancy and breastfeeding. While the women may smoke less, the patches provide a steady **blood level of nicotine** (21 mg patch is equal to 17 cigarettes daily) that can still affect the growing fetus and result in low birth weight and preterm birth. Some authorities believe that nicotine gum or lozenges, which allow nicotine levels to fall between use, may be safer.

Antiretroviral drugs used for treatment of HIV/AIDS should continue during pregnancy for those already taking drugs because stopping increases risk of increased viral load and transmission to the fetus. Those who have not been treated should be encouraged to start a regimen of combination

antiretroviral therapy (ART) as soon as the pregnancy is diagnosed to reduce risk of fetal transmission. When selecting drugs, antiretroviral drug-resistance studies should be carried out. Mothers with HIV/AIDS should not breastfeed.

NAS and Withdrawal Associated with Maternal Substance Abuse

Neonatal abstinence syndrome (NAS) includes the manifestations of withdrawal that a neonate undergoes after exposure to drugs while *in utero*. These may vary somewhat depending on the type and extent of substance abuse, which may include prescription narcotics, heroin, antidepressants, and benzodiazepines. NAS is more readily treated if the mother's substance abuse was controlled with drugs such as methadone and buprenorphine. Buprenorphine causes less severe NAS than methadone. Substance abuse may result in *in utero* growth restriction, abruptio placentae, fetal cardiac arrhythmias, preterm labor and delivery, and fetal death. Neonates often have low birth weight, small head circumference, tremors, seizures, diarrhea, and hypertonic reflexes. They may feed poorly, so they may need high-caloric formula, and may cry excessively and sleep poorly. The infant may receive drugs (morphine, methadone, and buprenorphine) to relieve withdrawal symptoms. Dehydrated infants (from diarrhea) may require IV fluids. Swaddling, kangaroo care, and maintaining a quiet dimly lit environment may help to soothe the infant.

Psychotropic Medications During Pregnancy

Commonly used **psychotropic medications** may pose risks to the fetus and newborn, so risks and benefits should be discussed with the physician. Typical medications include:

- **Benzodiazepines** (alprazolam, lorazepam, diazepam, clonazepam): Study results have been inconsistent in regards to whether benzodiazepines cause birth defect or development/behavior problems, but the neonate may have withdrawal symptoms, such as dyspnea, tremors, jitters, excessive crying, and difficulty sleeping. Combining benzodiazepines with diphenhydramine may result in increased rate of stillbirths.
- **Buspirone**: Little data regarding pregnancy available, but classified as a Class B drug.
- **SSRIs** (fluoxetine, sertraline, citalopram, paroxetine, escitalopram): May cause persistent pulmonary hypertension of the newborn if taken during the last 50% of the pregnancy. Paroxetine (Paxil®) may result in congenital heart disease. Withdrawal symptoms in neonate may occur within 2 days of delivery and may be similar to those of benzodiazepines.
- **SNRIs** (venlafaxine, duloxetine): Similar to SSRIs although withdrawal symptoms are less pronounced.

Common Postpartal Problems and Complications

Urinary Problems

Bladder retention, inability to initiate urine flow or completely empty the bladder, is common after delivery because of **periurethral edema**. **Dysuria** is usually transitory. Mothers should be encouraged to try to urinate within the first hour after delivery. The mother should empty the bladder at least every 4 to 6 hours, and the bladder should not be palpable. Warm water poured over the perineum or a warm shower may help relax muscles enough to promote urination. The time and amount of voiding should be recorded. Normal volume for each urination is 300 to 400 mL. Smaller amounts may indicate dehydration or incomplete bladder emptying, which may be verified by ultrasound. Repeated catheterization >2 times in 24 hours should be avoided. If the mother is still unable to urinate after straight catheterizations, then an indwelling catheter with prophylactic administration of ampicillin may be considered.

Constipation

Slowed GI motility often results in constipation in the postpartal period, especially if the mother is reluctant to bear down because of an episiotomy. If the mother holds a clean pad against the episiotomy and applies firm pressure while bearing down, this may alleviate discomfort. Adequate fluids and dietary fiber help promote evacuation. Stool softeners are often prescribed, but laxatives (other than fiber laxatives) and enemas should be avoided if possible.

Hemorrhoids

Pressure on veins in the rectum and anus during pregnancy and delivery may cause hemorrhoids. Usually, these begin in the days after delivery, but constipation may worsen them, so measures used to prevent constipation may help promote healing. Sitz baths and application of witch hazel pads may relieve discomfort. Other comfort measures include anesthetic ointments, manual replacement of hemorrhoids, and side-lying position.

Hunger

Mothers often feel very hungry after giving birth and may enjoy a light meal. If the mother had a C-section, she may be limited to clear liquids initially but should be progressed to a **regular diet** as soon as possible.

Thirst

Because fluids are lost during delivery, the mother often experiences marked thirst, alleviated by providing ample **oral fluids** to replace those lost. If the mother had a C- section and is receiving IVs, the rate of replacement must be adequate.

Chill

Postpartal chill immediately after delivery is common and may relate to neurological or vasomotor changes. The mother should be covered with a warmed **blanket** and offered warm **liquids**.

Diaphoresis

Perspiration increases during the puerperium to help eliminate excess fluid and waste products, and the mother may wake up drenched in sweat at night. The mother should be provided with a dry gown and linens and protected from chilling.

AFTERPAINS

With a first pregnancy, the uterus usually remains contracted after delivery, but with subsequent pregnancies or complications, such as hydramnios or retention of clots or placental tissue, the uterus may alternate between contraction and relaxation, causing severe cramp-like afterpains in the 2 to3 days after delivery. If the mother receives oxytocin to stimulate contractions, this may increase discomfort. Breastfeeding naturally stimulates release of oxytocin, so nursing may cause afterpains. **Analgesic agents** such as acetaminophen or ibuprofen an hour before nursing and at bedtime may relieve discomfort.

FLATULENCE

The GI tract is sluggish after birth because of hormonal changes and decreased muscle tone. Flatulence is common, especially after C-section. This is alleviated by early ambulation, turning from side to side, avoiding carbonated beverages, and taking antiflatulent medications.

PERINEAL EDEMA/PAIN

Bruising and swelling of the perineum are common because of birth trauma, although excessive bruising may indicate hematoma. Small hematomas resolve over time, but large collections of blood may need to be drained. Gentle palpation of an episiotomy incision should cause minimal tenderness. If the incision is warmer than surrounding tissue, or redness or indurated areas appear, these changes may indicate an infection that requires antibiotics. Swelling may be reduced by applying an ice pack. A sitz bath may relieve perineal discomfort after episiotomy.

FATIGUE/SLEEP DISTURBANCE

Fatigue is common after delivery, but it sometimes becomes chronic and is associated with **sleep disturbance**. Because the baby must be fed around the clock, the mother is rarely able to sleep more than 3 hours at a time. During this period, the mother should be encouraged to nap frequently when the infant sleeps and to increase activity. Family support is critical. If the mother is breastfeeding, she can pump and have someone else to do occasional feedings.

POSTPARTUM BLUES

Adjustment reaction with depressed mood, more commonly referred to as **postpartum blues,** is a mild depression that occurs in 50 to 80% of women after childbirth. Onset is usually ≤5 days postpartum and duration is typically 2 to 3 days, but it may persist for up to 10 days in some women. *Symptoms* include mild insomnia, anger, mood swings, fatigue, irritability, impaired concentration, depressed affect, and frequent episodic tearfulness. The cause is not clear but may relate to changes in hormones and psychological adjustments to parenting. Because mothers often are discharged on the first or second day postpartum, symptoms may not appear until after discharge, so mothers and family should be advised about the symptoms and encouraged to seek help if the symptoms persist, suggesting a more serious depression. About 20% of women experiencing postpartum blues progress to **postpartum depression**. Mothers should be reassured and supported during this period.

CARE OF MOTHER WITH HIV/AIDS

Mothers infected with **HIV/AIDS** who are **asymptomatic** prior to pregnancy usually have no added risk for acceleration of their disease, but increased risk occurs if the **CD-4 count** was already low. Because about half of neonatal infections occur during birth and delivery, the HIV/AIDS mother may have an elective C- section at 38 weeks. Routine care should be provided, always using standard precautions to avoid contact with blood or other body fluids. The mother is at increased postpartal risk of hemorrhage, urinary and endometrial/pelvic infections, and poor wound healing, and requires careful evaluation for complications. The mother should be educated about all aspects of her disease and its implications and about the need for follow-up care for both her and her infant. Mothers should be advised not to breastfeed as the virus may be transmitted through human milk. Prior to discharge, the mother should receive referrals to social agencies that can provide support.

Spinal Headaches Following Spinal Block

Spinal headaches may occur following a spinal block for delivery when **cerebrospinal fluid (CSF)** leaks from the meninges, usually within a few hours up to 48 hours. The headaches may persist for a few hours to over a week. Sitting and standing results in pain from the reduced volume of CSF creating traction on pain-sensitive CNS structures. Some women experience associated dizziness, nausea, and vomiting. Spinal headache can be prevented and treated by keeping the woman flat in supine position for several hours and increasing hydration. Some find relief from administration of caffeine, a vasoconstrictor. If the pain is severe or persistent, an epidural blood patch is applied to the epidural space. (A small volume of blood is obtained from the mother [without coagulation] and then injected into the epidural space at the same site.) Relief is usually achieved immediately. If pain persists after the blood patch, then further testing and evaluation is needed to determine another cause, such as cerebral thrombosis.

Obstetrical Lacerations

Risk factors for **obstetrical (vaginal/perineal) lacerations** include fetal macrosomia, precipitous labor and delivery, fetal malpresentation, and forceps- and vacuum-assisted delivery. Lacerations often occur in the **anterior vaginal wall** near the urethra but are usually superficial and heal without intervention. Longitudinal lacerations are most common with forceps- or vacuum-assisted delivery and occur in the upper or middle third of the vagina, often extending into underlying tissue and posing the risk of hemorrhage. Tearing may be prevented by allowing labor to progress slowly, delivering in side-lying position, avoiding assisted delivery, and utilizing an episiotomy if tearing appears imminent. **Classifications** of obstetrical laceration:

Degree	Description
First	Laceration of vaginal mucosa or perineal skin but not underlying tissues.
Second	Laceration extends to underlying subcutaneous tissues but not rectal sphincter or rectal mucosa
Third	Laceration extends though rectal sphincter but not rectal mucosa.
Fourth	Laceration extends through rectal mucosa.

Patient Education

Educational Needs of New Mothers

The **educational needs** of the new mother and family vary depending on age, background, education, experience, and expectations. The needs of the adolescent mother with no experience may be quite different from those of the multiparous mother. Assessing individual needs can be difficult in the short time women are usually hospitalized, so education should cover a wide range of topics. A checklist of topics may be a helpful starting point for the mother to indicate her needs. Because mothers are usually fatigued for the first 24 to 48 hours, teaching after that time is most effective, but many mothers leave the hospital on the second day. Demonstration with return demonstration is an effective method to ensure that a mother can carry out tasks, but education should anticipate other needs and concerns that may arise. Mothers often have concerns about a variety of issues, such as childcare, contraception, and resuming sexual relations. Pamphlets, website information, or videos that can be sent home with the mother are very helpful.

Principles of Adult Learning

Adults have a wealth of life and/or employment experiences. Their attitudes toward education may vary considerably. There are, however, some **principles of adult learning** and typical characteristics of adult learners that an instructor should consider when planning strategies for teaching patients and families.

Practical/goal-oriented	Provide overviews or summaries and examples. Use collaborative discussions with problem-solving exercises. Remain organized with the goal in mind.
Self-directed	Provide active involvement, asking for input. Allow different options toward achieving the goal. Give responsibilities.
Knowledgeable	Show respect for life experiences/ education. Validate knowledge and ask for feedback. Relate new material to information with which they are familiar.
Relevancy-oriented	Explain how information will be applied. Clearly identify objectives.
Motivated	Provide certificates of achievement, if possible, or other tangible reward.

Visual-Auditory-Kinesthetic Model of Cognitive Learning

Not all people are aware of their preferred **learning style.** A range of teaching materials and methods that relates to all 3 learning preferences—visual, auditory, kinesthetic—and are appropriate for different ages and should be available. Part of assessment for teaching involves choosing the right approach, based on observation and feedback. Presenting learners with different options often gives a clue to their preferred learning style. Some people have a combined learning style.

Visual learners learn best by seeing and reading.	Provide written directions, picture guides, or demonstrate procedures. Use charts and diagrams. Provide photos, videos.
Auditory learners learn best by listening and talking.	Plan extra time to discuss and answer questions. Provide audiotapes. Explain procedures while demonstrating and have learner repeat.
Kinesthetic learners learn best by handling, doing, and practicing.	Provide hands-on experience throughout teaching. Encourage handling of supplies/equipment. Allow learner to demonstrate. Minimize instructions and allow person to explore equipment and procedures.

Readability

Studies have indicated that learning is more effective if oral presentations and/or demonstrations are supplemented with reading materials, such as handouts. **Readability** (the grade level of material) is a concern because many patients and families may have limited English skills or low literacy, and it can be difficult for the nurse to assess people's reading level. The average American reads effectively at the sixth to eighth grade level, regardless of education achieved, but many health education materials are written at a much higher level. Additionally, research indicates that even people with much higher reading skills learn medical and health information most effectively when the material is presented at the sixth to eighth grade level. Therefore, patient education materials and consent forms should not be written at higher than the sixth to eighth grade level. Readability index calculators are available on the Internet to assist in preparing materials by giving an approximation of grade level and difficulty for those without expertise in teaching reading.

Postpartum Self-Care

Preparing the mother for **postpartum self-care** requires evaluating the mother's understanding of self-care activities as well as the needs of the infant. Educational topics include:

- **Physical care** of breasts and perineum.
- Methods of dealing with **complications**, such as afterpains and constipation.
- **Nutritional needs**, including discussion of cultural preferences
- **Psychological adaptations**: Mothers are often passive during the first 24 hours, with some quiet and others talkative. By 12 hours after birth, most mothers begin to assume responsibility for the child and their own care. Some may feel overwhelmed and require additional support.
- **Attachment**: Methods of improving attachment should be reviewed. Some women may be disappointed because of gender or the infant's appearance, but with support, most women feel attachment within 1 to 2 days.
- **Postpartum blues**: Mothers should be apprised that postpartum blues is common and made aware of danger signs of depression.

Contraception

Oral Contraceptives

Many methods of **birth control** are available, including condoms, intrauterine devices, spermicides, and barriers, such as diaphragms, sponges, and cervical caps, but hormonal contraceptives are commonly used. There are 2 types of **oral contraceptives**, but there are many different brands with differing amounts of hormones.

- **Combined** (estrogen [ethinyl estradiol] and progestin): These may be *monophasic* (constant doses), *biphasic* (constant estrogen but increased progestin on day 10, or *triphasic* (varying doses of both).
- **Progestin only**: These have fewer side effects than combined forms, but can increase estrogen levels and incidence of thrombosis.

Oral contraceptives are **contraindicated** for those who smoke or have evidence or history of breast cancer, coronary artery disease, or elevated cholesterol, because they are associated with increased risk of thrombosis. Common *side effects* (depending upon the particular drug) include an increase in acne, facial hair growth, weight increase, rash or itching, amenorrhea, decrease in libido, headache, nausea, and breakthrough bleeding. Changing to a different contraceptive may alleviate symptoms.

Injectable, Ring, and Patch Contraceptives

Newer methods of contraception include injectable, ring, and patch contraceptives. One primary advantage is that the woman does not need to remember to take pills, but risks are similar to oral contraceptives.

- **NuvaRing®** is a ring that in inserted vaginally and left in place about the cervix for 3 weeks. It is removed for the fourth week, during which there may be withdrawal bleeding. It is as effective as oral contraceptives.
- **OrthoEvra®** is a small adhesive patch that is applied to the torso, chest (excluding the breasts), arms, or thighs every week for 3 weeks; the fourth week is patch free. It is as effective as oral contraceptives.
- **Depo Provera®** is injectable medroxyprogesterone acetate that is given every 13 weeks. It is contraindicated with a history of deep vein thrombosis or smoking. It may relieve symptoms of endometriosis.

Emergency Contraception

Females who have had unprotected sexual intercourse, whether consensual or rape, and are at risk for pregnancy may desire **emergency contraception.** Emergency contraception inhibits ovulation and prevents pregnancy, rather than aborting a pregnancy. Emergency contraceptives have been marketed for use ≤72 hours after unprotected intercourse, but recent studies indicate they are effective for ≤120 hours.

Plan B Next Choice (Levonorgestrel)	The first pill (0.75 mg) must be taken ≤120 hours (5 days) after unprotected intercourse, and the second (also 0.75 mg), 12 hours later.
Plan B One-step (Levonorgestrel)	One pill (1.5 mg) only is taken ≤120 hours (5 days) after unprotected intercourse. This is now used more commonly than Plan B.
EllaOne (Ulipristal acetate)	One pill (30 mg) is taken ≤120 hours (5 days) after unprotected intercourse (FDA-approved for sale in US in August 2010).

A follow-up pregnancy test should be done if the person does not menstruate within 3 weeks, as the failure rate is about 1.5%. Side effects include nausea (relieved by taking medication with meals or with an antiemetic), breast tenderness, and irregular bleeding.

Contraceptive Devices

Male and Female Condom

These are more effective if used with **spermicide**, but **nonoxynol-9 (N-9)** should be avoided because it interferes with protection against sexually transmitted diseases. Patients should have instruction in proper use to avoid semen leaking from the male condom. Condoms are 80 to 90% effective.

Intrauterine Device

IUDs are usually T-shaped and are inserted through the cervix into the uterus (with the attached string palpable at the cervical opening). IUDs prevent pregnancy by causing a local **inflammatory response** that prevents **fertilization**. Some are plastic, but ParaGard® is copper, which has antisperm effects and can be left in place for up to 10 years. Mirena® releases levonorgestrel, a synthetic progestin, and can be left in place for 5 years. It can be used with smokers, but there may be some side effects because of the hormone: acne, increased facial hair, and thickening of cervical mucosa. IUDs are 95 to 99% effective. Adverse effects of IUDs include abnormal bleeding, discharge, or infection.

Diaphragm

This round device has a flexible supporting ring and a dome-like latex cup, so assessment of the patient for latex allergy is necessary. The concave surface, which faces the cervix, is coated with **spermicide** before the diaphragm is inserted. The diaphragm is fitted to the individual using sized fitting rings during a pelvic exam so it seats properly below cervix and is held in place by vaginal muscles. Diaphragms range in size from 50 to 90 mm. They should not be placed more than 2 hours prior to intercourse because spermicide loses effectiveness. Diaphragms are left in place for at least 6 hours after intercourse, but not more than 12 hours. Each act of intercourse requires additional insertion of spermicide vaginally. The diaphragm should be washed with soap and water after use, and inspected under bright light for tears or holes prior to each use. The diaphragm is 85 to 95% effective if used properly. Changes in weight or pregnancy can alter size requirements, so diaphragms should be **refitted** when either of these has occurred.

Cervical Cap

This latex cap is smaller than the diaphragm (22 to35 mm) and more cone-shaped. It fits about the cervix rather than below it. Like the diaphragm, it is used with **spermicide**. It may cause **cervical irritation**, so women may need Pap smears more frequently (every 3 months), but it has the advantage of being able to stay in place for up to 48 hours. Leaving it in for long periods increases the risk of vaginitis and toxic shock syndrome. Cervical caps do not require additional spermicide for each act of intercourse and are 85 to 95% effective.

Contraceptive Sponge

This is a donut-shaped, spongy barrier device that is impregnated with **nonoxynol-9 (N-9)**, so it is 85 to 95% effective. It does not protect against **STDs**. The sponge has a concave central indentation on one side that fits over the cervix to act as a barrier. The outside has a string for easy removal. The sponge is left in place for 6 hours after intercourse, but not >30 hours.

Contraceptive Practices

Coitus Interruptus

This requires withdrawing the penis from the vagina prior to **ejaculation**. It is a frequently used method of birth control, especially among teenagers, but it is completely unreliable as sperm may leak prior to ejaculation.

Rhythm Methods

Using rhythm methods requires determining when the woman **ovulates** and abstaining from sex during the **fertile phase**. Pregnancy rates are about 40%, so this method is only advised if couples are disciplined, monitor their cycles carefully, and are willing to abstain from sex for long periods during each cycle. This method is often used because of religious restrictions against artificial birth control. Ovulation detection kits (such as Ovulindex®) are available over the counter. They detect the enzyme guaiacol peroxidase in cervical mucosa. This indicates ovulation will occur in about 6 days. These kits, however, are more reliable for those attempting to become pregnant than to avoid pregnancy.

Sterilization Procedures

Vasectomy

The male's **vas deferens** are clipped or severed and then tied or sealed under local anesthetic. The procedure is done with one central puncture or bilateral incisions. Other birth control methods must be used for 4 to 6 weeks. It may take up to 36 ejaculations to clear remaining sperm. A sperm count is done at 6 weeks, with follow-up at 6 and 12 months to check for recanalization that might restore fertility. Discomfort is usually minimal. *Complications* include infection, pain, hematoma, and recurrent epididymitis. Reversal techniques are 30 to 85% effective.

Tubal Ligation

Tubal ligation seals the fallopian tubes to prevent conception. Various methods are available, including clipping, silicone rings, cauterization, and surgical cutting and realigning. Tubal ligation is often done during C-section or shortly after vaginal birth because the tubes are easier to isolate after pregnancy. Complications include infection, pain, perforated or burned bowel, and hemorrhage. Reversal techniques are 45 to 80% effective.

Maternal Nutrition During Postpartal Period

The maternal **postpartum diet** should be nutritionally well balanced. Because many women are **anemic** after delivery, foods high in **iron** (red meats, organ meats, green leafy vegetables) or fortified with iron (cereals) should be included daily. Mothers taking iron supplementation should avoid taking the supplement with dairy products, as calcium may interfere with absorption. Dairy products may be taken at other times. Mothers, especially those ≤24, need 4 daily servings of **high calcium foods**, such as milk. **Vitamin C** helps absorption of iron, so diet should include broccoli, oranges, potatoes, and tomatoes. Adequate dietary **fiber and fluids** (2 to 3 L daily) help to prevent constipation. Adequate **protein** (about 60 g for most people) and vitamin C help to promote healing. Because mothers are fatigued, they should try to include foods that require minimum preparation but should avoid fast foods, which are often high in saturated fat and sodium. Breastfeeding mothers need about 500 additional calories daily.

Lactation

Anatomy of Lactation

The breasts are mammary glands involved in **lactation** (production of milk). During pregnancy, progesterone stimulates the growth of **alveoli** (milk glands), which produce milk. The breasts usually increase in size by about 8 weeks of pregnancy. Veins become more prominent on the breasts as circulation increases. Estrogen causes the **ductal system** that leads from the alveoli to the nipple to grow and expand. The areola and nipple darken and enlarge, and the Montgomery tubercles (small raised glands in the areola), which secrete an antibacterial lubricating substance, increase in size. By the end of the first trimester, the alveoli begin to produce **colostrum**. During the last trimester, the breasts enlarge and the alveoli increase in size. After delivery of the placenta, estrogen and progesterone levels fall and **prolactin**, which promotes milk production, increases. Nursing stimulates production of both prolactin and oxytocin, which contracts cells lining the ducts, causing the **letdown** reflex. As the alveoli produce milk, it flows through the ducts into the **lactiferous sinuses**, small sacs below the areola.

Human Milk

Human milk has immunologic benefits that formulas lack, resulting in decreased morbidity in breastfed infants. Human milk contains these important substances:

- **Antibodies**: Secretory IgA to provide protection from respiratory, enteric, and viral pathogens.
- **Primary nutrients:** Protein with whey-to-casein ratio of 60:40 (including IgM, IgG, lactoferrin, lysozyme, casein [40%], and fibronectin), carbohydrate (about 40% of total calories), and fat (free fatty acids).
- **Secondary nutrients**:
  - Nucleotides
  - Vitamins A, C, D, E; vitamin D content ≤25 IU/L; supplement if ≤2 months of age
  - Enzymes: anti-inflammatory and antibacterial properties, including lipase, which breaks down fat
  - Growth factors
  - Hormones: prolactin, cortisol, thyroxine, insulin, and erythropoietin
  - Cells: beta-lymphocytes, macrophages (90%), neutrophil, T-lymphocytes, cytokines, interleukin 1b, 6, 8, 10, 12 (both inflammatory and anti-inflammatory properties)

Maternal Nutritional Needs While Breastfeeding

Nutritional needs while breastfeeding include a nutritious, well-balanced diet with adequate protein and complex carbohydrates: fruits, vegetables, and whole grains. Mothers who are breastfeeding need a caloric intake of about 2500 to 2800 per day or about 500 calories more than a normal diet. Even mothers who are overweight should avoid trying to cut calories for the first 6 weeks, as doing so may impact milk production. Eating 3 meals with 2 snacks, spreading intake throughout the day, is usually better than eating 2 or 3 large meals. Most foods do not affect the infant, so mothers can generally enjoy the same foods they ate before and during pregnancy. However, if the infant develops diarrhea or stomach upset after certain foods, the mother should avoid these. Because of concerns about mercury in fish, canned light tuna should be limited to 8 ounces a week, and mothers should completely avoid fish with high levels of mercury, including shark, swordfish, king mackerel, and tilefish (also called golden or white snapper), tuna steak (fresh or frozen), orange roughy, Spanish mackerel, marlin, and grouper.

Normal Breastfeeding

Hormonal changes with birth stimulate the breasts to increase milk production in preparation for **breastfeeding**. The mother may feel some increased fullness. On gentle palpation, the breasts should feel full but not hard, and may be slightly tender. The mother should be advised to avoid sleeping in the prone position, as this compresses the breasts and increases the risk of complications, such as clogged milk ducts. Breastfeeding should begin immediately or within 30 to 60 minutes of birth. **Colostrum** does not pose a danger to the neonate, even if aspirated, and nursing promotes maternal bonding with the infant, as well as contraction of the uterus. Colostrum, produced the first 2 to 4 days, is thick and yellow and produced only in teaspoons, but this is adequate for the neonate, whose stomach capacity the first day is only 5 to 7 mL. Colostrum provides both antibodies and protein. By day 3, **transitional milk** is thinning and the stomach capacity is 1 ounce. By day 7, when **mature milk** is starting to come in, the neonate's stomach capacity is 1.5 to 2 ounces.

Benefits of Human Milk

Human milk is the food of choice for newborn infants. **Colostrum**, produced during the first few days after birth, is scant, thick, yellowish, and high in protein and antibody content. Colostrum stimulates the passage of meconium. **Transitional milk** (days 3 to 14) is thinner and white, with a composition closer to that of mature milk. By the second week, most mothers produce 23 to 27 ounces of bluish-white **mature human milk**. Most neonates nurse every 1 to 3 hours for 20 to 40 minutes.

- Human milk provides appropriate amounts of carbohydrate, protein, fat, vitamins, minerals, enzymes, and trace elements.
- It contains maternal antibodies that help bolster the infant's immature immune system.
- Breastfed babies have reduced risks of eczema, asthma, obesity, and elevated cholesterol later in life.
- Breastfeeding enhances the bond between the mother and the infant by physical contact and promotes recognition of communication signals.
- The maternal cost is an extra 500 calories a day and extra water.
- There is no chance of causing kidney damage by mixing formula incorrectly.

Breastfeeding Positioning

During nursing, the baby should be turned toward the mother, with the face tilted up toward the mother's so they can make eye contact, and the mouth slightly below the nipple, which is pointed toward the baby's upper lip or nostrils. There are several **positions** that work well for nursing.

- **Cradle**: The baby is cradled in the arm on the nursing side with the arm supported by a pillow. The mother uses the opposite hand to guide the nipple, and positions the infant toward her.
- **Cross-cradle:** The hand on the side of the breast used is free to guide the breast while the opposite arm crosses over the baby with the hand supporting the baby's head.
- **Football**: The infant is tucked under the arm on the nursing side with the arm supporting the baby's back and the hand supporting the head.
- **Side-lying:** This position is similar to the cradle hold but the mother is reclining on her side, so there is no pressure on the abdomen. Infant is cradled by the arm on the nursing side.

Latching On

Once the infant is in position, the mother should grasp the breast using a C-hold or U-hold (to make the breast more firm) and lean toward the baby, guiding the nipple toward the infant's mouth. Brushing the nipple against the infant's mouth usually causes the infant to open the mouth and lunge toward the breast. Then, the mother guides the nipple into the infant's mouth while pulling the infant toward the breast. The infant's lower lip should be low on the areola so the baby **latches** on to both the areola and the nipple.

Problems Associated with Latch-on

Most **problems associated with latch-on** result from poor maternal technique and are easily resolved with demonstration and support:

- **Infant latching on to the end of the nipple,** resulting in pain and limited milk flow: The mother should learn to brush the nipple against the infant's lips until the baby opens the mouth completely before inserting the nipple.
- **Infant's mouth on just the nipple and not areola**: The mother should use a C-grip or U-grip to guide the nipple into the infant's mouth, making sure that most of the areola (1-1.5 inches) is covered by the infant's mouth.
- **Inverted nipples**, making latching on difficult: If the nipple is so flat that the infant cannot easily latch on, using a silicone nipple shield for the first few minutes may help to elongate the nipple, at which point the shield should be removed because the shield doesn't allow adequate breast stimulation, and the infant must work harder to suckle.

Letdown

Suckling stimulates nerves in the areola and nipple, increasing production of prolactin and oxytocin, which in turn stimulate contraction of cells about the areola, causing milk to be ejected in a "let-down" (milk-ejection) reflex, which is sometimes associated with a tingling sensation, usually within a few minutes of nursing. It may take up to 2 weeks before letdown is efficient.

Suck-Swallow Sequence

A neonate usually **sucks** and then **swallows** when the mouth becomes full. Each suck usually fills the mouth, a **suck to swallow ratio** of 1:1. Infants do not breathe while swallowing, so a 1:1 ratio means the child must breathe quickly, resulting in a rapid suck-hold breath and swallow-breathe sequence. During a swallow, the soft palate rises to block access to the nasal passages, the larynx rises, and the epiglottis covers the airway to prevent aspiration. If milk flow is inadequate, the child may need to suck twice for each swallow (2:1). If the flow is too fast, the child may need to swallow twice or more for each suck (1:2) and some milk may run down the pharynx and into the airway, resulting in aspiration. Or, the child may need to swallow so rapidly there is no time to breathe, and apnea may occur. A newborn usually sucks twice a second for about a minute and then about once per second as the milk flow increases.

Sucking and Swallowing Disorders

Sucking and swallowing disorders are very common in the preterm infant because of immaturity (coordination of sucking and swallowing occurs at 33-36 weeks) but may be caused in term infants by a number of conditions, including trisomy 21, FAS, cleft palate, central nervous system disorders (anoxia, hydrocephalus), congenital infection (rubella, cytomegalovirus), respiratory disorders (apnea, pneumonia, RDS, and cardiac or ENT anomalies. Typical characteristics of swallowing disorders include:

- Silent aspiration (not associated with cough or clearing airway).
- Laryngeal penetration (associated with lack of pharyngeal response).
- Nasopharyngeal reflux (especially common in preterm infants and may trigger apnea).

Pneumonia frequently develops in infants with sucking and swallowing disorders, so diagnosing the cause is critical. Observation is not sufficient because of the frequency of silent aspiration. Feeding infants in the upright position can reduce nasopharyngeal reflux. Tests include radiographic (video fluoroscopy) or fiberoptic evaluation of swallowing.

Breastfeeding

Frequency and Duration

Most infants initially nurse every 1 to 3 hours, but during **growth spurts** (2 to 3 weeks, 6 weeks, 3 months, and 6 months), the infant may nurse every half to one hour for 2 to 3 days, stimulating the breasts to increase production. Nursing usually takes 20 to 45 minutes, with 15 to 20 minutes on each side. Nursing should begin on the last breast used. Infants may nurse more frequently in the late afternoon and evening. Infants should be fed every 3 hours until they regain their birth weight, even if the infant must be awakened. Infants vary in **demand schedules**. Some eat 5 to10 times over a 3-hour period and then sleep for about 4 hours. The schedule is less important than assuring that the child nurses **8 to 12 times** in 24 hours and appears satisfied. By 8 to 12 weeks, infants begin sleeping longer at night. Some may sleep through the night at 4 months, while others continue to nurse at night.

Feeding Cues

The infant gives a number of **feeding cues** to show hunger. Mothers should be taught to recognize these cues, as it's more difficult for a frantically hungry baby to latch on. These are some indications that the infant is hungry:

- Licking the lips.
- Sucking motions of the mouth.
- Rooting or bobbing of the head.
- Keeping hands in fists.
- Bringing hands near mouth or face.
- Turning the head toward and trying to suck on a finger stroking the baby's cheek or lower lip.
- Crying (usually the last indication).

Infants who are consistently not receiving adequate nutrition usually appear sleepy and listless. They often stop gaining weight or lose weight. Skin turgor may be poor. Urinary output and stools decrease. The infant may appear disinterested in nursing. On the other hand, an infant who is satisfied usually stops sucking and may turn the head away from the breast or resist nursing. The infant will appear relaxed and may doze. Some infants take short breaks while nursing and then resume.

Nipple Shields

Silicone **nipple shields**, which fit over the mother's nipple and areola, are sometimes used if a mother's nipples are inverted or flat, but they should not be used with cracked nipples if the mother can tolerate feeding. The breast does not receive adequate stimulation if the infant feeds with the shield in place, so milk production decreases and the baby may not be able to get adequate nutrition. Also, because the silicone nipple feels different from the breast, the infant may be reluctant to wean from the shield. If it is absolutely necessary to use a nipple shield for a flat or inverted nipple, it should be used only for the first few minutes, as even a flat nipple will usually elongate during that time. Then the rest of the feeding can be done without the shield.

Supplemental Nursing System

Supplemental nursing systems allow the mother to provide supplemental nutrients or medication to the infant while breastfeeding. A typical system has a container for the liquid supplement and a tubing system with a tubing clamp to adjust flow. The tubing is taped to the breast and the end extends about a quarter-inch past the end of the nipple on the top, so the baby encloses both the nipple and the tubing in the mouth when nursing. The tubing should be under the baby's upper lip. Once the baby begins to nurse, the clamp is released so the supplement begins to flow. The bottom of the container is usually positioned level with the breast or slightly lower, so the child must suckle in order to gain the supplement. If the container is higher than the breast, the solution may flow too freely and may choke the child.

Expressing and Storing Human Milk

A mother can **express and store milk** for her infant if the infant is unable to nurse or if she must be separated from the infant. The most efficient method is to use a **bilateral electric breast pump**. The **pulsatile electric pump** provides adequate stimulation in the early postpartum period to establish and maintain the mother's milk supply, usually emptying the breasts within 15 to 20 minutes. If the child is not nursing, the pump should be used at least 8 times in each 24-hour period. Other methods of expressing milk include manual expression and use of a hand pump. Electric pumps usually have collection systems, so the milk flows into a bottle that can be used for feeding. Human milk can be stored for later use using the following guidelines:

- **Room temperature**: 4 hours.
- **Refrigerated**: ≤7 days (best used within 48 hours).
- **Frozen**: in the freezer compartment of the refrigerator for 2 weeks, 3 to 4 months in a separate-door freezer-refrigerator, and 6 months in a deep freezer at 0 °C.

Maternal Attachment Process

By the time of birth, most mothers have developed an emotional connection with their infants and demonstrate a number of typical steps in the **maternal attachment process**.

- **Touching:** The mother usually begins by lightly touching the infant's extremities with her fingertips and running her palm over the baby's trunk. This exploration of the infant can proceed very quickly in minutes, or be more tentative and take days. Early skin-to-skin contact with the infant tends to accelerate this process.
- **En face positioning:** The mother increases the amount of face-to-face eye contact with the infant, typically holding the infant close to her face and responding to eye contact by speaking in a sing-song high-pitched tone (baby talk).
- **Responding:** The mother tends to respond verbally to sounds the infant makes. Initially, the mother may feel separate and distant from the child, especially if she doesn't feel an immediate bond, and she should be reassured that these feelings are normal.

Maternal Illness and Contraindications to Nursing

Some maternal **contraindications** to breastfeeding include:

- Infection with HIV/AIDS.
- Use of antiretroviral medications.
- Active untreated tuberculosis.
- Infection with human T-cell lymphotropic virus (II or II).
- Illicit drug use.
- Use of chemotherapeutic agents.
- Radiation therapy (may require only interruption during treatment).
- Use of other medications that pass into the milk and may harm the child.
- Presence of herpes on the breast.
- Presence of varicella lesions on the breast (may resume after lesions crust).

Additionally, infants with galactosemia cannot tolerate lactose, which is present in human milk. Mothers who are ill or become pregnant while nursing should be evaluated on an individual basis to determine if they should continue to breastfeed their infants. Mothers with psychiatric disorders, such as schizophrenia or postpartum depression/psychosis, may be unable to breastfeed because of emotional disturbance or medications used to treat these conditions.

Complications of Breastfeeding

Engorgement

Production of milk sometimes outstrips demand in the first 2 to 3 days as the mother is starting to nurse, and the breasts become **engorged** (enlarged, taut, and painful). The mother should be reassured that this is normal and can be relieved, as new mothers may feel they should stop nursing or be afraid they are doing some-thing wrong. Nursing frequently (every 2 to 3 hours) and gently massaging the breast toward the nipple during nursing should reduce engorgement. If the areola is hard, some milk should be manually expressed to soften the areola before the infant latches on. Breast pumps and heat (except in a shower) may increase engorgement. Cold compresses, acetaminophen, or ibuprofen may provide relief. Engorgement usually recedes within 24 to 48 hours.

Insufficient Milk

Only about 1.5% of women are actually physiologically unable to produce **sufficient milk** for an infant. In almost all cases, the mother is simply not nursing correctly or frequently enough to stimulate milk production.

Blocked Milk Duct

A palpable, localized lump or an area of hard, swollen erythematous tissue usually indicates a **blocked duct**. Causes include nursing the baby in the same position or wearing a constricting or poorly-fitting bra. While painful, blocked ducts generally open within 24 to 48 hours, with symptoms receding, as opposed to mastitis which tends to worsen. Massaging the affected area while breastfeeding, manually expressing the breast during a warm shower, applying heat to the area, and using a breast pump to completely empty the breast after feeding may alleviate the blockage. Additionally, while breastfeeding on the affected side, the infant should be positioned so the chin points toward the blocked area, usually using the football position. If blockage is not alleviated, blocked milk ducts may progress to **mastitis**.

Mastitis

Indications that the breast has become infected (**mastitis**) with bacteria include induration, swelling, erythema, increasing fever, and acute pain. Without prompt treatment, painful abscesses may form. The infected area may be localized, sometimes appearing similar to blocked milk duct, or generalized, encompassing the whole breast. The mother may have chills and flu-like symptoms before obvious inflammation of the breast. Usually, the mother becomes infected from the infant, most commonly with *Staphylococcus aureus,* so breastfeeding does not endanger the neonate. Treatment includes antibiotics—usually penicillin G, dicloxacillin, or erythromycin—and nursing, pumping, or expressing on the affected side to prevent abscess formation. Applying heat or massaging the breasts in a warm shower may increase circulation. Pain relief includes alternating warm and cold compresses, and acetaminophen or ibuprofen.

Cracked Nipples

Nipples often become sore when the mother begins breastfeeding, but this typically lessens in a few days. However, **cracked nipples** may lead to infection. These are some of the causes:

- The baby latching on improperly to just the nipple and not the areola. Use of drying lotions or soaps
- Use of a breast pump with too much suction
- Monilial infection from thrush in the baby's mouth

Sometimes changing the baby's **position** or rotating positions during nursing may reduce discomfort. Nursing should begin on the least sore nipple, as the infant nurses more strongly at first. The breasts should be cleansed only with water and a small amount of human milk applied to the nipple after nursing, unless the baby has thrush. One hundred percent USP modified **lanolin** (Lansinoh® or PureLan®) applied to the nipples may promote healing. It does not need to be removed for breastfeeding. Acetaminophen or ibuprofen may be taken 30 minutes before nursing. Nipple shields should be avoided if possible, as they interfere with latching on.

Impact of Drugs on Breastfeeding

Virtually all drugs are excreted to some degree (usually 1-2% of maternal dose) in the **human milk**. Drugs that are highly protein-bound or have molecular weight >200 pass less easily into human milk than lipid-soluble drugs. Human milk is slightly acidic compared to plasma, so compounds that are weakly alkaline may be present in human milk in larger amounts than in plasma. Mothers should be advised to take medications after breastfeeding to minimize transfer. Some medications have adverse effects on infants:

- **Opiates***:* Sedation.
- **Aspirin**: Risk of Reye's syndrome.
- **Antibiotics**: Penicillins may cause diarrhea; tetracycline, stained/mottled teeth, and chloramphenicol, gray baby syndrome.
- **Antifungals**: GI symptoms, such as diarrhea, vomiting; blood dyscrasias.
- **Cardiovascular drugs***:* Reserpine may cause diarrhea, bradycardia, lethargy, and respiratory distress; propanolol may cause respiratory depression, bradycardia, or hypoglycemia.
- **Psychotherapeutic agents***:* Sedation, poor feeding. Lithium may cause cyanosis and hypoventilation.
- **Ethanol**: Lethargy, drowsiness, depressed motor development.

Perinatal Substance Abuse and Newborn Feeding

Mothers who engage in **substance abuse** should not breastfeed if they:

- Use large quantities of **vasoconstrictive stimulants**, such as amphetamines or cocaine
- Drink >8 servings of **alcohol** daily or engage in binge drinking.
- Take sedating **opioids**, such as heroin, or benzodiazepines.

Despite concerns, many mothers continue to breastfeed while engaging in substance abuse. In that case, mothers should be educated about their drug of choice and the effects on infants, and on methods to breastfeed as safely as possible. Some **safeguards** include:

- Stopping injection drug use.
- Using drugs only after breastfeeding and using drugs during times the child sleeps longest.
- Expressing milk during periods of drug use to maintain milk supply.
- Pumping extra milk during "safe" times to provide feedings to the infant during times of drug use.
- Avoiding breastfeeding during the time the drug is most active, breastfeeding only after the blood level of the drug peaks (e.g., alcohol peaks in 30 to 90 minutes, so avoid breastfeeding for 1 to 2 hours for every 2 standard drinks ingested).

Maternal/Newborn Separation

Maternal/newborn separation should be avoided as much as possible, as it interferes with bonding and causes distress to the neonate. In some cases, such as with caesarean section or premature birth, some separation is necessary, but nursing staff should facilitate contact. Babies who are held with skin-to-skin contact often cry less and nurse better. In many facilities, immediate skin-to-skin contact occurs after vaginal and caesarean delivery, with the mother encouraged to hold and nurse the child during the initial assessment. Mothers should be encouraged to utilize rooming-in and should be with their babies at all times for the first few days, as this facilitates bonding and helps the mother learn to recognize the baby's cues. Additionally, mothers who room-in around the clock are more likely to breastfeed exclusively.

Maternal Attachment/Bonding Phases

Acquaintance

During the acquaintance period, the first few days, responding helps the mother to recognize **clues** the child is giving about needs, such as hunger. The mother's ability to respond to those needs strengthens the bond and helps her gain confidence in her parenting ability. During this time, the infant is also learning to recognize **routines**, such as nursing when held toward the breast.

Mutual Regulation

During this phase, which may vary in duration, the mother is learning to **balance** the needs of the infant against her own needs, and she may have some negative feelings, such as resenting her lack of sleep or feeling frustration with the infant's crying. The mother may be afraid to express any negative feelings, fearful that people will think she is a "bad" mother, but these feelings are normal until the mother and infant reach a mutual balance. The ability of the mother and infant to recognize each other's cues and respond to them is termed **reciprocity**.

Psychosocial and Ethical Issues

Maternal Attachment/Bonding Assessment

Assessment of maternal attachment/bonding should be done prior to discharge so that any issues and needed interventions can be discussed. In doing the assessment, the nurse evaluates the mother's

- Progression in touching and face-to-face eye contact with extended times and indications of attraction, such as verbally responding to the infant and cuddling the infant. If there has been no progression, the nurse should assess contributing environmental, cultural, and social factors that may be interfering.
- Consistency in caring for the infant and seeking knowledge about and validation of her infant care; adjusting care to the needs of the infant. Sensitivity to infant's needs, such as recognizing discomfort or hunger quickly and exhibiting pleasure at infant's response to her efforts.
- Pleasure in the infant, expressed by calling the infant by name, noting family traits/characteristics, showing overt happiness. If the mother shows displeasure or apathy, this may indicate poor attachment, but might also indicate that the mother is experiencing pain or weakness.

Paternal and Sibling/Family Bonding

Paternal attachment, referred to as engrossment, occurs in many ways similar to maternal attachment. The father may feel pride and wonderment at the child and develop a strong sense of nurturing. Early and frequent contact with the infant promotes engrossment, so the nurse should ensure that the father is not overlooked after delivery but is able to hold, touch, and respond to the child as soon as possible.

Sibling and family attachment are important. Siblings should be allowed to visit the mother and infant as early as possible and be encouraged to hold or care for the infant as appropriate for their ages. Siblings sometimes feel left out or overshadowed by the new infant, so it's important that the parents take time to talk to the siblings and give them attention as well. Grandparents and other family members also form attachments to the infant and should be included.

Barriers to Parent-Infant Interaction

There are many **barriers to parent-infant interaction**, especially with preterm infants or those with genetic disabilities or birth defects that require prolonged hospitalization or treatment. Barriers include:

- **Physical separation:** When the infant cannot be held or fed, when the child is transported to a different facility outside of the area, or when the mother is discharged and the infant remains hospitalized, this prevents attachment.
- **Lack of clear understanding of handicaps and/or developmental problems:** Lack of infant response is sometimes interpreted as rejection, and parents may be frightened by abnormalities.
- **Attitude of medical staff:** Negative attitudes may cause the parent to grieve rather than attach to the child. Staff members need to encourage the parents to become involved in the child's care and to provide stimulation. Staff often needs to demonstrate care to parents, who may be intimidated by the infant's condition and medical needs.
- **Environmental overload:** The equipment (alarms, ventilators, monitors) and environmental constraints (no chairs) may overwhelm parents.

FAMILY TYPES

The following are some of the different types of families:

- **Nuclear** – This **husband-wife-children** model was once the most common family type but is no longer the norm. In this model, the husband is the provider, and the mother stays home to care for the children. This makes up only about **7%** of current American families.
- **Dual career/dual earner** – This model, where **both parents work**, is the most common in American society, affecting about **66%** of two-parent families. One parent may work more than another, or both may work fulltime. There may be disparities in income that affect family dynamics.
- **Childless** – Ten to fifteen percent have no children because of **infertility** or **choice**.
- **Extended** – These may include **multigenerational families** or **shared households** with friends, parents, or other relatives. Childcare responsibilities may be shared or primarily assumed by an extended family member, such as a grandparent.
- **Extended kin network** – Two or more nuclear families live close together, share goods and services, and support each other, including sharing childcare. This model is common in the Hispanic community.

SINGLE-PARENT

This is one of the fastest growing family models. Typically, the mother is the single parent, but in some cases, it is the father. The single parent may be widowed, divorced, or separated, but more commonly, has never married. In cases of divorce or abandonment, the child may have minimal or no contact with one parent, often the father. Single parents often face difficulties in trying to **support and care for a child** and may suffer **economic hardship**.

STEPPARENT

Because of the high rate of divorce, stepparent families are common. This can result in **stress** and **conflict** when a new child enters the picture. There may be jealousy and resentment on the part of siblings and estranged family members. In some cases, families can work together to achieve harmony and provide added support to children.

BINUCLEAR/CO-PARENTING

In this model, children share time between two primarily nuclear families because of **joint custody agreements**. While this may at times result in conflict, the child benefits from having a continued relationship with both parents.

COHABITING

Unmarried heterosexual couples live together. The relationships within this model may vary, with some similar to the nuclear family. In some cases, people are in committed relationships and may avoid marriage because of economic or personal reasons. A planned child may strengthen the relationship, but an unplanned child may cause conflict.

GAY/LESBIAN

Whether gays and lesbians marry or cohabit, they create families in **non-traditional ways**. For example, lesbians may use sperm donors. Gay couples often adopt. Children in these families may face social pressures because of their parents' lifestyles.

PREPARATION OF SIBLINGS FOR BIRTH OF INFANT

Preparation of siblings prior to the birth of an infant can decrease anxiety and sibling rivalry by helping the children feel that they are participants in the process and are valued. Children should be prepared for physical changes in the mother, changing family dynamics, and infant care. Formal classes may be available of children ages 3 to12 to help them identify and express their concerns, and to teach them about pregnancy and childcare. Booklets, books, and videos are also available. The parent/teacher may use dolls to demonstrate childcare and allow the children to practice holding and caring for the baby. When possible, children should have contact with an infant, such as that of a friend or family member. Children may help to decorate the infant's room or prepare a "welcome" gift, such as a drawing or toy. Children should be told who will care for them during labor and delivery and should visit the mother and infant as soon after delivery as possible.

Preparation of Grandparents

Grandparents may vary widely in their feelings about a pregnancy. For example, the parents of a pregnant adolescent may feel anger and despair, while the parents of a mature married parent may be thrilled. Grandparents can provide significant support and should be included in planning early in the pregnancy, but the parents should keep clear **boundaries** when it comes to decision-making. In some cases, there may be conflicts between the grandparents and the parents regarding religious or cultural practices. While it may be difficult to confront these issues, it's better to deal with them during the **pregnancy** than after delivery. The parents should state their desires and plans openly, giving their reasons. Grandparents may benefit from classes or a review of current standards and practices in relation to pregnancy, delivery, and breastfeeding.

Cultural/Lifestyle Factors Affecting Family Integration

Values

Values based on attitudes, ideas, and beliefs often connect family members to common **goals**. However, these values may be influenced by many **external factors**, such as education, social norms, and attitudes of peers, other family, and coworkers, so values may change and this may impact family integration.

Roles

In some families, roles are clearly defined by **gender** and **task** (homemaker and breadwinner), but the roles blur or are **shared** in many families, and in some cases, the father becomes the primary caregiver while the mother works. Other common roles include peacemaker, nurturer, and social planner. How these roles are perceived and actualized affects the manner in which a child is integrated into the family.

Decision-Making

Family power structures vary widely, but in many families, **power** rests with one person who makes ultimate decisions and whose opinions affect other family members. In many traditional cultures (Latino, Asian, Middle Eastern) power lies with the father, a grandparent, or another family member. However, in American society, this may vary because of diversity. Power may be **shared** or it may rest with either the mother or the father.

Socioeconomic

Employment trends, marriage rates, and economic trends all affect **family integration**. Many people have become unemployed and are unable to support their families, resulting in severe **stress**, which may be exacerbated by the arrival of a new child. The divorce rate is high, leaving many parents with inadequate funds to support a child. Even if both parents are employed, the cost of living continues to escalate, including the cost of caring for a child.

Intimate Partner Violence

Prevalence Amongst Pregnant Women

Up to 25% of women in the United States have suffered **intimate partner violence (IPV)**, and 45% of women who are victims of IPV continue to be abused during pregnancy, and in some cases, violence starts with pregnancy or escalates, especially if the partner resents the pregnancy. All pregnant women should be routinely screened for IPV by asking directly about abuse when the partner is absent as women may be rightfully fearful. The risk to the fetus is high, especially if the partner targets the abdomen as this can cause placental injury and placental abruption. IPV during pregnancy is associated with greater risk of low-birth weight, preterm birth, and neonatal mortality. Risk factors for IPV during pregnancy include recent immigrants (especially from cultures in which violence toward women is common), history of child abuse, prior IPV, substance abuse, history of depression/suicide attempts, young age (<24), low education, and unplanned pregnancy. In >50% of cases of IPV, the children are also at risk of abuse.

Signs and Symptoms

Injuries consistent with intimate partner violence/abuse:

- **Characteristic injuries**
  - Ruptured eardrum.
  - Rectal/genital injury—burns, bites, trauma.
  - Scrapes and bruises about the neck, face, head, trunk, arms.
  - Cuts, bruises, and fractures of the face.
  - Pregnant women often have injuries in multiple body areas, especially the abdomen, breasts, and genitalia.
- **Patterns of injuries**
  - Bathing suit pattern—injuries on parts of body that are usually covered with clothing as the perpetrator abuses but hides evidence of abuse.
  - Head and neck injuries (50%).
- **Abusive injuries (rarely attributable to accidents)**
  - Bites, bruises, rope and cigarette burns, welts in the outline of weapons (belt marks)
  - Bilateral injuries of arms/legs.
- **Defensive injuries**
  - Back of the body injury from being attacked while crouched on the floor face down.
  - Soles of the feet from kicking at perpetrator.
  - Ulnar aspect of hand or palm from blocking blows.

Assessment for and Response to Domestic/Dating Violence

Assessment for intimate partner violence should be done for all patients, regardless of background, lifestyle, or signs of abuse. The nurse should be informed about IPV and aware or risk factors, typical injuries, and danger signs. The interview should be conducted in private (or with children <3 years old). The office, bathrooms, and examining rooms should have information about IPV posted prominently. Brochures and information should be available to give to patients. Patients may present with a variety of physical complaints, such as headache, pain, palpitations, numbness, or pelvic pain. They are often depressed and may appear suicidal and may be isolated from friends and family. Victims of IPV often exhibit fear of perpetrator (such as a parent, spouse, boyfriend, or girlfriend) and may report injury inconsistent with symptoms. If a patient admits to injuries from IPV, the first question should be, "Is the person who hurt you here?" because security may need to be called. It's important to remain supportive and nonjudgmental and to provide information and assistance.

Relinquishing Child for Adoption

A mother relinquishing her child for **adoption** may have feelings of ambivalence and sadness. Many who relinquish their infants for adoption are young and/or unmarried. Adoptions may be closed or open, so procedures will vary. In some open adoptions, the adoptive parent(s) may accompany the mother and participate in the birth, with the birth mother relinquishing the child immediately after birth. In this case, the adoptive parents should be treated as the actual parents of the child, while staff should recognize the needs of the birth mother and provide for her emotional and physical support. In other cases, the child is first relinquished to an agency, such as Social Services, which then places the child. If possible, prior to the birth, the birth mother should indicate how she wants to handle the birth. Some want to hold and spend time with the child; others do not. The birth mother should be in a single room, rather than with other mothers, to protect her privacy.

Factors That Influence Grief

The emotions that individuals and families experience with the loss or severe illness/disability of an infant are varied and dependent on many factors that influence grief.

- **Cultural influences**: Different cultures have their own practices and beliefs concerning sickness, death, and dying, and varying rituals and ceremonies for processing loss.
- **Family system**: The family's composition, the roles of its various members, and its economic circumstances affect its expression of grief. A large family with extended community support processes grief differently from a single mother living far from home.
- **Siblings**: The impact on other children in the family must be considered, in addition to the impact on the parents.
- **History of loss**: Many diseases have a genetic component, and this may not be the first child to be affected.

Review Video: Patient Treatment and Grief
Visit mometrix.com/academy and enter code: 648794

Review Video: Coping with a Disability
Visit mometrix.com/academy and enter code: 630500

Stages of Grief

Grief is a normal response to the death or severe illness/abnormality of an infant or fetus. How a person deals with grief is very personal, and each person will grieve differently. Elisabeth Kubler-Ross identified **five stages of grief** in *On Death and Dying* (1969). A person may not go through each stage but usually goes through two of the five stages:

- **Denial**: The parents may be resistive to information and unable to accept that a child is dying/impaired or believe that the child is not theirs. They may act stunned, immobile, or detached and may be unable to respond appropriately or remember what's said, often repeatedly asking the same questions.
- **Anger**: As reality becomes clear, parents may react with pronounced anger, directed inward or outward. Women, especially, may blame themselves and self-anger may lead to severe depression and guilt, assuming they are to blame because of some action before or during pregnancy. Outward anger, more common in men, may be expressed as overt hostility. (Continued)

- **Bargaining**: This involves if-then thinking (often directed at a deity): "If I go to church every way, then God will prevent this." Parents may change doctors, trying to change the outcome.
- **Depression**: As the parents begin to accept the loss, they may become depressed, feeling no one understands and overwhelmed with sadness. They may be tearful or crying and may withdraw or ask to be left alone.
- **Acceptance**: This final stage represents a form of resolution and often occurs outside of the medical environment after months. Parents are able to resume their normal activities and lose the constant preoccupation with their child. They are able to think of the child without severe pain. With a disabled child, acceptance may be delayed because of daily challenges and reminders.

Supporting Parents/Family of Dying Infants

Parents/families of dying infants often do not receive adequate support from nursing staff, who may feel unprepared for dealing with parents'/families' grief and are unsure of how to provide comfort, but parents/families are in desperate need of this **support**. Below are some guidelines for providing support to the parents/family of a dying infant **prior to the time of death**:

- Stay with the family and sit quietly, allowing them to talk, cry, or interact if they desire.
- Avoid platitudes: "His suffering will be over soon."
- Avoid judgmental reactions to what family members say or do, and realize that anger, fear, guilt, and irrational behavior are normal responses to acute grief and stress.
- Show caring by touching the infant and encouraging family to do the same.
- Touching hands, arms, or shoulders of family members can provide comfort, but follow clues of the family.
- Provide referrals to support groups, if available.

Time of Death

Below are some guidelines for providing support to the parents/family of a dying infant **at the time of death**:

- Reassure the family that all measures have been taken to ensure the infant's comfort.
- Express personal feeling of loss: "She was such a sweet baby, and I'll miss her," and allow the family to express feelings and memories.
- Provide information about what is happening during the dying process, explaining death rales, Cheyne-Stokes respirations, and so forth.
- Alert family members to imminent death if they are not present.
- Assist in contacting clergy/spiritual advisors.
- Respect feelings and needs of parents, siblings, and other family members.

After Death

Below are some guidelines for providing support to the parents/family of a dying infant **after the infant has died**:

- Encourage parents/family members to stay with the infant as long as they wish, to hold the infant and/or say goodbye.
- Use the infant's name when talking to the family.
- Assist them in making arrangements, such as contacting a funeral home.
- If an autopsy is required, discuss with the family and explain when it will take place.
- If organ donation is to occur, assist the family in making arrangements.
- Encourage family members to grieve and express emotions.
- Send a card or condolence note.

Types of Grief

Anticipatory grief occurs when a child is diagnosed with a terminal illness. The parent begins to mourn over the loss of the child before he or she expires.

Incongruent grief occurs when the mother and the father are "out of synch" in their grieving process, stressing their relationship. It may be due to the differences in how men and women grieve, or it may be because the woman typically bonds with the infant during the pregnancy, while the father bonds after the child is born.

Delayed grief occurs when the grieving process is postponed months to years after the loss of a child. Initially, the parent may not be able to grieve appropriately, because of an inability to cope, or the pressing need to care for other family members.

Gender Differences in Grieving

When faced with the death of a child, **men and women** generally grieve differently.

- **Women** are often more expressive about their loss and more emotional. They are more likely to look for support from others. **Men** often grieve in a more solitary and cognitive manner. They are generally more oriented to fact-gathering or problem-solving.
- The bond that develops between a pregnant woman and the developing fetus is unique and generally very intense. The father often forms a stronger bond after the birth of the child.

When one parent does not grieve in the same fashion as the other (**incongruent grieving**) this may be a source of conflict in their marriage. How a person acts on the outside is not always a true indicator of how that person is feeling on the inside.

Bioethics

Bioethics is a branch of ethics that involves making sure that the medical treatment given is the most **morally correct choice**, given the different options that might be available and the differences inherent in the varied levels of treatment. In the acute/critical care unit, if the patients, parents, and the staff are in agreement when it comes to values and decision-making, then no ethical dilemma exists; however, when there is a difference in value beliefs between the patients/parents and the staff, there is a **bioethical dilemma** that must be resolved. Sometimes discussion and explanation can resolve differences, but at times, the institution's ethics committee must be brought in to resolve the conflict. The primary goal of bioethics is to determine the most morally correct action using the set of circumstances given.

Ethical Terms

Beneficence and Nonmaleficence

Beneficence is an ethical principle that involves performing actions that are for the purpose of benefitting another person. In the care of a neonate, any procedure or treatment should be done with the ultimate goal of benefitting the infant, and any actions that are not beneficial should be reconsidered. As the infant ages and/or condition changes, procedures need to be continually reevaluated to determine if they are still of benefit.

Nonmaleficence is an ethical principle that means healthcare workers should provide care in a manner that does not cause direct intentional harm to the patient:

- The actual act must be good or morally neutral.
- The intent must be only for a good effect.
- A bad effect cannot serve as the means to get to a good effect.
- A good effect must have more benefit than a bad effect has harm.

Autonomy and Justice

Autonomy is the ethical principle that the individual has the right to make decisions about his/her own care. In the case of neonates, the infant cannot make autonomous decisions, so the parents serve as the legal decision maker. The nurse must keep the parents fully informed so that they can exercise their autonomy in informed decision-making.

Justice is the ethical principle that relates to the distribution of the limited resources of healthcare benefits to the members of society. These resources must be distributed fairly. This issue may arise if there is only one bed left and two delivering mothers. Justice comes into play in deciding which mother should stay and which should be transported or otherwise cared for. The decision should be made according to what is best or most just for the patients and not colored by personal bias.

Confidentiality

Confidentiality is obligatory in a professional-patient relationship. Nurses are under an obligation to protect the information they possess concerning the patient and family. Care should be taken to safeguard that information and provide the **privacy** that the family deserves. This is accomplished through the use of required passwords when family members call for information about the patient and through the limitation of who is allowed to visit. There may be times when confidentiality must be broken to save the life of a patient, but those circumstances are rare. The nurse must make all efforts to safeguard patient records and identification. Computerized record keeping should be done in such a way that the screen is not visible to others, and paper records must be secured.

Newborn Feeding and Nutrition

Fat-Soluble Vitamins in Formulas

Vitamins found in formulas are organic nutrients required in small amounts to maintain growth and normal metabolism. **Fat-soluble vitamins** include:

- **Vitamin A:** Important for growth and development of tissues and in proper functioning of the immune system. Vitamin A supplementation in extremely low birth weight infants has been shown to reduce the incidence of bronchopulmonary dysplasia.
- **Vitamin D***:* Required for adequate calcium and phosphorus absorption. Vitamin D deficiency leads to rickets (soft bones, bowed legs).
- **Vitamin E:** An antioxidant that is limited in preterm infants, making them susceptible to developing hemolytic anemia without proper supplementation.
- **Vitamin K***:* Important in the clotting process. Infants receive an injection of Vitamin K shortly after birth to prevent hemorrhagic disease of the newborn.

Excessive fat-soluble vitamins A and D are toxic because they accumulate in adipose tissue and the liver. Water-soluble vitamins include thiamine (B_1), riboflavin (B_2), niacin (B_3), pantothenate (B_5), pyridoxine (B_6), cobalamin (B_{12}), C, biotin, and folic acid. Excessive water-soluble vitamins are excreted in the urine.

Neonatal Nutritional Needs

Caloric Requirements

The **caloric needs** of a neonate (pre-term or term) depend on postnatal age, activity, current weight, growth rate, thermal environment, and route of nutritional intake. Cold stress increases caloric requirements. Infants who receive parenteral nutrition need fewer calories, as they do not have any fecal loss, and the nutrients are not absorbed by the gastrointestinal tract. These are the general requirements for adequate growth:

- **Full term infant**: 100 to 120 cal/kg/day
- **Premature infants**: 110 to 160 cal/kg/day
- Infants who are recovering from **surgery** or have a **chronic illness**, such as bronchopulmonary dysplasia (BPD): ≤180 cal/kg/day

Unfortified formulas and most human milk supply 20 calories per ounce. To ingest 120 cal/kg/day, an infant needs to ingest 6 ounces/kg/day of unfortified formula or human milk. Special formulas designed for premature infants and fortifiers that can be added to human milk provide higher calorie contents per ounce (22 to 24 calories per ounce).

Protein, Fat, and Carbohydrate Requirements

Requirements for protein, fats, and carbohydrates are as follows:

- **Protein:** Neonates require adequate protein to sustain growth, the amount depending on gestational age. A **positive nitrogen balance** exists when the intake of protein meets or exceeds the infant's requirements. A negative protein balance occurs when protein is provided in inadequate amounts, leading to catabolism (muscle breakdown). Premature neonates have higher protein requirements than full term infants:
    - Full term: 2 to 2.5 g/kg/day
    - Preterm: 3.5 to 4 g/kg/day
- **Carbohydrates**: One gram provides 3.4 calories. Carbohydrates should provide approximately 40 to 50% of total daily calories. Lactose is the predominant carbohydrate. Premature infants may be deficient in the enzyme lactase (enzyme that breaks down lactose), so premature infant formulas utilize lesser amounts of lactose, combined with glucose polymers.
- **Fat**: One gram provides 9 calories. Lipids should supply approximately 40 to 52% of total daily calories. Common sources of lipids include palm, soybean, coconut, and safflower oils. Premature infant formulas have a higher percentage of fat supplied as medium-chain triglycerides (MCT). MCTs can be absorbed without pancreatic lipase or bile salts, which are deficient in premature infants.

Iron Supplementation

All formula-fed term infants should receive **iron-fortified formulas**. Breastfed term infants should be given **iron supplementation** when they are several months old. The **premature infant** is especially susceptible to iron deficiency because of the lack of maternal iron transfer during the third trimester and the multiple blood samplings that occur with the extensive monitoring of the premature infant. To minimize the risk of iron deficiency anemia, premature infants fed human milk should be started on iron supplementation once they receive full enteral feeds. Studies have shown that premature infants fed a premature formula have better iron stores when that formula is supplemented with 15 mg/L of iron compared to those receiving formula with 3 mg/L of iron.

Infant Formulas

A wide variety of **infant formulas** are available, but the 3 primary types include:

- **Cow-milk based formulas** (Enfamil®, Similac®, Good Start®): These are appropriate for most infants. These are enriched with various components, including vitamins, minerals, iron, tyrosine, phenylalanine, and carnitine.
- **Soy-based formulas** (Isomil®, Soyalac®, ProSobee®, Nursoy®): These are appropriate for infants with primary lactose deficiency or galactosemia and those allergic to cow-milk-based formulas.
- **Therapeutic formulas** (Nutramigen®, Pregestimil®): Many preparations are available to meet special needs.

Formula may be purchased in ready-to-feed bottles or cans that require no preparation, liquid concentrate, or powder. Concentrate and powder require the addition of water, so a clean water supply and the ability to measure correctly are necessary to avoid inadequate or unsafe nutrition. Babies who are bottle-fed with formula usually feed less frequently than those who are breastfed. Neonates usually take 2 to 3 ounces of formula every 3 to 4 hours. Neonates require approximately 2.5 ounces of formula for each pound (0.5kg) of weight within each 24-hour period.

Pros and Cons of Soy Formulas

Energy Source	Soy Formulas	Cow's Milk Formulas
Carbohydrate	Sucrose	Lactose
Protein	Soy isolate from the soy bean	Whey and casein in various ratios (similar to human milk)
Pros of Soy Use		**Cons of Soy Use**
Soy is appropriate for use in infants with: Hereditary galactosemia and hereditary lactase deficiency. Documented IgE mediated allergy to cow's milk protein. Temporary lactase deficiency that may occur after infectious gastroenteritis. Parents who are seeking a vegetarian-based diet.		Soy cannot be used for premature infants weighing less than 1,800 grams because it results in: Less weight gain. Less linear growth. Increased risk for developing osteopenia. Elevated levels of alkaline phosphatase. Elevated levels of aluminum. Phytoestrogens found in soy formulas may alter normal endocrine patterns of the infant.

Therapeutic Infant Formulas

Pregestimil® is a hypoallergenic formula specially designed for infants with malabsorption caused by gastrointestinal or hepatobiliary disease. It provides hydrolyzed (predigested) protein that is easier to digest. The majority of the fats are in the form of medium-chain triglycerides (MCT). MCTs are easier to digest than other fats.

Similac® PM 60/40 is a cow's-milk-based formula that has a low phosphorus content and low renal solute load. It is designed for infants with impaired renal function or with hypocalcemia due to hyperphosphatemia. It has a whey-to-casein ratio of 60:40.

Nutramigen® Lipil is a hypoallergenic formula designed for infants sensitive to the intact protein found in cow's-milk-based formula. The proteins are hydrolyzed (digested) and easier to absorb. Cow's-milk protein allergy is an indication for use of this formula. It contains docosahexaenoic (DHA) acid and arachidonic acid (ARA) that are also found in human milk. DHA and ARA are omega 3 and 6 fatty acids that support normal brain, eye, and nerve development.

Special Preterm Formulas

Preterm formulas are designed with the special requirements of the premature infant in mind. These infants often have an increased caloric requirement to meet growth expectations. Preterm formulas differ from full term formulas because they provide:

- 24 cal/ounce as opposed to the 20 cal/ounce found in human milk and formulas for full term infants.
- Increased levels of protein, vitamins, and minerals, particularly increased amounts of vitamin D, calcium, and phosphorus to prevent osteopenia of prematurity.
- Less lactose than term formulas, so they are less likely to cause diarrhea.

Human milk can be "fortified" with the addition of human milk fortifiers (HMF) to achieve the same results. Infants are typically switched to a transitional or cow milk-based formula prior to discharge.

Supplementary or Complementary Feeding

Supplementary or complementary feeding with breastfed babies is usually discouraged because it may weaken the suckling reflex or cause the child to lose interest in breastfeeding, especially if a bottle is offered before breastfeeding is well established. To breastfeed, the child must latch on differently to the breast than to a bottle nipple, with the mouth opened more widely for the breast. Additionally, the tongue moves front to back when nursing (expressing milk) and up and down (squeezing the nipple) when feeding from a bottle. Changing from one to the other can be confusing for the infant, and some cannot adjust. Once the infant nurses well—usually after about 4 weeks—mothers who want to pump for supplementary feedings may try to slowly introduce the bottle. Neonates do not need water and should not be given juice or sugar water.

Newborn Assessment and Management

Transition to Extrauterine Life

Cold Stress/Hypothermia

Cold stress/hypothermia in the neonate is a body temperature measurement of less than 36.5 °C rectally with associated symptoms. Preterm neonates are especially vulnerable to cold stress, as they have limited ability to intrinsically create or conserve body heat. They do not shiver, have limited ability to constrict superficial blood vessels and have limited amounts of both subcutaneous and brown fat. Signs of cold stress include:

- Body is cool to touch.
- Central cyanosis and acrocyanosis.
- Mottling of skin.
- Poor feeding, weak suck, increased gastric residuals, and abdominal distension.
- Bradycardia.
- Shallow respirations with tachypnea.
- Restlessness and irritability.
- Apnea.
- Lethargy and decreased activity.
- Weak cry.
- Hypoglycemia.
- Central nervous system depression with hypotonia.
- Edema.

Thermoregulation

There are a number of steps in the **treatment of hypothermia**:

1. Determine if the cause of hypothermia is from an abnormal physiological process in the infant or from environmental conditions.
2. Rewarm the infant slowly, because too rapid rewarming may result in apnea or hypotension.
3. Maintain the ambient temperature at 1 to 1.5 °C higher than the infant's temperature. Oxygen consumption is not elevated when the difference between the skin temperature and the environmental air temperature is less than 1.5 °C.
4. Increase the air temperature by approximately 1 °C every hour until the infant's temperature is in the normal range and stable.
5. Warm IV fluids with a blood-warming device prior to infusion, to enhance warming of the child.
6. Closely monitor the infant's blood glucose levels, vital signs, and urinary output during rewarming.

Neutral Thermal Environment

A **neutral thermal environment** (NTE) is a place in which the infant's body temperature is maintained within a normal range without alterations in metabolic rate or increased oxygen consumption (i.e., environmental temperature in which oxygen consumption and glucose consumption are lowest). Infants who are in an NTE are not utilizing energy to maintain their body temperature in the normal range. Just because an infant has a normal body temperature does not mean he/she is in an NTE. The infant may still be utilizing mechanisms, such as non-shivering thermogenesis, to maintain body temperatures, as evidenced by increased oxygen consumption and poor weight gain over time. Charts are commercially available that outline the appropriate NTE for infants based on current weight and birth weight.

Incubators

The goal of placing an infant in an **incubator** is to provide a neutral thermal environment (NTE) that places minimal stress on the infant. Most incubators are rigid, box-like structures like an Isolette, in which an infant is kept in a controlled environment to receive medical care. The infant is allowed to grow and mature here before being transitioned to the more "uncontrolled" environment of an open crib. Features that incubators possess that enhance the production of an NTE include a heater, a fan to circulate warmed air, and a humidity control. They also usually have a way to increase the oxygen content of the environment and ports to allow for nursing care without removing the infant. A servo-control is used in conjunction with a temperature-sensing thermistor that is attached to the infant to help regulate the infant's temperature within a set range. Some incubators may have double walls that lessen radiant heat loss. Infants who are in need of close monitoring are not placed in an incubator, but instead are placed under a radiant warmer with minimal covering. This allows the nurse to monitor the infant's skin color and breathing patterns more closely.

Radiant Warmers

Radiant warmers are devices that provide overhead heat directly to the infant. Radiant heaters provide an area for direct observation and free access to the infant, which is very useful in the initial evaluation and resuscitation (if necessary) of the newborn, or for procedures such as intubation or line placement. Radiant heat devices work best if the room temperature is kept above 25 °C. Two problems related to radiant warmers include:

- Promote dehydration if an infant is placed under them for a prolonged amount of time, especially if the infant is premature.
- Risk overheating the infant or cause first-degree burns.

Temperature sensors must be appropriately placed and the infant's temperature monitored frequently to ensure the infant is not being over or under heated.

Heat Transfer Mechanisms

Heat transfer mechanisms to consider when caring for a neonate, especially a premature one: conduction and convection:

- **Conduction**: The transfer of heat between solid objects of different temperatures in contact with each other. Heat is transferred from the body of the infant to a cold surface it may come into contact with, such as a scale. Care should be taken to make sure the scales are warmed before use. Conduction can also be used to warm the infant by placing a warmed blanket next to the skin.
- **Convection**: The transfer of heat through air currents moving around and across an infant's body. Incubators use convection of warm air being pumped into the incubator to keep an infant warm. Heat can be lost this way if a cool draft is allowed near the infant.
- **Radiation**: Heat transferred between two objects not in contact with each other. This is the transfer of heat through emission of infrared rays. Radiant warming beds use this mechanism to warm the infant. Heat loss occurs when an infant is in an incubator and the walls of the incubator are cooler than body temperature. The neonate in an incubator with this situation will lose body heat through radiation from his body to the cooler walls, despite the warm air being pumped in.
- **Evaporation**: Loss of heat occurs when moisture evaporates from the surface of the skin. Evaporation is the result of conversion of liquid into a vapor and is a major concern at birth, as a wet infant can experience a 3-degree drop in body temperature in only about 10 minutes. Thus, it is critical to dry the neonate at birth, and to replace wet linens with warm and dry ones.

Minimizing Heat Loss

At delivery, **minimize heat loss** while evaluating the newborn by following these steps:

- Dry the infant thoroughly (including hair) to minimize evaporative heat loss, and remove wet towels.
- Place a cap on the infant's head, as the head is the most significant area of heat loss.
- When the infant is to be weighed, cover the scales with a warm cloth to minimize conductive heat loss.
- Place infant in a warm environment such as:
    - Skin-to-skin contact with mother, and cover them with a warm blanket.
    - Bundled in warm blankets and given to mother to hold.
    - Underneath a preheated warmer for further evaluation or resuscitation.

Minimizing heat loss is especially important if the newborn is premature or has intrauterine growth restriction, but full-term newborns also suffer if they become chilled.

Kangaroo Care

Dr. Edgar Ray invented **kangaroo care** in the late 1970's in Bogotá, Columbia, when morbidity and mortality rates rose in his NICU, but he had limited technological resources. Kangaroo Care consists of placing the infant, after drying and warming, in minimal clothing in an upright position on the mother's bare chest between her breasts. This allows for skin-to-skin contact with the infant's head next to the mother's heart. A precipitous drop was noted in premature infant mortality after this method of care was instigated. The concept is to provide the neonate with closeness similar to that experienced with the mother while in the womb. Kangaroo care is maintained for as long as the neonate allows. Preterm infants attached to ventilators and IV infusions also benefit from kangaroo care. There are physiological and psychological benefits for both the neonate and the mother.

Enhanced bonding between the neonate and the mother, shorter hospital stays, low cost, and decreased morbidity and mortality are all documented benefits.

The following are specific benefits of kangaroo care for the mother, the neonate, and the institution:

- **Mother's Benefits**
  - Enhanced bonding with the infant.
  - Increased production of milk with higher rates of successful breastfeeding.
  - Increased confidence in caring for the infant.
  - Increased opportunity for teaching and assessing maternal care by nursing staff.
- **Neonate's Benefits**
  - Regulation of temperature, heart and respiratory rates.
  - Calming effect with decreased stress.
  - Decreased episodes of apnea.
  - Increased weight gain.
  - Enhanced bonding with the mother.
  - Fewer nosocomial infections.
- **Institutional Benefits**
  - Earlier discharge from hospital.
  - Decreased morbidity and mortality (especially in developing countries).
  - Decreased use of financial resources.

NST

Non-shivering thermogenesis (NST) is the major route of rapid increase of body temperature in response to cold stress in the term neonate. NST is the oxidation of brown fat to create heat. Brown adipose tissue contains a high concentration of stored triglycerides, a rich capillary network, and is controlled by the sympathetic nervous system. Brown fat cells have a rich supply of mitochondria that are unique, in that when fat is metabolized ATP is not produced, but instead heat is created. Temperature regulation is controlled by the posterior hypothalamus. When a cold body temperature is detected, the posterior hypothalamus responds by triggering the adrenal glands to release norepinephrine and the pituitary gland to release thyroxine. Both norepinephrine and thyroxine stimulate NST. Brown adipose production begins around 26 to 28 weeks of gestation and continues until 3 to 5 weeks after delivery. Premature infants have limited amounts of brown fat and limited ability to create heat via NST.

Skin Temperature Probes

Skin temperature probes are often used to monitor the temperature of the infant in an Isolette or radiant warmer. Incorrect placement of the probe can alter the reading, causing the warming device to deliver too much or too little heat. The temperature probe should not be placed over a bony area of the body or over an area where brown adipose tissue is abundant. Brown adipose tissue is abundant around the neck, the midscapular region of the back, the mediastinum and organs in the thoracic cavity, kidneys, and adrenal glands. A common probe placement area for an infant who is supine is over the liver. If the probe is not making good skin contact, it will indicate that the infant is cold, and the warmer will deliver increased amounts of heat, possibly causing hyperthermia. If the probe is underneath the infant, it may indicate an artificially warm temperature and decrease heat to the infant, causing hypothermia.

Stress Related to Light

Light is a necessary component of caring for both the sick and healthy neonate in the delivery room and nursery. Adequate lighting is required to evaluate the at-risk neonate, to assess color, to complete procedures such as intubation, or to give medications. Light discourages the growth of pathogens. However, constant bright light interferes with the development of natural diurnal rhythms because it arouses the central nervous system and stresses the infant. Controlling light helps to stabilize the infant. Some simple methods to protect the neonate from light over-stimulation and to establish a normal sleep cycle include:

- Reducing overhead light levels when direct visualization is not necessary.
- Covering incubator hoods to reduce light entering the incubator.
- Dimming the lights at night to help establish a natural day/night pattern (circadian rhythm).

Stress Related to Noise

Excessive **noise** causes agitation in both term and especially preterm neonates. The preterm neonate has less ability to self-calm, and over-stimulation results in decompensation, as demonstrated by increased oxygen requirements and increased apnea and bradycardia episodes. The American Academy of Pediatrics (AAP) recommends noise levels in the nursery and NICU be kept at **≤45 decibels**. A normal speaking voice is between 50 to 60 decibels. Noise levels above 80 to 85 decibels damage the cochlea and cause hearing loss in adults. To keep noise acceptably low:

- Turn radios/TVs off or down.
- Designate a daily quiet time.
- Close incubator portholes gently, because closing a plastic porthole can spike the decibel level more than 80 dB.
- *Whisper* — avoid speaking loudly.
- Remove bubbling water from ventilator tubing.
- Educate parents about the deleterious effects of over-stimulating their infant with loud noises.

Environmental Stressors and "Time Out"

Premature neonates have a very limited ability to deal with **environmental stressors,** but these stressors can affect all neonates. Signs of stress in neonates include:

- Color changes, such as mottling or cyanosis.
- Episodes of apnea and bradycardia.
- Activity changes, such as tremors, twitches, frantic activity, arching, and gaze averting.
- Flaccid posture (sagging trunk, extremities and face).
- Easy fatigability.

When the infant shows signs of stress, a **"time out"** recovery period is indicated:

- Stop the activity causing the stress.
- Reduce unnecessary stimuli, e.g., lower the lights and postpone non-essential manipulation of the neonate.
- Give the neonate a chance to calm or soothe himself.
- Bundle the neonate and place him/her in a comforting, side-lying position with the shoulders drawn forward and the hands brought to midline.

Laboratory Findings

Microbiological Testing

Neonates with exposure to microbiological agents before, during, or after birth may require **microbiological testing:**

- Blood cultures are done to isolate causative agents in order to begin appropriate antibiotic treatment.
- In some cases, microbiological testing of expressed human milk may be indicated.
- Microscopic examination of urine and urine culture may be done to identify urinary pathogens.
- Stool cultures may be done to identify GI pathogens.
- Tracheal secretions may be cultured to identify pathogens causing pneumonia, especially in infants who are ventilated. The findings should be reviewed along with chest radiographs to ensure that positive findings don't just represent tracheal colonization alone.
- Gram stain and scraping of conjunctiva may be done to identify gonococcal conjunctivitis.
- Skin culture may be indicated for the infant with a skin infection.

Clinical Laboratory Urine Tests

Urine testing includes:

- **pH** should range from 4.5 to 9.0. An alkaline (high) pH can be caused by urinary tract infections, diarrhea, or kidney infection. An acidic (low) pH may reflect lung disease, hyperglycemia, or diarrhea with dehydration.
- **Specific gravity** ranges from 1.001 to 1.040 (usually about 1.015).

About 2% of full-term infants have asymptomatic bacteriuria, but this increases to about 10% for preterm infants. However, the urinalysis alone is not an effective test to determine if an infant has a urinary tract infection because the neonate's urine usually contains leukocytes (≥25/mm3 in males and ≥50/mm3 in females), and urine cultures of infants <3 days often show poor results, even in the presence of infection, so blood cultures (and in some cases cultures of CSF) should be done if infection is suspected as neonates are more likely to develop kidney infections and sepsis from cystitis than older infants. The most common infective agent is *Escherichia coli* although *Candida* and *Staphylococcus* are common with prolonged hospitalization.

ABGs

Arterial blood gases (ABGs) are monitored to assess effectiveness of oxygenation, ventilation, and acid-base status, and to determine oxygen flow rates. Partial pressure of a gas is that exerted by each gas in a mixture of gases, proportional to its concentration, based on total atmospheric pressure of 760 mm Hg at sea level. Normal values for children include:

- Acidity/alkalinity (pH): 7.26-7.44.
- Partial pressure of carbon dioxide ($PaCO_2$): 35-45 mm Hg.
- Partial pressure of oxygen (PaO_2): >80 mg Hg.
- Bicarbonate concentration (HCO_3): 22-28 mEq/L.
- Oxygen saturation (SaO_2): >92-95%.

The relationship between these elements, particularly the $PaCO_2$ and the PaO_2 indicates respiratory status. For example, $PaCO_2$ >55 and the PaO_2 <60 in an infant previously in good health indicates respiratory failure. There are many issues to consider. Ventilator management may require a higher $PaCO_2$ to prevent barotrauma and a lower PaO_2 to reduce oxygen toxicity. Premature infants may need lower PaO_2 to prevent retinopathy of prematurity.

Invasive Blood Gas Monitoring

Invasive blood gas monitoring options include the following:

- **Arterial blood gas (ABG)** is the most informative measurement of blood gas status. If an infant has an umbilical artery catheter, it is easily obtained by aspirating 1-2 mL of blood.
- **Venous blood gas (VBG)** is easier to obtain if an arterial catheter is not in place. In order to compare the values in the VBG with an ABG, make the following calculations:
    - Add 0.05 to the pH of the VBG.
    - Subtract 5-10 mmHg from the PCO_2 of the VBG.
- **Capillary Blood Gas (CBG)** can be obtained with a heel stick, without a venous or arterial line, but the values obtained in a CBG are the least accurate and are rarely useful. The oxygen status of the neonate (reflected in the PO_2) can be estimated by clinical evaluation of the neonate and a noninvasive pulse oximeter reading.

Clinical Laboratory Tests for Red Blood Cells

Red blood cells (RBCs or erythrocytes) are biconcave disks that contain hemoglobin (95% of mass), which carries oxygen throughout the body. The heme portion of the cell contains iron, which binds to the oxygen. RBCs live about 120 days in adults but this is reduced 20-25% in neonates and 50% in preterm infants. The RBCs are destroyed and their hemoglobin is recycled or excreted. Normal values of red blood cell count vary by age:

- Neonate: 4.1-6.1 million per mm^3.
- 2-6 mos: 3.8-5.6 million per mm^3.

The most common disorders of RBCs are those that interfere with production, leading to various types of anemia:

- Blood loss.
- Hemolysis.
- Bone marrow failure.

The morphology of RBCs may vary depending upon the type of anemia:

- Size: Normocytes, microcytes, macrocytes.
- Shape: Spherocytes (round), poikilocytes (irregular), drepanocytes (sickled).
- Color (reflecting concentration of hemoglobin: Normochromic, hypochromic.

Laboratory Findings

Several different tests are used to evaluate the condition and production of **red blood cells** in addition to the red blood cell count:

Test	Normal values	Discussion
Hemoglobin	Neonate: 14.5 to 22.5 g/dl 2 months: 9.0 to 14.0 g/dl	Carries oxygen. Decreased in anemia and increased in polycythemia.
Hematocrit	Neonate: 48 to 69%; 3 days: 44 to 75% 2 months: 28 to 42%	Indicates the proportion of RBCs in a liter of blood (usually about 3 times the hemoglobin number).
Mean corpuscular volume (MCV)	Neonate: 95 to 121 μm^3 0.5 to 2 years: 70-86 μm^3	Indicates the size of RBCs and can differentiate types of anemia. For adults, <80 is microcytic and >100 is macrocytic, but this varies with age.
Reticulocyte count	0.5 to 1.5% of total RBCs	Measures marrow production and should rise with anemia.
Platelets	150,000 to 400,000	Essential for clotting. May increase to >1 million during acute infection or with iron deficiency anemia.

Clinical Laboratory Tests for WBCs

Leukocytes are white blood cells (WBCs). Normal total values vary according to age. The differential is the percentage of each type of WBC out of the total. The differential will shift with infection or allergies, but should return to normal values:

Item	Neonate	1 day	2 weeks	1 month
WBCs ($X\ 10^3/\ mm^3$)	9.0-30.0	9.4-34.0	5.0-20.0	5.0-19.5.
Myelocytes	0%	0%	0%	0%
Neutrophils (bands)	9.1%	9.2%	5.5%	4.5%
Neutrophils (segs)	52%	52%	34%	30%
Lymphocytes	31%	31%	48%	56%
Monocytes	5.8%	5.8%	8.8%	6.5%
Eosinophils	2.2%	2.0%	3.1%	2.8%
Basophils	0.6%	0.5%	0.4%	0.5%

Neonatal Physical Assessment and Gestational Age

Neonate Physical Assessment

The neonate should undergo three different types of **physical assessment**:

- **Immediate**: The first examination is done in the delivery room to determine the need for resuscitation or other intervention. This includes the APGAR assessment.
- **1-4 hours after birth:** The second examination includes gestational age assessment, which must be completed within 24 hours for accuracy, and brief physical assessment to determine if there are any problems that might place the infant at risk. This includes assessment of respiratory and cardiac status, cord color, skin color, and movement. The Modified Ballard scoring system is often used.
- **≥24 hours after birth (or prior to discharge):** The final examination should include a complete physical and behavioral assessment that includes all systems and evaluation of reflexes. All weights and measurements are taken and reviewed. This exam requires observation, palpation, and auscultation. In some cases, instead of a separate examination at 1-4 hours, only this complete physical examination is completed.

Rapid Assessment

A **rapid assessment** should be performed within seconds of birth to determine if the infant is breathing and crying, if the amniotic fluid is clear, if there is appropriate muscle tone, and if the infant is at term. If any of these conditions are not met, then the child should be placed under radiant heat, and further resuscitation should be performed. The basic steps to **resuscitation** include:

- Drying and warming the infant
- Positioning the infant and clearing the airway, if necessary
- Stimulating and repositioning the infant

The **respiration and heart rate** of the child should be evaluated throughout the initial procedures:

- Rate and character of respirations noted and chest wall movement observed
- Heart rate assessed with stethoscope or by measuring the pulse rate at the base of the umbilical cord (should be >100 bpm)

APGAR Delivery Room Assessment

Dr. Virginia Apgar developed the **APGAR** test in 1952. APGAR stands for **A**ppearance, **P**ulse, **G**rimace, **A**ctivity, and **R**espiration. The APGAR is the first test given to a newborn. It is used as a quick evaluation of a newborn's physical condition to determine if any emergency medical care is needed and is administered 1 minute and 5 minutes after birth. The test is administered more than once, as the baby's condition may change rapidly. It may be administered for a third time 10 minutes after birth if needed. The baby is rated on the five subscales and scores added together. A total score of ≥7 is a sign of good health.

Sign	0	1	2
Appearance (Skin Color)	Cyanotic or pallor over entire body	Normal, except for the extremities	Entire body normal
Pulse (Heart Rate)	Absent	<100 bpm	>100 bpm
Grimace (Reflex Irritability)	Unresponsive	Grimace	Infant sneezes, coughs, and recoils
Activity (Muscle Tone)	Absent	Flexed limbs	Infant moves freely
Respiration (Breathing Rate and Effort)	Absent	Bradypnea, dyspnea	Good breathing and crying

LGA

Large for gestational age (LGA) infants are those whose weight places them above the 90th percentile for their gestational age. The main pathologic cause for LGA is maternal diabetes (either gestational diabetes or diabetes mellitus). Infants exposed to elevated levels of glucose produce elevated amounts of insulin, which has an anabolic effect on the developing fetus, causing macrosomia (large body). Poor control of diabetes during pregnancy generally results in a larger infant with these common health problems:

- Delivery complications (shoulder dystocia, clavicle fracture, prolonged vaginal exit requiring use of forceps or Caesarian section, and perinatal asphyxia).
- Abnormal blood test results (hypoglycemia developing within 1-2 hours of birth, hyperbilirubinemia, hypocalcemia, hypomagnesemia, hyperviscosity [thickened blood] secondary to polycythemia [elevated platelets]).
- Jaundice.
- Feeding intolerance.
- Lethargy.
- Respiratory distress.
- Birth defects.

SGA

Small for gestational age (SGA) infants are those whose weight places them below the 10th percentile for their gestational age. SGA is also called dysmaturity and intrauterine growth restriction. SGA babies commonly aspirate meconium, and have a low APGAR score, asphyxia, hypoglycemia, and polycythemia. Common causes of SGA include:

- Multiple gestation (twins, triplets, quadruplets).
- Constitutional SGA because both parents are small.
- Many genetic defects, such as trisomy 18 (Edwards syndrome), Down syndrome, and Turner syndrome.
- Placental malfunction or misplacement (inadequate fetal nutrition from reduced blood flow, sepsis, placenta previa, or abruptio placentae).
- Maternal disease (pre-eclampsia; high blood pressure; malnutrition; advanced diabetes mellitus; chronic kidney, heart, or respiratory disease; and anemia).
- Infections such as cytomegalovirus, toxoplasmosis, and rubella.
- Maternal tobacco, illegal drug, or alcohol use during pregnancy.
- Birth defects.

Birth Weight and Gestational Age Acronyms

These terms do not take into account the estimated gestational age of the infant:

- **ELBW (Extremely Low Birth Weight)**: birth weight of less than 1,000 g (2.2 lb)
- **VLBW (Very Low Birth Weight)**: birth weight of less than 1,500 grams (3.3 lb)

The following terms take into account the estimated gestational age of the infant in comparison to the birth weight:

- **SGA (Small for Gestational Age)**: less than the tenth percentile for gestational age
- **AGA (Appropriate for Gestational Age)**: between the tenth and ninetieth percentiles for gestational age
- **LGA (Large for Gestational Age)**: greater than the ninetieth percentile for gestational age

Neonatal Physical Assessment

Modified Ballard Score

The **Modified Ballard Score** is used to estimate **maturity and gestational age** in newborn infants. It is most reliable when performed within the first 12 hours of life. The Ballard Score was modified to include evaluation of extremely premature infants with gestational ages as low as 20 weeks (score 10) and as high as 50 weeks (score 44). It scores 6 measurements of **neuromuscular maturity** and 6 signs of **physical maturity** on a scale of -1 to +4 or 5, depending upon the category.

The six Modified Ballard Score **neuromuscular measurements** are as follows:

1	Observation of the infant's **posture** while lying supine indicates the total amount of **muscle tone** the infant possesses. Increased amounts of flexion of the elbows and knees correlates with increased gestational age.
2	**Square window test** measures the resistance to stretching of **extensor muscles** in the infant's forearm. Increased ability for the tester to flex the infant's wrist correlates with greater gestational age.
3	**Arm recoil test** measures the tone of the **biceps muscles**. Increased amount of arm recoil (flexion by the infant after the infant's arms are extended) correlates with greater gestational age.
4	**Popliteal angle measurement** assesses the flexor tone of the **knee joint**. Increased resistance to flexion at the knee is associated with greater gestational age.
5	**Scarf sign test** measures the tone of **shoulder flexor muscles**. Increased resistance to movement of the infant's arm across the chest is associated with greater gestational age.
6	**Heel-to-ear test** measures the tone of **pelvic girdle muscles**. Increased resistance to movement of the infant's foot to its ear is associated with greater gestational age.

The six Modified Ballard Score **physical signs of maturity** are as follows:

1	**Skin**: Immature infants have thin, transparent skin. The vernix caseosa begins development at the beginning of the third trimester. Dried, cracked skin occurs as this protective coating disappears after the fortieth week.
2	**Lanugo**: Fine, usually unpigmented hairs begin to appear at 24 to 25 weeks of gestation and thin as the neonate matures.
3	**Plantar surface of feet**: Very immature infants have no creases on the soles of their feet. Creases develop first on the anterior portion, and more mature infants will have creases over the entire sole.
4	**Breast buds**: These are fatty tissue underneath the areola which increase in size as the fetus matures.
5	**Ears**: Increased cartilage content produces a more rigid pinna; ear recoil increases as the infant matures.
6	a) **Male genitalia**: The testes descend from the abdomen into the scrotum at 30 weeks of gestation, and the scrotum develops rugae as the fetus matures. b) **Female genitalia**: Initially, the female fetus has a large clitoris and small labia majora. As the fetus matures, the labia majora enlarge, while the clitoris shrinks.

Infants Born at 24 to 25 Weeks

The characteristics of infants born at 24 to 25 weeks are as follows:

Characteristic	Expected findings
Skin	Very thin with visible veins and absent or minimal vernix caseosa, as it is just beginning to be secreted at 20 weeks
Lanugo	Sparse
Feet	Plantar surfaces smooth; may be faint marks on the anterior surfaces
Areolae	Newly developing; breast buds are not yet present
Eyes	Open
Ears	No or very limited recoil
Posture	Immature, indicated by limited flexion of the limbs while infant is in supine position
Square window sign	Shows decreased flexion at the wrist of approximately 60 to 90°
Range of motion	Increased ROM (lone tone) when performing the popliteal angle, scarf sign, and heel-to-ear examinations
Arm recoil	Limited or no recoil

Postterm Infants (>42 Weeks)

Note: Many are normal in size and appearance, but some continue to grow in utero and weigh >4000 g and may exhibit postmaturity syndrome (about 5%), putting the infant at increased risk.

- Alert appearance (may indicated intrauterine hypoxia)
- Skin: loose, dry, cracking, parchment-like, lacking lanugo or vernix. May have meconium staining—yellow to green (indicating recent passage)
- Fingernails: long (sometimes with meconium staining)
- Scalp hair: long/thick.
- Body: long, thin (fat layers absent)
- Hypoglycemia from nutritional deprivation
- Hypothermia because of decreased brown fat and liver glycogen
- Meconium aspiration (risk increases with oligohydramnios), increasing risk of impaired gas exchange
- Polycythemia as response to hypoxia, increasing risk of impaired tissue perfusion
- Seizures resulting from hypoxia
- Cold stress (lack of fat stores)
- Congenital anomalies

Brazelton Neonatal Behavioral Assessment Scale

The **Brazelton Neonatal Behavioral Assessment Scale** is a multi-dimensional scale that is used to assess a neonate's state, temperament, and behavioral patterns. It includes assessment of 18 reflexes, 28 behaviors, and 6 other characteristics. It is usually completed on day 3 with an attempt to elicit the most positive response, usually when the infant is comforted and in a quiet dim room. Scoring correlates to the child's awake or sleep state. Infants are scored according to response in many areas, including:

- **Habituation**: Ability to diminish response to repeat stimuli.
- **Visual and auditory orientation***:* Ability to respond to stimuli, fixate, and follow a visual object.
- **Motor activity***:* Assessment of body tone in various activities.
- Variations: Changes in color, state, activity, alertness, and excitement during the exam.
- **Self-quieting activities***:* Frequency and speed of self-calming activities, such as sucking on hand, putting hand to mouth, focusing on object or sound.
- **Social behaviors***:* Ability to cuddle, engage, and enjoy physical contact.

Sleep States

Infants spend a high percentage of their time in **sleep states**. Sleep periods are divided into active sleep or quiet sleep by observing the infant's behavior:

- **Quiet sleep** is restorative and fosters anabolic growth. Quiet sleep is associated with increased cell mitosis and replication, lowered oxygen consumption, and the release of growth hormone. During quiet sleep, the infant appears relaxed, moves minimally, and breathes smoothly and regularly. The eyelids are still. The infant only responds to intense stimuli during quiet sleep.
- **Active sleep** is associated with processing and storing of information. Rapid eye movement (REM sleep) occurs during active sleep, but it is unknown if newborn infants are able to dream. During active sleep, the infant moves occasionally and breathes irregularly. Eye movements can be seen beneath the eyelids. Infants spend most of their sleep time in active sleep, and it usually precedes wakening.

Awake States

Infants have different levels of consciousness in the 4 **awake states**. Infants respond differently to outside stimuli and interaction from caregivers, depending on which state they are in:

- **Drowsy***:* This is characterized by variable activity, mild startles, and smooth movement. There is some facial movement. Eyes open and close, breathing is irregular, and response to stimuli may be delayed.
- **Quiet alert***:* The infant rarely moves, breathing is regular, and the infant focuses intently on individuals or objects that are within focal range, widening eyes. Face appears bright and alert, breathing is regular, and the infant focuses on stimuli.
- **Active alert***:* The infant moves frequently and has much facial movement although face not as bright and alert, eyes may have a dull glaze, breathing is irregular, and there are variable responses to outside stimuli.
- **Crying***:* Characterized by grimacing, eyes shut, irregular breathing, increased movement with color changes and marked response to both internal and external stimuli.

Neonatal Neurosensory Capabilities

The normal **neonatal neurosensory capabilities** are as follows:

Hearing	The neonate's crying after birth clears middle ear mucus and the eustachian tubes, and hearing becomes acute with hearing thresholds similar to adults and children. Because hearing deficit is one of the most common congenital abnormalities, all infants should be assessed for hearing.
Vision	The neonate's vision is about 10 to 30 times less acute than that of an adult, but the infant has peripheral vision, can fixate at 8 to14 inches, and can accommodate to large objects. The neonate is able to perceive shapes, colors, and faces.
Tactile sense	The neonate has a good sense of touch and reacts emotionally to tactile stimulation.
Smell	The neonate has a strong sense of smell after nasal passages clear and will react to the smell of milk or turn away from strong smells.
Pain	Neonates experience pain, and pain prevention/management should be part of neonatal care.

Universal Hearing Screening

Universal hearing screening is recommended by the AAP for all newborns. Hearing loss in neonates may occur because of genetic abnormalities, *in utero* infections with cytomegalovirus or rubella, meningitis, craniofacial abnormalities, or Usher's syndrome. Admission to the NICU for longer than two days increases the likelihood of hearing loss by tenfold, so all newborns should be screened for hearing loss — not just those with risk factors — prior to discharge. Undiagnosed hearing loss results in severe language and developmental delay. Identification and early intervention during the critical time period of language development decreases the morbidity associated with neonatal hearing loss. Reasons for screening include:

- An easy-to-use test is available with high degrees of sensitivity and specificity.
- Hearing loss is otherwise difficult to detect until language milestones have been missed
- Interventions are available to correct conditions.
- Early intervention results in improved outcome.
- The screening process can be performed in a cost-effective manner.

Assessment of Muscular Tone

Determining the quality of **muscle tone** in a neonate is an important part of neuromuscular assessment. The child is placed supine with the head in neutral position and the LRN Nurse moves body parts (arms, legs, head) to determine if the muscle tone is flaccid, jittery, or hypertonic. Neonates are slightly hypertonic so that some resistance should be felt to movement, such as when moving a leg or straightening an arm. Tone should be symmetric. The extremities are usually flexed and legs abducted to abdomen. This assessment allows the LRN Nurse to differentiate common fine tremors or jitteriness found in neonates from seizure activity or nervous system disorders that cause muscular twitching. Normal fine tremors are usually halted by holding or flexing the extremity while seizure activity or twitching does not resolve by holding

Assessment of Neonatal Sucking Reflex

Touching the roof of the neonate's mouth triggers **sucking**. The sucking reflex begins to appear at 32 weeks of gestation, but is not fully developed until 36 weeks. Premature neonates often have an immature or weak suck, and need additional patience and support to feed. Preterm neonates have difficulty coordinating sucking, swallowing and breathing simultaneously. Preterm neonates have immature neurological systems and less ability to handle external environmental stressors. Stressors include medically necessary and unavoidable frequent examinations, respiratory support from oxygen or a ventilator, administration of medications, light, noises of a busy NICU, or even oral feeds. As a neonate matures, the infants develop skills to self-soothe h when stressed. Some of these skills include nonnutritive sucking:

- Sucking of hands or fingers.
- Sucking on a pacifier.
- Sucking during sleep.

Neonatal Reflexes Assessment

Reflex	Eliciting reflex	Normal response	Discussion
Palmar grasping	Stroke the infant's palm.	The infant responds by grasping the finger.	Grasp reflex is stronger in premature infants and fades away at 2 to 3 months of age. Absence indicates CNS deficit or muscle injury.
Rooting	Stroke the side of the infant's cheek.	The infant turns the head in the direction of the touch, and opens mouth to feed.	Rooting reflex helps the infant find and latch onto the mother's breast.
Sucking	Touch the infant's mouth.	The infant sucks.	Premature infants may have an absent or weak suck reflex, as it usually develops around week 32 of gestation. Weak or absent reflex indicates CNS deficit or depression.
Moro (startle)	Make a loud sound or give the infant a gentle jolt.	The infant extends arms, legs, and neck, and then pulls back arms and legs. May also cry.	Moro reflex disappears at 5 to 6 months of age. Asymmetric response indicates peripheral nerve injury, or fracture of long bones, clavicle, or skull.
Blinking	Flash light at eyes.	Eyelids close.	Absence or delay may indicate cerebral palsy, hydrocephalus, and developmental delay.
Tonic neck (fencing)	With infant supine, turn head to one side.	Extremities flex on opposite side and extend on same side.	May be incomplete immediately after birth and should diminish by 4 months. Persistence >4 months may indicate neurological abnormalities.
Babinski (plantar)	Stroke the lateral aspect of the sole from heel to ball of foot.	Hyper-extension of all toes.	Persists until ≤2 years, after which the toes flex.
Trunk incurvation (Galant)	With infant prone, stroke down one side of the spine (1 inch from spine).	Pelvis turns to stimulated side.	Absence indicates CNS depression or lesion of spinal cord. Should disappear by 4 months.
Tongue extrusion	Touch tip of tongue.	Neonate pushes tongue out of mouth.	Continuous or repetitive extrusion indicates CNS abnormalities or seizure activity.

Review Video: Tonic Neck Response
Visit mometrix.com/academy and enter code: 421866

Systems Review

Neonatal Appearance and Measurements

Head	Disproportionately large for body
Body	Long
Extremities	Short and in flexed position (feet usually dorsiflexed after breech birth)
Hands	Clenched
Neck	Short with chin resting on chest
Abdomen	Prominent
Hips	Narrow
Chest	Rounded
Weight	2500 to 4000 g (average about 3400); physiologic weight loss of 5 to 10% for full term and 15% for preterm
Length	45 to 55 cm (average 50 cm)
Head circumference	32 to 38 cm (usually 2 cm greater than chest circumference)
Chest circumference	30 to 36 cm

Neonatal Vital Signs

Temperature	Drops rapidly (skin temperature falls 0.3 °C/minute) after birth with exposure to ambient room temperature but stabilizes within 8 to 12 hours (measured for 3 minutes by axillary method; range from 36.3-37.0 °C)
Blood pressure	56 to 77/33 to 50 mm Hg
Pulse	120 to120 bpm awake; 100 bpm asleep; 180 bmp crying
Respiration	30 to 60 per minute

Normal Neonatal Cardiac Rates

Normal cardiac rates can vary widely from one neonate to another, so it's important to understand the normal range in order to determine if the infant has an abnormal pulse. Rates will also vary depending upon whether the infant is awake, sleeping, or active. Pulse rate should be taken with a stethoscope, because the pulse may be difficult to palpate or count accurately manually. The neonatal **point of maximal intensity (PMI)** is located at the intersection between the 4th intercostal space and the midclavicular line (versus the adult PMI located at the 5th intercostal). Additionally, this allows for assessment of heart murmurs.

Newborn infant	At rest: 100 to 180 Asleep: 80 to 160 Active/sick: ≤220
1 to 12 weeks	At rest: 100 to 220 Asleep: 80 to 200 Active/sick: ≤220

Monitoring of heart rate is particularly important as alterations of heart rate occur with periods of apnea. A period of apnea is usually followed by decreased heart rate, as well as decreased oxygen saturation. Respiratory rates should be monitored as well as heart rate. **Color** should be noted. Pink coloring indicates good perfusion. Generalized mottling or central cyanosis should be investigated further.

Infant Blood Pressure

Normal **blood pressure** values for **term infant**:

- Systolic-56-77 mm Hg.
- Diastolic 33-50 mm Hg.
- MAP 42-60 mm Hg.
- Hypertension: Systolic >90 and diastolic >60.

Normal values for **preterm infant:** In a preterm infant, systolic and diastolic values will vary depending on the gestational age and size of the infant. A preterm infant should have a mean arterial pressure that is a number matching the gestational age in weeks of that infant. For example, an infant born at 28 weeks gestation should have a MAP of 28.

- Hypertension: Systolic >80 and diastolic >50.

Proper **fit of the blood pressure cuff** is imperative to obtain an accurate reading. One must measure the width of the infant's arm in the area that the cuff will be applied. Once this measurement is obtained, the cuff should be approximately 25% wider than this measurement. A cuff too small results in BP reading too high and too large results in BP reading too low.

Neonatal Cardiac Assessment

S1

S1 is the heart sound heard as the mitral and tricuspid valves close at the beginning of the contraction of the ventricle (systole). S1 is easiest to hear if the stethoscope is placed at the fourth intercostal space while the infant is supine and calm. If the S1 heard is louder than normal, that means **cardiac output** and **blood flow** are higher than normal. The conditions that can cause this are:

- Patent ductus arteriosus
- Ventricular septal defect
- Tetralogy of Fallot

If the S1 heard is softer or quieter than normal, this is an indication of **lowered cardiac output**, which could cause these problems:

- Congestive heart failure
- Myocarditis

S2

S2 is the sound heard when the pulmonic valve and the aortic valve close at the end of the contraction of the ventricles (systole). S2 is easiest to hear at the upper left border of the sternum. S2 is normally split, as the aortic valve closes slightly ahead of the pulmonic valve. In the presence of a cardiac defect, the S2 split becomes widener (the difference in time between the closing of the aortic and pulmonic valve becomes greater). Conditions that cause a **widened S2 split** include:

- Atrial septal defect
- Tetralogy of Fallot
- Pulmonary stenosis
- Ebstein anomaly

Conditions that cause **no split** in the S2 (the two valves close at the same time, or one is not closing) include:

- Pulmonary or aortic atresia
- Aortic or pulmonary stenosis
- Persistent pulmonary hypertension

Peripheral Pulses

Peripheral pulses, usually palpated at the brachial or femoral arteries, are graded according to **strength**. Peripheral pulses may be difficult to palpate in a neonate and should not be relied upon for cardiac assessment. Pulses should always be verified by auscultation:

- 0 = absent
- 1+ = weak
- 2+ = weak to average
- 3+ = strong
- 4+ = bounding

Weak pulses are noted in conditions that cause a decrease in cardiac output. Some of these conditions include:

- Any defect resulting in obstructed blood flow leaving the left ventricle
- Failure of the heart muscle itself
- Shock

Bounding pulses (4+) are noted when there is too much blood coming from the aorta. Some of the conditions that would cause this are:

- Patent ductus arteriosus
- Aortic insufficiency
- Shunts

Cardiopulmonary Monitoring

Cardiopulmonary monitoring includes electrocardiogram (ECG) and respiratory sensors. Usually 3 chest ECG leads that record the electrical activity of the heart and sense respiratory movement are placed, and the patterns are recorded on a visual screen. Many computerized monitors have memory capability so that data can be analyzed out of real time. They can also be set to record certain events, such as periods of apnea. Alarm thresholds are set, so that an alarm indicates dangerous changes. Apnea alarms should be both visual and auditory. False alarms may occur and should be thoroughly evaluated for cause, such as loose leads or movement. Home monitors include records of compliance so that a review of data shows the time the monitor was actually in use. Home monitors are used for infants at risk for SIDS. Because of interference problems that might provide inaccurate readings, monitors should never be used as a sole evaluation of cardiopulmonary status. Observation and examination must be used to verify the infant's condition.

Neonatal Chest and Respiratory Assessment

The neonate's **chest and respiratory status** should be evaluated by observation and auscultation. The chest should be symmetric and the ribs flexible. The xiphoid process may protrude slightly. Breasts are sometimes engorged, and the nipples may secrete small amounts of white fluid. Accessory nipples may be noted. Pulmonary function assessment should include anterior and posterior auscultation. Abdominal movement should synchronize with respirations. Periodic breathing is common, but apneic periods should be <20 seconds or they can result in cyanosis or bradycardia. The **Silverman-Anderson Index** is used to evaluate respiratory status. A score of 0 indicates normal findings, and higher scores indicate respiratory distress.

Characteristic	**0**	**1**	**2**
Chest/abdomen	Rise to-gether with inspiration	Rising abdomen with sinking or lagging upper chest	See-saw movement
Intercostals	No retraction	Minimal retraction	Pronounced retraction
Xiphoid process	No retraction	Minimal retraction	Pronounced retraction
Nasal flaring	None	Minimal flaring	Pronounced flaring
Grunt (expiratory)	None	Grunt heard with auscultation	Audible grunt

Neonatal Pulse Oximetry

Pulse oximetry is a means of monitoring the saturation level of the **hemoglobin** in the blood. For example, a reading of 98% indicates that 98% of the hemoglobin available is bound to oxygen or saturated with oxygen. A machine uses infrared light to read the hemoglobin. Several things can affect the accuracy of this reading.

- The **perfusion status** of the neonate. If the infant is suffering from a condition that results in poor perfusion (hypovolemia, hypotension, etc.), the pulse oximetry reading will be inaccurate, as the machine will have difficulty reading the blood.
- **Phototherapy** used for jaundice will also cause inaccurate readings, because like the tool used in pulse oximetry, it is a light.
- Use of **dopamine**, a potent vasoconstricting drug that causes problems reading the blood for oxygen levels if the veins are constricted, affecting blood flow.

Pulse oximetry is now a recommended screening tool for congenital heart defects. While not diagnostic, it provides information that can either rule out congenital heart defects, or trigger further investigation.

NEONATAL GASTROINTESTINAL ASSESSMENT

As the neonate breathes, air enters the **GI system**—first the stomach and then the intestines—within 2 to 12 hours, and enters the colon within 24 hours. Bowel sounds are usually present within 30 to 60 minutes of birth. The stomach has a capacity of about 50 to 60 mL and empties intermittently, usually beginning a few minutes after feeding begins and continuing for 2 to 4 hours after; however, because of immaturity of the cardiac sphincter, the neonate may regurgitate the first few feedings. If regurgitation becomes continuous, further evaluation is indicated. Infants produce little saliva until the salivary glands mature in about 3 months. Term neonates usually pass **meconium** within 8 to24 hours, although they may not do so for 48 hours. First meconium is thick, dark, and tarry. **Transitional stools** for the next few days are usually brown to green, after which the child should pass normal stools. Stools of breastfed babies are usually yellow-gold and mushy, and those of formula fed babies are pale yellow and pasty.

NEONATAL ABDOMINAL AND RECTAL ASSESSMENT

The **abdomen** should be soft, symmetric, and rounded. A distended abdomen with engorged vessels may indicate GI abnormalities. Bowel sounds (present about an hour after birth) should be auscultated prior to palpation. The liver is usually palpable 1 to 2 cm below the right coastal margin, and the tip of the spleen may be palpable in preterm infants only in the left lateral upper quadrant. It should not extend >1 cm below the costal margin. The umbilical cord should be white or blue-white, with two umbilical arteries and one umbilical vein observed and no discharge or bleeding. Presence of only one umbilical artery is associated with GI/GU congenital anomalies. Green/yellow discoloration may indicate meconium staining. The abdomen should be examined carefully for hernias while the infant is at rest and crying.

The **rectal area** should be examined to determine if the anus is present and patent. Meconium is usually passed within 24 hours of birth. Soft swelling in the femoral area may indicate hernia or undescended testicle.

NEONATE SKIN APPEARANCE

Newborns' skin appearance depends on the development and thickening of their dermis, epidermis, and vernix caseosa. When skin develops during week 15 of gestation, it is initially thin and translucent. By week 20, vernix caseosa production begins. Vernix is a thick, waxy substance secreted by the sebaceous glands and mixed with sloughed-off skin cells, often described as "cheesy." The stratum corneum (protective top layer of the epidermis) develops from weeks 20-24. The epidermis continues to develop and thicken, and is able to form a water barrier by week 32. Near term, the vernix washes away and the skin becomes more wrinkled without its protection:

Gestational Age	Skin Appearance
24-26 weeks	Translucent, red, many visible blood vessels, and scant vernix
35-40 weeks	Deep cracks, no visible blood vessels, and thick vernix
42-44 weeks	Dry, peeling skin, no vernix, and loss of subcutaneous fat

NEONATAL INTEGUMENTARY ASSESSMENT

SKIN CHARACTERISTICS

Color	Skin colors vary with race, but all should be pink-tinged to some degree, as skin pigmentation is slight after birth.
Birth-marks	Asian, African-American, and other dark-skinned infants may have *Mongolian spots* (blue-black discoloration) on the buttocks and dorsal area. *Nevus flammeus* (port-wine stain) is a demarcated unraised red-purple lesion caused by capillaries below the epidermis. *Nevus vasculosus* (strawberry mark) is a capillary hemangioma, a raised, demarcated, dark red lesion.
Acrocyanosis	Slight cyanosis of the hands and feet during the first 2 to 6 hours after birth, especially if chilled. Color returns rapidly when skin blanched.
Mottling	Common for hours to weeks after birth and may relate to prolonged periods of apnea or chilling.
Harlequin sign	Deep color on one side of body only for 1 to 20 minutes. Usually transient.
Erythema toxicum	Perifollicular lesions (1 to 3 mm), white or yellow with pustule; appears suddenly over body (except palms and soles). Usually transient. Cause unknown.
Milia	Small raised white spots on face from exposed sebaceous glands. Transient.

CAFÉ AU LAIT SPOTS

Café au lait spots (CAL) are flat skin lesions with increased melanin content and regular or irregular borders. If the CAL spots are faint, use of a Wood lamp to make them easier to see. Fewer than 3 café au lait spots have no clinical significance. However, 6 or more café au lait spots with a diameter larger than 5 mm occur in 95% of patients with **neurofibromatosis type 1 (NF1)**, a disorder of chromosome 17. Lisch nodules on the irises and Crowe's sign (freckles on the axillae and inguinal area) corroborate the diagnosis of NF1. The pediatrician must be alerted that this child should receive future monitoring for the symptoms that occur with NF1, such as bowed legs, rib lesions, scoliosis, neurofibromas, glaucoma, and corneal opacification. Café au lait spots are also associated with tuberous sclerosis, McCune-Albright syndrome, ataxia telangiectasia, Gaucher disease, basal cell nevus syndrome, and Fanconi anemia. Eighteen percent of infants affected with CAL are African American, 3% are Hispanic, and 0.3% are white.

CUTIS MARMORATA

Cutis marmorata is a disorder in which the infant's skin mottles or marbles when exposed to cold, because the **superficial blood vessels** dilate and contract at the same time. Cutis marmorata occurs in 50% of infants during the first few months of life because of immature vascular and neurological systems. In areas where vessels contract, the skin appears white or pale, and in areas where vessels dilate, the skin is pink or red. The infant's skin color returns to normal when he or she is rewarmed. Cutis marmorata poses no threat to the infant and resolves as the baby matures. Down syndrome babies are prone to cutis marmorata. **Cutis marmorata telangiectatica congenital (CMTC)** is a rare variant with the same appearance, but the skin does not return to normal with rewarming and ulcers form. Infants with CMTC often have undergrowth or overgrowth of the involved limb. The mother may have been exposed to a teratogen or had high hCG during pregnancy. The infant may have Sturge-Weber or Klippel-Trenaunay syndromes.

HEMANGIOMA

Hemangioma is a bright red vascular tumor that occurs in 1-3% of neonates, especially in girls, preterm infants <1500 g, and those whose mothers had chorionic villus sampling. The head and neck are the most common sites. Hemangiomas may initially appear as a faint telangiectasia or red macule, but they proliferate rapidly during the first year after which they go through a slow involution in which they decrease in size, usually complete in 95% by adolescence. Hemangiomas may be superficial, deep, or mixed and may involve skin as well as organs. Complications, such as airway compromise, vision problem, ulceration, renal abnormalities, imperforate anus, and skeletal anomalies may occur as the hemangioma grows, depending upon adjacent structures. Imaging of hemangiomas is indicated only in infants that display evidence or possibility of underlying structural abnormalities. *Treatment* may include just monitoring or systemic or localized treatment with corticosteroids to slow proliferation. Oral propranolol is the first-line therapy for infantile hemangiomas in infants age 5 weeks to 5 months. Pulsed dye laser treatment is a common treatment to reduce proliferation.

Erythema Toxicum

Erythema toxicum is a skin eruption of erythematous papules, vesicles, and sometimes pustules that is essentially benign and occurs in ≥50% of newborns. It is a generalized rash that resembles that of herpes simplex, occurring on the face, limbs, and trunk (everywhere except the palms and soles of the feet). It usually occurs 2-3 days after birth. The lesions are surrounded by mottled erythematous halo of about 0.5 to 1.5 cm. Individual lesions often appear and resolve within hours but new lesions occur. Lesions may be limited to a few on the face or may cover the body. Erythema toxicum is often associated with eosinophilia and occurs in the first few weeks of life before the immune system matures, so it is hypothesized the rash may be an allergic response. The rash usually resolves in about 2 weeks without treatment.

Neonatal Pustular Melanosis

Neonatal pustular melanosis is a benign rash (vesicles and macules) that is present at birth is about 2.2% of white infants and 4.4% of black. Usually, in preterm infants, vesicles (2-4 mm) with milky fluid are present at birth and rupture, leaving a halo of white scaly tissue and a pigmented macule at the center. Erythema is not associated with this rash. Full-term infants may exhibit only the macular stage as the vesicles ruptured prior to birth. The pigmented discoloration fades with time but may persist for ≤3 months. The cause of neonatal pustular melanosis is not known. The rash may be localized and sparse or profuse (beneath chin, neck, upper chest, upper back, and buttocks). No treatment is indicated and there appears to be no long-term sequelae, but the lesions must be differentiated from congenital herpes infection, especially if erythema is evident.

Subcutaneous Fat Necrosis

Subcutaneous fat necrosis is a nodular skin lesion disorder that usually occurs ≤6 weeks of birth in full-term or post-term infants caused by necrosis of subcutaneous fatty tissue. Onset is usually between days 2-21. Subcutaneous fat necrosis is commonly associated with hypothermia, trauma to tissue from forceps, neonatal stress (various causes) and hypercalcemia. Single or multiple lesions may develop, ranging in size from about 1 cm to many centimeters with erythema obvious over lesions. Lesions are usually rubbery and often distributed across the buttocks, upper legs, shoulders, upper back, upper extremities, and cheeks. In some cases, fluctuant lesions may open and drain or require aspiration. The lesions usually resolve over time with no treatment. Serum calcium should be monitored and hypercalcemia evaluated for cause and treated as necessary.

Port Wine Stain

Port wine stain (capillary angioma) is a birthmark comprised of dilated capillaries below the epidermis. The lesion is usually on the face or neck and is light pink at birth but darkens with age. The lesion alone is benign but it may be an indication of other disorders, such as Sturge-Weber syndrome (neurological disorder with seizures, paralysis, and glaucoma) or Klippel-Trenaunay-

Weber syndrome (disorder with hypertrophy of bones and soft tissue as well as varicose veins and multiple port wine stains), so the infant should be evaluated and have an eye examination, especially if the lesion is on the eyelids as this is associated with glaucoma. Over time the capillary angioma may thicken and form nodules, so early treatment is advisable. The most common treatment is laser therapy, which destroys the capillaries without damaging other tissue, usually done in infancy to prevent psychological trauma and to prevent changes in the skin, such as thickening.

Ecchymosis, Petechiae, Hyperpigmentation, and Hypopigmentation

Ecchymosis (large blue-purple discolored bruising) and **petechiae** (pinpoint <1mm hemorrhagic areas) may be the result of birth trauma, particularly difficult births, breech births, or forceps-assisted birth and is most noticeable on the presenting part. These types of bruising usually fade within 24-48 hours, but if they persist, they may indicate underlying pathology. Ecchymosis and petechiae can indicate clotting disorders and bleeding in the tissue, such as can occur with DIC. They may also be evidence of thrombocytopenia (especially diffuse petechiae) and vitamin K deficiency.

Hypopigmentation may be caused by a number of disorders, including PKU, Addison's disease, vitiligo, albinism, and herpes simplex virus. It may also result from post-inflammatory changes **Hyperpigmentation**, while rare in the newborn, can occur with severe toxoplasmosis infection, Addison's disease, liver disease, porphyria, pellagra, sprue, lentiginosis, and melanism. Untreated syphilitic lesions may cause hypo- or hyperpigmentation after regression.

Neonatal Musculoskeletal Assessment

The **musculoskeletal system** should be assessed for muscle tone. Maintenance of fetal position or limp tone may indicate hypoxia, CNS abnormalities, or hypoglycemia. Joint movement should be spontaneous with good muscle tone. Spasticity or floppiness indicates cerebral palsy or other disorder. Jitteriness may indicate hypoglycemia or hypocalcemia.

Extremities should be short, flexed, and able to move symmetrically through range of motion, but without full extension. Arms/legs should be equal in length with feet and hands of normal size (5 digits each). Feet are flat. Hips should abduct to >60°. Cyanosis or clubbing of nails indicates cardiac anomalies, and yellow-green discoloration indicates meconium staining.

The **back and spine** are examined with the infant in a prone position. The spine should be straight, without a sacral or lumbar curve, which develops only after the child begins to sit. Obvious anomalies, such as spina bifida, and indications of a pilonidal dimple, skin lesions, or tufts of hair that may indicate abnormalities should be noted. C-shaped spine may indicate spina bifida occulta, and lumbar lordosis may indicate myelomeningocele.

Congenital Hip Dislocation

Congenital hip dislocation, also known as **developmental dysplasia of the hip or DDH**, is hip instability resulting from misalignment of the **femoral head** and **acetabulum**. Hip instability may present as dislocation, subluxation, or acetabular dysplasia (abnormal structural development of the joint). *Symptoms* may not be evident until after the neonatal period. The condition tends to worsen as the child grows. Involvement of the left hip is more common than the right. There appears to be a genetic tendency and an association with breech birth. Signs at ≤3 months include:

- Positive Barlow's test (Pressing on the knees to apply pressure to the head of the femur when hips are flexed causes posterior subluxation.)
- Positive Ortolani test (Hips rotated through range of motion cause click at abduction as femoral head slips.)

The AAFP recommends against using imaging for universal screening of DDH, but rather screening high-risk infants who are between 6 weeks and 6 months of age with a physical assessment that is otherwise normal. Radiography for the screening of DDH should be reserved only for children 4 months of age or older in this category.

Referral to an orthopedist is indicated for application of **Pavlik harness** for infants <3 months of age. Per AAFP guidelines, avoid tightly swaddling the legs and extending or adducting the hips.

METATARSUS ADDUCTUS

Metatarsus adductus ("toeing in") is the most common congenital disorder of the foot, occurring in about 1:1000 births. Metatarsus adductus is a convex curve turning the forefoot inward at the tarsometatarsal joint. Metatarsus adductus occurs equally in males and females and is common among siblings. It is believed the condition may be related to position in the uterus, and it is often associated with oligohydramnios. About 50% have bilateral metatarsus adductus and 10-15% have hip dysplasia as well. In most cases, simple stretching exercises are the only needed therapy, and most cases resolve by 3 months. If the curvature is >15°, serial casting, changed about 1 time weekly, may be necessary to maintain the foot in the correct position. Braces or special orthopedic shoes may be used after casting is completed.

TALIPES EQUINOVARUS

Talipes equinovarus (clubfoot) is a congenital abnormality of the foot that involves 3 types of deformities:

- The midfoot is directly inferiorly (equinus).
- The hindfoot turns inward (varus).
- The forefoot adducts toward the hell and then turns superiorly in partial supination.

Typically, the foot is small, the Achilles tendon shortened, and the lower leg muscles atrophied. The condition begins during the first trimester, so the foot position is very rigid at birth. Clubfoot occurs in about 1:1000 births with a male to female ratio of 2:1. About 50% of cases are bilateral. Cases vary in severity and some may be associated with other abnormalities, such as myelomeningocele. Diagnosis is often made on ultrasound (16-20 weeks) or at birth. The cause is unclear, but there appears to be a genetic component. Treatment is by long leg serial casting (changed every 1-2 weeks) begun shortly after birth. In some cases, surgery may be required (at 3-12 months) followed by casting and bracing.

Tibial Bowing

Tibial bowing is deviation of the **tibial diaphysis**. There are 3 different types, determined by the direction of the deformity.

- **Anterolateral bowing** is associated with neurofibromatosis and may either be present at birth or become obvious over time. Treatment is with orthosis from above the knee to below the ankle. Surgery is not done, as it can cause pseudoarthrosis.
- **Anteromedial bowing** is associated with fibular hemimelia (aplasia or hypoplasia). In past times, amputation was common, because it causes a 3-inch length discrepancy in leg length at maturity; however, limb-lengthening procedures are often done now.
- **Posteromedial bowing** is associated with a calcaneovalgus deformity (flexible flatfoot). There may be muscle weakness and inequality in limb length (1 to 5 cm at birth). While angular deformities usually resolve over time, the medial bowing often remains, resulting in problems associated with a shortened limb, so limb-lengthening procedures may be considered later.

Scoliosis

Scoliosis is a lateral (S-shaped) spinal curvature >10°. Curvature >30° produces marked deformity. The curvature of scoliosis may be structural or compensatory. Congenital scoliosis is increasing because of survival of infants with preterm birth. About 10% of congenital scoliosis relates to abnormalities of the intervertebral/vertebral bodies, affecting the growth of the trunk, most commonly hemivertebra. The male to female ratio is 2.5:1 with about a third of the curvatures at the upper thoracic level with decreasing incidence down the spine (5% at lumbosacral area). Thoracolumbar curvatures carry the worst prognosis. About 20-50% of cases have other spinal cord abnormalities, and 30-60% of these have other anomalies, such as VATER syndrome. Impairment of pulmonary function is a major complication. Bracing is a successful treatment for <10% of cases, but it may be used early to prevent further curvature in preparation for later surgery.

Achondroplasia

Achondroplasia is the most common cause of **dwarfism**, in which bone growth is inhibited as the result of an abnormal gene on **chromosome 4**. Achondroplasia can be inherited in an autosomal dominant fashion, but the majority of cases (75 to 80%) occur because of spontaneous mutations. Clinical features of achondroplasia apparent at birth include a long narrow torso with short arms and legs. The proximal segment of the limbs (upper arms and thighs) is disproportionately short. The head is large, with frontal bossing and midface hypoplasia. A small hump (gibbus) may be present in the mid-to-lower back. Mild, generalized hypotonia may be present. Monitor the infant's head size for the development of hydrocephalus. The pediatrician may order a skeletal survey to identify many of skeletal features associated with achondroplasia and to help confirm the diagnosis.

Osteogenesis Imperfecta

Osteogenesis imperfecta (OI) is a genetic disorder of collagen synthesis that results in brittle, easily fractured bones. OI occurs in 1 in 20,000 live births. Collagen is a major component of bone that gives it both strength and flexibility. Infants with OI either produce defective collagen or deficient amounts of collagen. Four different types of OI have been identified, with symptoms ranging from very mild to lethality in the neonatal period. *Common features* of OI include:

- Brittle bones that fracture easily (fractures may be present at birth).
- Bowing of long bones.
- Shortened limbs.
- Discolored, brittle teeth.
- Blue sclera.
- Skeletal deformities, including scoliosis.
- Respiratory difficulties.
- Weak muscles.

Generally, OI is inherited in a dominant fashion, but a new mutation may cause the disorder in approximately 25% of cases. Parents of children diagnosed with OI must be instructed on correct methods of handling, bathing, and placing their child in the crib to sleep to minimize trauma and the development of fractures.

Birth Injuries

Clavicular Fracture

Clavicular fracture is the most common injury during birth. This fracture usually does not affect respiration. Breech delivery increases risk for rib fractures: The larger the infant, the more likely to suffer one or more fractured ribs. These fractures may not cause any noticeable symptoms. If there are multiple rib fractures, the infant will show signs of pain when moved or picked up and may develop difficulty breathing that could indicate atelectasis from the fracture. Premature infants can also develop rib fractures after birth from simple handling and chest physiotherapy due to the extremely fragile nature of these bones. A chest x-ray makes the diagnosis of rib fracture. . The infant should be evaluated for other signs of traumatic injury, given acetaminophen for pain, and the infant's arm immobilized with a figure-8 clavicle strap with the baby's shoulder elevated above heart level. The mother should be taught to carry the baby by supporting the back and shoulder. The clavicle heals in about four weeks.

Cranial Nerve Trauma

Injury to cranial nerves can occur during birth (the recurrent laryngeal nerve is the most common) caused by compression of the head against the sacrum during birth or from the use of forceps. Symptoms relate to the specific type of nerve injury but may present as temporary or permanent paralysis. Often asymmetry, drooping of eye or mouth, or failure of the eyelid to close is noted, especially when the infant cries. Traumatic injury to nerves usually resolves over time, beginning by the end of the first week but symptoms may persist to some degree for months. An open eye must be protected by the use of synthetic tears and patching to prevent damage. Those with injury to the laryngeal nerve may have dyspnea and dysphagia and may require small frequent feedings or enteral feedings until the condition resolves. In most cases, treatment is symptomatic with careful observation so that complications can be treated promptly.

Brachial Plexus Trauma

Trauma to the **brachial plexus** may cause a full term infant to hold his/her arm adducted and internally rotated after a delivery complicated by shoulder dystocia. There is movement in the hands. One to 3 infants per 1,000 live births suffer trauma to the brachial plexus. The brachial plexus is a collection of nerve tissue located in the shoulder area that is the pathway for nerves traveling from the spine to the arm and shoulder. These nerves control the movement of the shoulder and arm. Most commonly, the upper portion of this plexus is damaged, leading to weak arm muscles (Erb's palsy). When examined, the infant holds the arm adducted and internally rotated. The startle reflex is abnormal on the affected side, but the grasp reflex is normal. If the lower portion of the plexus is damaged, the hand is paralyzed also, and the grasp reflex is absent (Klumpke's paralysis). Most infants recover fully, but recovery depends on the degree of damage to the brachial plexus (complete tear vs. stretching).

Head Assessment

Caput Succedaneum and Cephalohematoma

Caput succedaneum and **cephalohematoma** are both examples of head molding resulting from head trauma during birthing. They can be observed during the newborn period and appear similar on physical examination because the neonate's head is swollen:

- **Caput succedaneum** is more common. It is a collection of fluid beneath the skin, but superficial to the periosteum. It often occurs when the head presses against the dilating cervix during the birth process. Vacuum assisted deliveries also contribute to caput succedaneum. The swelling crosses suture lines. Complications are rare. Swelling usually resolves over several days.
- **Cephalohematoma** occurs when blood vessels between the skull and the periosteum rupture, causing a subperiosteal collection of blood. The swelling appears several hours after birth. It does not cross suture lines. Complications such as anemia or hypovolemia may occur if the amount of bleeding is large. The blood will eventually be resorbed and may cause jaundice secondary to break down of red blood cells.

Craniotabes

Craniotabes is an area of softened skull found in 30% of newborns. It is softer and more pliable than surrounding tissue and gives way when pressure is applied, as though one is pushing on a ping-pong ball. It is more common in premature infants, but can also be found in full term infants. Usually, craniotabes occurs in the posterior occipital or posterior parietal bones or along the suture lines. Craniotabes is considered to be a normal finding that requires no treatment because it usually resolves by one month of age. Craniotabes may persist longer when it is positioned along a suture line. No work-up is required, but the infant should be carefully examined for indications of disease-related causes of craniotabes, including other conditions that effect bone growth or hardness, such as rickets, syphilis, marasmus, or osteogenesis imperfecta.

Fontanels

The newborn has 8 skull bones and 14 facial bones. Their adjoining edges are bone sutures. Soft spots where the skull flexes along sutures to exit the vagina are **fontanels**. The newborn has 6 fontanels:

- Diamond-shaped anterior fontanel (AF): 2.1 cm
- Triangular posterior fontanel (PF)
- Sphenoid fontanels (2)
- Mastoid fontanels (2)

The AF is the largest and most informative during clinical examination. Fontanels **bulge** when the newborn cries, vomits, lies down, or has hydrocephalus, intracranial tumor, hemorrhage, or meningitis. Fontanels should return to normal when the NNP holds the baby head up and the infant is calm. **Depressed fontanels** indicate the newborn is dehydrated. Conditions associated with an abnormally large AF include hypothyroidism, Down syndrome, achondroplasia, rickets, and increased intracranial pressure. Infants with Down syndrome may have an extra fontanel between the AF and posterior fontanel.

Assessments of the Eyes, Nose, Neck, and Throat

The appearance and movement of the **face** should be symmetric in the neonate and a number of different characteristics examined:

Eyes	Usually blue to blue/grey with white to bluish-white sclera. Small conjunctival hemorrhages and transient strabismus or squint may be evident. Pupils should be equal and reactive. Red retinal reflex should be present. Tears are usually absent during crying. Eye blink test causes lids to close.
Nose	Infants usually breathe through nose and should be able to breathe easily if mouth is closed. If not, the child should be examined for choanal atresia. Sense of smell is determined if the infant turns toward milk source or away from strong smells, such as alcohol.
Neck	The infant should be able to hold head up slightly while prone, but the head lags when lifted from the supine position because of weak muscles. Neck rigidity may indicate injury to sternocleidomastoid injury.
Throat	The palate should be highly arched, mucous membranes moist, and uvula midline (if bifid, this can indicate submucosal cleft). The infant should exhibit the sucking, rooting, gag, and extrusion reflexes.

Assessment of the Nose

If the nurse is unable to pass a suctioning tube through the nares, the infant may have **choanal atresia,** a rare condition that occurs in approximately 1 in 10,000 live births. It occurs in females twice as often as males. The choana are the two openings in the posterior nares that connect the nasal passages with the nasopharynx. Newborns are obligate nasal breathers. Successful nose breathing requires air to pass through the choana, so if these openings fail to form during fetal development, the infant must become a **mouth breather**. If atresia occurs only on one side (unilaterally), the infant may have no symptoms. The infant with **bilateral choanal atresia** has periods of respiratory distress and cyanosis that are alleviated by crying. Bilateral choanal atresia often becomes a medical emergency requiring intubation.

Assessment of Mouth

Neonatal Assessment of Mouth (*Press gloved finger against tongue to open mouth.*):

Lips	Should be pink, normal-shaped, and symmetric. Thin upper lip with smooth philtrum and short palpebral fissures may indicate fetal alcohol syndrome.
Sucking	Sucking (symmetrical) should occur if lips are touched. Asymmetric movement of the mouth may indicate injury to facial nerve.
Gums	Examined for precocious teeth and Epstein's pearls (keratin-containing cysts).
Tongue	Examined for ridge of frenulum tissue on underside (tongue-tied), although this is not clipped, and evidence of protrusion or hypertrophy, which can indicate various disorders, such as Down syndrome and hypothyroidism. Bluish swelling of the frenulum may indicate mucus/salivary gland retention cyst.
Mucus membranes	Examined for color and moisture, as cyanosis may indicate respiratory distress and dryness or dehydration. Excessive salivation and drooling may indicate esophageal atresia. White patches on mucus membranes/tongue indicate infection with *Candida albicans.*

Assessment of Ears

Position	The insertion point of the top of the ear should be parallel to the inner and outer canthus of the eye. Low-set ears may relate to a number of disorders, such as trisomy 13 and trisomy 18, intellectual disability, and various other disorders.
Shape/size	Ears should be proportionate to head size and symmetric.
Pliability	Ear should be soft and pliable. Cartilage is lacking in premature infants, and the pinna is soft. Cartilage should be firm by 38 to 40 weeks with 2/3 of pinna curving inward.
Hearing	Hearing may be initially assessed by observing response to sudden loud sound. Evoked otoacoustic emissions (EOAE) and auditory brainstem response (ABR) are used for universal hearing screening.
Tympanic membrane	Usually not examined with otoscope because of occlusion with vernix and blood after birth, but should appear gray-white and vascular.

Screenings for Hearing Loss

Otoacoustic emissions (OAE) are sounds generated by the cochlea. They are a measure of the integrity of the middle and inner ear, or more specifically, the outer hair cells of the cochlea. The audiologist measures OAE by inserting a probe into the infant's external auditory canal and stimulating the cochlea with several clicking noises. The audiologist uses a microphone to measure the OAE sent off by the cochlea.

Auditory brainstem response (ABR) examination measures the brain's reaction to sound (middle and inner ear and nerve pathway). The audiologist places electrodes on the infant's scalp, positions a device that makes sounds outside the ear, and measures the brain's response to the sound. Measured waveforms are compared to the normal, expected pattern. Both of these hearing examinations are scored as pass or fail. If the infant fails an audiology screening examination, further testing should be conducted by an **otorhinolaryngologist** (ENT doctor) to confirm if a problem truly exists, and if so, the nature of the hearing loss.

Review Video: Hearing Loss
Visit mometrix.com/academy and enter code: 539029

Cataracts

Cataracts, partial or complete opacity of the lens of one or both eyes preventing refraction of light onto the retina, can be either congenital or acquired and is associated with prenatal infections, such as rubella and CMV), hypocalcemia, or drug exposure. It can be related to trauma, systemic corticosteroids, genetic defects (albinism, Down syndrome) and prematurity. Clouding of the lens is not always obvious to the naked eye, so careful visual evaluations should be done for those children at risk.

Treatment depends upon the extent of the cataracts and whether they are unilateral or bilateral. Early diagnosis is important because surgical repair ≤2 months is the most successful with visual acuity in 55% at 20/40. The opaque lens is removed and the child uses corrective lenses or a lens is implanted. Antibiotic or steroid drops may be used after surgery.

Retinopathy of Prematurity

Retinopathy of prematurity (ROP), an abnormal vascular proliferative disease of the immature retina, is associated with infants born ≤31 week and <1500 g (50-70% of infants whose birth weight is <1,250 grams), especially those receiving oxygen therapy, and is a preventable cause of blindness in neonates. Retinal vascularization begins at around 16 weeks' gestation and is not complete until the infant is full term. Premature birth interrupts this normal progression. Exposure of these infants to hyperoxia causes reduction in their production of retinal vascular endothelial growth factor and vasoconstriction. Initially, oxygen can be supplied to the retina from the underlying choroid capillary bed. Over time, the retina becomes thicker and outgrows this blood supply. Hypoxia of the retina triggers neovascularity (disorganized growth of new blood vessels) and is accompanied by scar tissue. Contracting scars can cause retinal detachment. ROP may regress or progress and require treatment, such as cryotherapy, photocoagulation, or scleral buckling. Untreated ROP causes acuity defects, refractive errors, strabismus, glaucoma, retinal detachment, or blindness.

STRABISMUS

Strabismus occurs when the muscles of the eyes are not coordinated so that one eye deviates from the axis of the other. Strabismus may be congenital or acquired or associated with other disorders, such as albinism. *Deviations* include:

- **Phoria** is intermittent deviation but the child can focus eyes and maintain alignment for periods when looking at an object.
- **Tropia** is consistent or intermittent deviation in which the child is unable to maintain alignment of the eyes.
- Both phorias and tropias may be *hyper* (up), *hypo* (down), *exo* (out), *eso* (in toward nose), or *cyclo* (rotational).
- **Esotropia** is both eyes turning inwards (cross eyes) and *exotropia* is both eyes turning outward (wall eyes).

Treatment <24 months reduces *amblyopia* (reduced vision):

- Occlusion therapy: Patching or eye drops to blur vision in one eye.
- Surgical repair of rectus muscle.

NYSTAGMUS AND BLEPHAROPTOSIS

Nystagmus is **involuntary rhythmic movements** of one or both eyes, with horizontal, vertical, or circular movements, sometimes accompanied by rhythmic movements of the head. Nystagmus is common in neonates and should resolve in a few weeks, but may indicate pathology if it persists. It is often associated with albinism, CNS abnormalities, or diseases of the ear or retina, and sudden onset is cause for concern. There is no specific treatment other than to identify and treat underlying causes.

Blepharoptosis is drooping of one or both upper **eyelids** and may be congenital (autosomal dominant), with defective development of the levator muscles or cranial nerve III, or acquired as the result of trauma or infection. If vision is affected, surgical repair is done early to avoid amblyopia. If vision is unaffected, surgical repair is deferred until the child is 3 or older.

Conjunctivitis

Conjunctivitis is inflammation of the conjunctiva of the eye from bacteria, viruses, or chemical irritants. If infectious conjunctivitis occurs <30 days of birth, it is referred to as **ophthalmia neonatorum** and is commonly acquired during delivery:

- Pathogenic agents include *Chlamydia trachomatis, Neisseria gonorrhea,* and herpesvirus. It can also be caused by chemical irritants, such as silver nitrate (the reason it is no longer routinely used for eye prophylaxis).
- Antibiotic drops or ointment (typically erythromycin ointment) is applied to the newborns eyes to prevent conjunctivitis. Intravenous acyclovir is given to infants exposed to herpesvirus.

Untreated, gonococcal conjunctivitis usually develops in ≤5 days of birth and is characterized by purulent discharge and inflammation. It is treated with IV antibiotics (benzylpenicillin or cefotaxime). Chlamydial conjunctivitis develops at 3-14 days and is characterized by watery discharge and less inflammation that gonococcal conjunctivitis. It is treated with IV erythromycin and topical tetracycline.

Nasolacrimal Obstruction

The nasolacrimal duct system is usually mature by the eighth month of gestation, but in some cases, abnormalities such as fistula of the lacrimal sac, atresia, or lack of valves can cause malfunction or **nasolacrimal obstruction.** Nasolacrimal obstruction occurs in only 2 to 4% of newborns, but incidence is much higher in those with trisomy 21 (Down syndrome) at 22 to 36%. Nasolacrimal obstruction is often associated with eye anomalies (20%) or systemic anomalies (25%). *Diagnostic* tests include a dye disappearance test (most effective) and fluorescein drops in each eye (should clear in 5 minutes). Most cases (90%) of congenital obstruction resolve within a year without treatment, although some physicians recommend digital massage. If infection occurs, topical antibiotics are indicated. If obstruction persists, surgical repair (probing, intubation, dilatation) may be indicated.

Microtia

Microtia means tiny ears. Microtia is a congenital deformity of the outer ear that ranges from a slightly small pinna to complete absence of the external ear and the external auditory canal. Microtia can involve one or both ears, and is usually not seen on prenatal ultrasound, but is discovered at birth. Microtia has four grades:

- **Grade I**: The ear is smaller, but still has identifiable structures (pinna, helix, and antihelix). The external ear canal is present, but is often narrowed.
- **Grade II:** The pinna is smaller and less developed than in Grade I. The external auditory canal is closed off.
- **Grade III**: The external ear is essentially absent, except for a small remnant of tissue. This is the most common type of microtia.
- **Grade IV**: Total absence of the external ear and external auditory canal, also called anotia.

Infants with microtia usually have conductive hearing loss in the affected ear. Reconstruction of the affected ear is generally begun when the child is 4 to 6 years old, and will require a hearing aid if conductive hearing loss is present.

Types of Hearing Loss

The neonate may have a number of different **types of hearing loss**:

- **Sensorineural** hearing loss may be mild or severe and occurs when the cochlea (sound receptor in the inner ear) is impaired by a genetic syndrome; *in utero* infections like rubella; postnatal meningitis; or ototoxic medication, such as aminoglycoside antibiotics or the diuretic furosemide, which damage the cochlea.
- **Conductive** hearing loss occurs from an abnormality in the sound conduction system in the outer and middle ears (external ear canal, tympanic membrane, and auditory ossicles). Congenital cholesteatoma is an example of conductive hearing loss.
- **Mixed** hearing loss occurs when an infant has a component of both sensorineural and conductive hearing loss.
- **Central** hearing loss is rare and occurs when defects or damage of the auditory nervous pathway or auditory brain centers are present in infants with kernicterus, episodes of hypoxia, or intraventricular hemorrhage.

Orofacial Clefts

Cleft lip (CL), **cleft lip with cleft palate** (CLP), and **cleft palate** (CP) are orofacial clefts, which can be a part of a more complex syndrome or isolated anomalies:

- **CL** occurs when the medial nasal and maxillary processes fail to merge during the fifth week of embryological development. The cleft is generally at the junction of the central and lateral parts of the upper lip and may be on the left or right side. If the cleft extends into the maxilla, it may be accompanied by a cleft palate and be deemed a CLP. Surgical repair is usually at 10 weeks.
- **CP** occurs when the palatal shelves of the maxillary bone fail to fuse. Fusion usually begins at the eighth week and continues until the twelfth week of embryological development. A spectrum of CP exists. Bifid uvula is the mildest form. Clefting of the soft palate is more severe. A complete CP (most severe form) involves clefting of the uvula, soft palate, and hard palate. Surgical repair usually begins at about 4 months.

Feeding Infants with Cleft Lip or Cleft Palate

Infants with severe **cleft lip and palate** may require enteral feedings, but many can be fed with a bottle or breast. An infant with an isolated cleft palate has difficulty creating negative pressure within the oral cavity, so breastfeeding is more of a challenge than bottle-feeding, but the infant can still breastfeed. To overcome the pressure problems, the infant must learn to squeeze the milk out of the nipple by compressing it between the remaining palate and the tongue. The mother should be taught to seal the cleft with her breast by positioning the infant with the cleft uppermost. The mother may also use her finger to seal the cleft while breastfeeding. For infants with a bilateral cleft, breastfeeding is usually impossible. The mother can express her milk into a bottle, so the infant still benefits from her antibodies. The goals are to have appropriate weight gain in the infant, minimize aspiration, and reduce the incidence of ear infections.

Laboratory Tests for Thyroid Hormones

The **thyroid gland** produces hormones critical for metabolism and growth. They are amino acids that contain iodine and are stored in the thyroid until needed by the body. The thyroid gland takes iodide from the blood and utilizes it to produce hormones. Thyroid hormone production is controlled by the thyroid stimulating hormone (TSH) produced by the pituitary gland and the thyrotropin-releasing hormone (TRH) produced by the hypothalamus. Together, the thyroid hormones increase metabolic rate and protein and bone turnover. They are necessary for the growth and development of the fetus and infant. Thyroid hormones include:

- **Thyroxine** (T_4) is a weak hormone that maintains the body metabolism in a steady state.
  - Neonate: 10-36 pmol/L.
- **Triiodothyronine** (T_3) is about 5 times stronger than thyroxine and can respond quickly to metabolic needs.
  - All ages: 4.0-7.4 pmol/L.
- **Thyrocalcitonin** is secreted in response to serum calcium levels and reduces the serum level of calcium and phosphate by increasing deposits in bones, aiding ossification and bone development.
  - Male: <19 ng/L.
  - Female: <14 ng/L.

Neonatal Genitourinary Assessment

Urinary Output

Genitourinary assessment requires evaluation of **urinary output**. The neonate's bladder volume is 6 to 44 mL, and many neonates void immediately after birth, although the small amount of urine may be overlooked. About 92% void within 24 hours and 99% by 48 hours. Neonates with **edema** may have higher urinary output as edema recedes. In the first 2 days, most infants void 2 to 6 times daily, with an output averaging about 15 mL/kg/day. After this, the infant should urinate 5 to 25 times per day, with volume increasing to 25 mL/kg/day. Urine may appear cloudy because of mucus, and initial voidings have high **specific gravity**, but specific gravity returns to normal levels when the child feeds. Pink stains, referred to as "brick dust spots" often show on the diapers, but these **urate deposits** are of no concern. Female infants may exhibit **pseudomenstruation**—slight bleeding—as maternal hormones are withdrawn.

External Genitalia

Female	The clitoris varies in size. By term, the labia major should cover the labia minor and clitoris. The clitoris and labia may be quite edematous, somewhat altering their appearance. The urethral opening should be behind the clitoris. A hymenal tag should be evident at the posterior vagina. If no tag is evident, then the infant should be examined for vaginal agenesis.
Male	The testes should be within the scrotal sac, which appears pendulous and covered with rugae. The scrotum may be edematous. The testes should be palpable and equal in size. The penis and the urethra should be in the correct position with an adherent prepuce that covers the glans and should not retract. Smegma may be present about the glans. Epithelial pearls (tiny, firm white lesions) may occur on the end of the prepuce. The penis may be erect at times.

Potter Syndrome

Potter syndrome is a congenital disorder, related to oligohydramnios or anhydramnios that results from **renal disease**, such as bilateral renal agenesis (BRA), other urinary obstruction, or amniotic sac rupture. There are 5 different **classifications** of Potter syndrome:

- **Classic**: BRA present
- **Type I**: autosomal recessive polycystic kidney disease
- **Type II**: one kidney missing and the other abnormal
- **Type III**: autosomal dominant polycystic kidney disease
- **Type IV**: hydronephrosis from obstruction (rarely causes death)

The lack of amniotic fluid causes the fetus to be compressed by the uterus, resulting in a number of **physical manifestations**:

- Potter's facies: parrot-beak nose, micrognathia, low-set ears, flattened nose, wide-set eyes, and skin fold from edge of eye across cheek
- Clubfeet, tibial bowing, or fused legs (sirenomelia)
- Genitourinary and gynecological abnormalities (small bladder, absence or abnormality of reproductive organs)
- Pulmonary abnormalities (underdeveloped alveoli)
- Diaphragmatic hernia

Treatment is supportive and symptomatic, but survival is extremely rare for most types.

VATER/VACTERL Syndrome

VATER syndrome, also known as **VACTERL** association, is an acronym for several different birth defects that often occur together. The letters in the acronym stand for:

- **V** – Vertebral defects (70%): Usually consist of smaller than normal vertebrae that may predispose the infant to develop scoliosis.
- **A** – Anal atresia or imperforate anus (55%): Often requires surgical correction at birth.
- **C** – Cardiovascular defects (75%): Common heart defects include ventral septal defect, atrial septal defect, and tetralogy of Fallot.
- **T** – Tracheoesophageal fistula (70%).
- **E** – Esophageal atresia (70%).
- **R** – Renal anomalies (in VATER it stands for Radial) (50%): Anomalies can be severe, including incomplete formation of the kidneys or obstruction of urine outflow.
- **L** – Limb anomalies (70%): Defects include absent or displaced thumbs, extra digits, fusion of digits, and forearm defects.

For VACTERL diagnosis, the infant must have 3 of 7 malformations. An infant with any one of these birth defects must also be evaluated for other defects in the association.

PKD

Polycystic kidney disease (PKD) is caused by renal cysts that develop from nephrons and can cause gross enlargement of kidneys. Cysts may be single or multiple (polycystic) and may involve one or both kidneys. There are 2 types of congenital PK.

- **Autosomal dominant** is the most common (90%), but symptoms are usually delayed until adulthood, although they can occur in infancy. Cysts may develop in any part of the nephron. It may progress to ESRD over time. Cysts may also form in the liver and pancreas. It is associated with cerebral artery aneurysms.
- **Autosomal recessive** is more rare and symptoms arise much earlier, sometimes in the fetus. It is always bilateral with enlarged kidneys.

Both types of PK often manifest with abdominal mass (sometimes bilateral flank), oliguria, ARF, Potter's facies (related to oligohydramnios), hypoplastic lungs, respiratory distress, and hypertension. These *treatments* cannot cure but can mitigate effects:

- Antihypertensives
- Antibiotics for infections
- Analgesia
- Growth hormone (autosomal recessive)
- Dialysis and transplantation (long term)

Posterior Urethral Valves

Posterior urethral valves are a urethral abnormality in males only in which urethral valves have narrow slit-like openings that impede urinary flow and allow reverse flow, damaging urinary organs, which swell and become engorged with urine. Thirty percent will develop long-term **kidney failure**. *Diagnosis* is by fetal ultrasound, voiding cystourethrogram (VCUG) to evaluate extent of valvular abnormality and other urinary defects, endoscopy to examine inside of urinary tract and take tissue samples, blood tests to assess kidney function and electrolytes.

Symptoms

Symptoms vary, depending upon severity, but may include:

- Small chest size with poor lung development and respiratory distress secondary to oligohydramnios (usually the most pressing clinical problem).
- Potter facies secondary to oligohydramnios.
- Limb deformities.
- Abdominal mass secondary to enlarged kidneys, bladder, or ascites.
- Sepsis, metabolic acidosis, and azotemia (increased blood levels of urea and other nitrogenous compounds)

Treatment

- **Medical management**:
  - Supportive care
  - Antibiotics
  - Electrolytes
  - Foley catheter
- **Surgical management**: Urinary diversion (usually closed after valve repair) and endoscopic ablation/resection to examine obstruction and remove valve leaflets.

Persistent Cloaca

Persistent cloaca is a condition in females with an **imperforate anus** and the rectum, vagina, and urethra forming a **single channel**, with a rectal fistula attached to the posterior wall of the channel. *Diagnosis* is made with a physical exam showing a single perineal opening. An abdominal mass (hydrocolpos— distended bladder) may occur. A voiding cystourethrogram (VCUG) will show bladder abnormalities if catheterization is possible.

Treatments include:

- **Colostomy**: Fecal diversion in neonate prevents fecal material from entering urinary system and causing infection.
- **Decompression of vagina**: Decompression prevents infection and scarring and relieves obstruction of urinary tract.
- **Posterior sagittal anorectovagino-urethroplasty (PSARVUP)**: This is usually done 2 months after colostomy. Rectum is separated from vagina, vagina is separated from urethra, urethra is reconstructed, vagina is reconstructed, and rectum is reconstructed with anoplasty.
- **Postoperative anal dilation**: Dilation begins 2 weeks after surgery until final size is reached.
- **Cystoscopy/ vaginoscopy**: Check for urethrovaginal fistula.
- **Colostomy removal**: Anastomosis of colon and rectum and colostomy removed.

Ambiguous Genitalia

If a neonate has **ambiguous genitalia,** then a complete examination should be performed with ultrasound to determine the gender of the child. In some cases, the child may be intersexed, but surgical sexual assignment/reassignment is now usually delayed until the child expresses a gender preference. Parents often need reassurance and support. Conditions related to ambiguous genitalia include:

- **Microphallus:** <2.5cm, often associated with hypospadias.
- **Clitoromegaly**: Rectal exam may help to palpate uterus, which is swollen at birth because of maternal hormones. This may be related to neurofibromatosis.
- **Congenital adrenal hyperplasia**: The fetus was exposed to masculinizing hormones during development. Females often exhibit enlarged clitoris or male-appearing genitalia partial or complete fusion of the labia, giving the appearance of a scrotum (but without testes).
- **Androgen insensitivity syndrome:** Genetically male neonates cannot respond to androgens and are born with external genitalia that range from typically male to typically female, depending upon the severity of the condition.
- **Ovotestes:** Both male and female genitalia and gonads are present.

Testicular Torsion

Testicular torsion is an emergent condition in which the testis rotates, twisting the spermatic cord and impairing circulation with resultant vascular engorgement and testicular ischemia. Testicular torsion is most common in boys 3-20, but it can occur in the neonatal period (70% prenatally). It is commonly associated with the congenital abnormality bell clapper deformity (the testes are situated transversely). In neonates, the testis may be undescended, predisposing it to torsion as it moves. The testis may not adhere adequately to the scrotal wall, so torsion often occurs at 7 to 10 days. Pain is usually acute and the neonate cries frantically. The scrotal area begins to swell. The cremasteric reflex (stroking the inner thigh causes retraction of the scrotum/testes) is lost with torsion. Diagnosis is made by testicular scan or sonogram. The torsion must be relieved within 6 hours to prevent further damage so the physician must be notified immediately. Manual reduction (sometimes effective) or surgical repair is done, with the testis then sutured into the correct position to the lateral scrotum to prevent recurrence.

EPISPADIAS

Epispadias is the urethral orifice in an abnormal position with a widened pubic bone. Epispadias often occurs with bladder exstrophy.

- In **boys,** the urethra may open on the top (dorsum), the sides, or the complete length of the penis. Boys may have a short, wide penis with abnormal chordee (curvature). It is 3 to5 times more common in males than females.
- In **girls,** the urethra, with a urethral cleft along its length, usually bifurcates the clitoris and labia, but may be in the abdomen.

Diagnosis is usually made on fetal ultrasound or at birth on examination. Surgical repair, usually during the first year, may include lengthening of the urethra in males, as well as bladder neck reconstruction. Multiple surgical procedures may be required to complete reconstruction for both males and females. Circumcision is delayed in males, as the foreskin may be used during the repair. Urinary diversion may be necessary if incontinence cannot be corrected

HYPOSPADIAS

Hypospadias occurs in one in 250 to 300 live male births. It is a congenital defect where the urethra opens onto the **anterior surface of the penis**, and not in its usual place at the tip. The urethral opening can be anywhere from the base of the penis to close to the tip on the ventral surface of the penis. Normal urine flow usually exits through this abnormally placed meatus. Hypospadias is classified into three different categories:

- **First degree,** in which the opening is on the glans
- **Second degree,** in which the opening is on the ventral surface of the shaft of the penis
- **Third degree,** in which the opening is on the perineum

No immediate management is required as long as the infant is able to void adequately. Surgical repair is usually performed later. Circumcision is delayed until the surgical repair of the hypospadias is performed, because the foreskin may be used during the repair.

UPJ OBSTRUCTIONS

Ureteropelvic junction (UPJ) obstruction is often discovered during prenatal ultrasounds, and is the most common cause of pediatric hydronephrosis (dilation of the renal pelvis). The most common cause of UPJ in the neonate is the lack of proper canalization of the renal pelvis during embryologic development. The obstruction can be mild or severe and may be asymptomatic in the newborn period. An abdominal mass may be the only sign of a UPJ obstruction with hydronephrosis in the newborn. Evaluate the UPJ obstruction early with renal ultrasound, voiding cystourethrogram, and a renal scan determine the degree of obstruction and the need for surgical correction. Another congenital anomaly occurs with UPJ obstruction in approximately 50% of cases and both kidneys should be evaluated. If the obstruction is severe enough, surgical correction via renal pyeloplasty is performed to prevent renal damage.

Inguinal Hernia and Hydrocele in Male Newborn

A mass in the male infant's scrotum may be an **inguinal hernia** or **hydrocele**. During fetal development, the testes migrate from the abdominal cavity into the scrotum through the inguinal canal. The processus vaginalis is a membrane surrounding the testes as they migrate, which normally seals shut and forms a thin band of tissue. When it does not seal properly, it leaves an opening between the abdominal cavity and the scrotum.

- An **inguinal hernia** is an extension of bowel through the inguinal canal, and possibly into the scrotum, that can be reduced (contents returned to the abdominal cavity) with gentle pressure.
- A **hydrocele** occurs when fluid enters the scrotum with the migrating testes. A soft, painless mass will be present that will not reduce (its size remains constant). **Unlike a hernia, a hydrocele will transilluminate**. A communicating hydrocele occurs when a small opening only allows fluid to enter the scrotal sac. This type of hydrocele will fluctuate in size throughout the day and is reducible.

Bladder Exstrophy

Bladder exstrophy is eversion of the posterior wall of the bladder through the anterior wall and through the lower abdominal wall with bladder and urethra exposed, a wide pubic arch, anterior displacement of the anus, renal disorders, and abnormalities of reproductive organs in both males and females. *Symptoms* include urinary and bowel problems related to specific anomalies. *Diagnosis* is by physical examination to assess abnormalities. Renal ultrasound is done to determine the number of kidneys and presence of hydroureteronephrosis. *Treatment* is in three stages.

- **First stage:**
  - Primary closure of bladder including ureteral stents and suprapubic urinary drainage; no ostomy necessary when done within 72 hours of birth.
  - Bilateral iliac ostomies after 72 hours because pelvic ring is not malleable.
  - Epispadias repair—may be done in first or second stage.
- **Second stage:**
  - Epispadias repair, usually between 6 and 12 months.
- **Final stage:**
  - Bladder neck reconstruction and reimplantation of ureters
  - Permanent urinary diversion: Required in 10 to 15% of cases

Vesicoureteral Reflux

Vesicoureteral reflux (VUR) is a condition in which urine from the bladder **backflows** into the ureters or kidneys. Normally, a valve exists at the junction of the ureters and the bladder, but in infants with VUR, this valve is defective. Prenatally, VUR may be diagnosed by an ultrasound showing dilated ureters or renal pelvis. Postnatally, an infant with VUR may have an abdominal mass, a urinary tract infection, or pyelonephritis. Nonspecific symptoms, such as respiratory distress, vomiting, failure to thrive, and renal failure may indicate pyelonephritis. VUR is more common in Caucasian children, and runs in families. It is more common if siblings have had VUR or if the parent has a history of VUR. Any infant with a history of a urinary tract infection or pyelonephritis should be evaluated for vesicoureteral reflux with a VCUG.

Newborn Care and Family Education

Safe Positioning for Infants

Infants should be placed on their **backs** for sleeping. Sleeping on the stomach increases risk of **sudden infant death syndrome (SIDS)**.

- Position the infant on the back when unattended or sleeping, but alternate the direction the head faces to prevent one side of the head from flattening (**positional molding**).
- Provide supervised time each day with the infant lying on the abdomen (only on firm surfaces) to strengthen head and neck muscles and to prevent positional molding.
- Hold the infant, rather than leaving in a carrier.
- Position baby in side-lying position, alternating from one side to the other, using specially designed supports to maintain the position.

Infant Car Seat

All infants, regardless of age, must be placed properly in an **infant car seat** during transit. Holding an infant while the car is in motion is not safe. Car seats should be new or in very good condition and fastened according to manufacturer's guidelines to ensure safety.

- Place the car seat in the back seat, and from any side airbags.
- Always securely buckle the child into the seat.
- Face the infant seat toward the rear of the car.
- Recline the seat so the infant's head does not fall forward.
- Place padding around (not under) the infant if the infant slouches to one side.
- Place blankets over the straps and buckles, not under.

Newborn Care for Special-Needs Neonate

Family involvement and education are vital for successful discharge of the **special-needs neonate** to ensure proper care. Bringing home a premature infant or one who has special needs is a daunting task for any parent, so preparation is essential.

- Educate the parents or guardian about appropriate care methods.
- Explain how to interpret the infant's cues concerning his needs and how to respond appropriately.
- Point out the different states of alertness during their infant's sleep and wake cycles. Identify the appropriate times and methods for infant interaction.
- Coach the parents to ensure that they perform each skill correctly and retain it. Observe interaction between the infant and parents in the nursery to help ensure continued wellness of the infant after discharge.
- Encourage kangaroo care immediately after birth for stable newborns, because it is an excellent method to foster bonding between the neonate and the mother. For neonates who require resuscitation and medical intervention, delay kangaroo care until the neonate is stable.
- If the parents are not ready, contact a social worker for follow-up.

Umbilical Cord Care

Education surrounding the **umbilical cord** should include the following information:

- Protect the cord from moisture, with top of diaper folded under the cord instead of covering it.
- If the cord becomes soiled, wash with mild soap and water, rinse, and dry. Swabbing with alcohol is still sometimes advised by physicians, but is no longer recommended and may increase skin irritation.
- Avoid covering the cord stump with clothing, which may cause irritation.
- Give the infant only sponge baths until the cord falls off in about 10 to 14 days.
- Report signs of infection, such as erythema, swelling, or purulent discharge.

Note: The umbilical cord changes color from grayish-brown to black as it dries and finally falls off in about 10 to 14 days.

Fecal Elimination

The first stool (**meconium**) is usually passed within 48 hours and is black and tarry looking. The stool then transitions to greenish as the baby nurses or takes formula, and by the third day, the stool is usually yellow or yellow-green for breastfed babies and yellow or light brown for formula-fed babies. Typically, babies have 2 to 3 stools daily by day 3 and ≥4 daily by day 5, but this may vary.

- Report abnormalities, such as bloody stools, watery stools, very hard stools, clay-colored or whitish stools, black stools (after meconium has passed), and "currant jelly" stools.
- Cleanse skin thoroughly after defecation with mild soap and water, plain water, or unscented baby wipes.
- Examine skin carefully for irritation.

Urinary Elimination

Urination is estimated according to the number of **wet diapers** in a 24-hour period. Typically, the infant has 1 wet diaper the first day, 2 the next, and so on until urination stabilizes at 6 to 8 wet diapers by about day 6.

- Check diaper frequently. Infants often urinate during or after feeding.
- Change diapers when wet, gently cleansing skin with mild soap and water, plain water, or unscented baby wipes.

Cradle Cap

Cradle cap may appear as scaly, crusted, or flaky skin on the scalp and other parts of the face. It is not contagious and usually clears by 1 or 2 months. It is not usually a sign of poor hygiene.

- Cleanse scalp or affected areas thoroughly, gently rubbing the area with a terry cloth or brushing to loosen crust or flakes.
- If persistent, try softening the crusts with olive oil, leave for 15 minutes, and then brush or gently comb to loosen crusts or flakes. Finally, wash with baby shampoo.

Diaper Rash

Diaper rash usually results from leaving the infant in soiled/wet diapers and/or not adequately cleansing the skin, although breastfed infants sometimes react to foods the mother has eaten. A rash may also indicate an allergic response to baby wipes or other products, such as lotions or creams. Antibiotics may cause diaper rash. In some cases, a **fungal infection** may occur, usually characterized by red weepy open areas. Purulent discharge may indicate infection.

- Change diapers as soon as possible when wet or soiled.
- Cleanse skin gently with water.
- Remove diaper and expose skin to air whenever possible.
- Apply barrier cream or ointment especially formulated for diaper rash to prevent or treat diaper rash.
- Contact physician if rash worsens and does not respond to treatment, as antifungals, cortisone, or topical antibiotics may be indicated.

BREASTFEEDING

Neonates should be fed on demand. Most newborns nurse every 2 to 3 hours or bottle-feed every 2 to 4 hours (8 to 12 times daily) for 20 to 40 minutes. Over time, the infant will establish a more regular feeding schedule, but this may vary widely.

- Try to recognize clues that the infant is hungry and nurse/feed before the infant begins crying frantically. Signs of hunger include licking, rooting, sucking, making fists, bringing hands to mouth, and bobbing the head.
- Stroke the infant's cheek or lower lip, and a hungry infant will usually turn and try to suck the finger.
- Monitor number of diapers and stools per day, as decrease to less than the average normal number may indicate dehydration and inadequate nursing/feeding.
- Observe the infant's behavior closely, as some infants nurse for a while and then nap at the breast or take a break before resuming nursing/feeding. A full baby often turns away from the breast/bottle, stops sucking, or resists feeding.

CHOKING OR GAGGING IN INFANT

Education regarding chocking/gagging should include the following:

- Ensure small hazardous items, such as pins and cotton balls or materials, such as baby powder are out of reach.
- DO NOT prop bottle for feeding.
- Burp infant regularly during feedings, whether breast or bottle.
- Keep baby in upright position with head elevated during feedings.
- Check nipple of bottle to ensure it is dripping and not running freely.
- If infant is choking, secure face down on forearm, tilted downward, and use the heel of the hand to thump in the mid-back. Repeat as necessary. If choking does not resolve with evidence of breathing immediately, call 911 and begin CPR.

Note: Prevention is important, as most **choking and gagging episodes** can be avoided.

Burping the Infant

Both breastfed and bottle-fed babies require **burping** because they swallow air when feeding, although bottle-fed babies tend to require more burping. Infants often show indications (grimacing, squirming, spitting up, and crying) that they are uncomfortable and need to burp.

- Burp the infant routinely after 2 or 3 ounces of formula or after nursing on one breast.
- Position the infant on the shoulder with a burp cloth under the infant's head and gently pat or rub the infant's back.
- Change to a different position if the baby doesn't burp. Try on the opposite shoulder or with the infant sitting on the lap supported by one hand while the other hand pats or rubs the infant's back.

Circumcision

Circumcision rates have dropped by 10% over the last 30 years, with about 58% of male infants now being **circumcised** in the United States. The American Academy of Pediatrics has confirmed that the benefits outweigh the risks, though they do not have a formal recommendation for circumcision and instead leave that decision up to the parents. Benefits including decreased risk of prostate cancer, urinary tract infections, and sexually transmitted diseases such as HIV. Most parents make their decision based on cultural or religious beliefs or the factor of cost, as some insurance companies and many Medicaid programs are not covering the cost of circumcision. While at one time infants were not thought to experience pain, it is now clear that they do, so circumcision should be done using a local anesthesia or topical EMLA cream. After circumcision, the end of the foreskin is typically swollen and red, and some small amount of bleeding may persist for 24 hours. Change the diaper immediately, because urine may cause pain to the open tissue. Cleanse the area gently with water and pat dry. Apply petroleum jelly gauze to the incision area as directed by individual physician. Avoid using soap or commercial cleansing products, such as baby wipes, until the circumcision heals. Report any change, such as increased swelling, redness, temperature, or purulent discharge.

Uncircumcised Penis

The infant's foreskin is different from the adult male's and does not **separate and retract** until the child is ≥5 years old.

- DO NOT attempt to retract the foreskin.
- DO NOT use cotton swabs to clean.
- Wash the penis with soap and water or just water during the routine bath.

Fontanels

The infant's fontanels (anterior and posterior) are covered by thick membranous tissue and should feel flat but firm.

- DO NOT be afraid to touch the fontanels or cleanse the scalp.
- Report **bulging** above the level of the skull, as this may indicate increased intracranial pressure.
- Report a **soft fontanel** that sinks below the level of the skull, as this may indicate dehydration.

Non-Nutritive Sucking

Nonnutritive sucking occurs when an infant sucks on an item such as a pacifier, or his/her own fist. Nonnutritive sucking is not associated with nutritional intake, but it is an important method of self-quieting and begins in the uterus at about 29 weeks of gestation. Extremely premature infants often lack basic neurodevelopmental capabilities, and cannot coordinate sucking, swallowing, and breathing simultaneously. Typically, the ability to suck and swallow in a coordinated fashion is not present until 32 to 34 weeks of gestation. Premature infants should be encouraged to perform non-nutritive sucking during the gavage feeding process if they can accomplish it. Benefits of nonnutritive sucking include:

- Improved digestion of enteral feeds because digestive enzyme release is stimulated.
- Facilitated development of coordinated nutritive sucking behavior.
- Calming of the distressed infant.

Bathing the Infant

The infant should receive **sponge baths** until the cord falls off at 10 to14 days, and then a bath in an **infant tub** (NOT in an adult tub). Mild soap/shampoo intended for babies or water alone may be used for the bath.

- Make sure the environmental temperature is warm.
- Fill tub with 2 to 3 inches of water.
- ALWAYS check water temperature to make sure it is warm and *not hot*.
- Set hot water heaters ≤120 °F to prevent inadvertent scalding.
- Support the baby during the bath with one arm under upper back to support the neck and head while holding the infant under the axillae.
- Pour water over the child with the free hand and use that hand to wash the hair and the body.
- Lift the baby from the tub and wrap in a towel to dry.
- Dry thoroughly, making sure all skin folds and crevices are dry to prevent irritation and rashes.
- Avoid use of lotions or creams.

Vitamin K

Vitamin K is essential for the synthesis of prothrombin, so it is necessary for **blood clotting**. Vitamin K is synthesized in the intestinal tract by *Escherichia coli,* but these bacteria are absent in the newborn, so newborns are routinely given an injection of vitamin K_1 (AquaMEPHYTON®), 0.5 to 1.0 parenterally or subcutaneously within an hour of birth to prevent hemorrhage. Vitamin K_1 promotes formation of clotting factors II, VII, IX and X. The preferred site for injection is the middle third of the vastus lateralis muscles of the thigh. The usual procedure is to cleanse the skin of the upper thigh with alcohol, allow to dry, and inject the solution with a 25-gauge, 5/8-inch needle held at a 90-degree angle to the skin. After aspiration, the solution is injected slowly; the tissue is massaged gently with the alcohol swab after the needle is withdrawn. Vitamin K_1 should be given prior to **circumcision**. Bleeding may occur on the second or third day after administration, resulting in bruising, bleeding (umbilical cord, nose, GI, circumcision). Vitamin K_1 may also increase **hyperbilirubinemia**.

Sucrose Analgesia

Sucrose analgesia (Sweet-Ease™) is used to relieve stress and discomfort in infants before and during medical procedures, such as heel sticks, IV insertion, injections, suctioning, and insertion of NG tubes. Sweet-Ease™, a commercially prepared product, is 24% sucrose in an oral solution into which a standard pacifier is dipped and given to the infant, usually 2 minutes before a procedure. The pacifier may be re-dipped every 2 minutes for a total of 4 times. If the infant cannot suck, 0.1 mL of solution is placed on the anterior tongue with a medical syringe with the same frequency. For more painful procedures, such as lumbar puncture and circumcision, sucrose analgesia may be used in conjunction with other forms of analgesia to provide comfort. Contraindications include: <32 weeks gestation, hyperglycemia, history of asphyxia or intolerance to feedings, critical illness, paralysis, opioid sedation, and infants NPO for surgery unless cleared by anesthesiologist.

Hepatitis B Vaccine

Hepatitis B is transmitted through blood and body fluids, including during birth; therefore, it is now recommended for all newborns as well as all those <18 and those in high risk groups >18 (drug users, men having sex with men, those with multiple sex partners, partners of those with HBV, and healthcare workers). Hepatitis B can cause serious liver disease leading to liver cancer. Three injections of monovalent HepB are required to confer immunity:

- Birth (within 12 hours).
- Between 1-2 months.
- ≥24 weeks.

Note: If combination vaccines are given after the birth dose then a dose at 4 months can be given.

If the mother is Hepatitis B positive, the child should be given both the monovalent HepB vaccination as well as HepB immune globulin within 12 hours of birth. Adverse reactions include local irritation and fever. Severe allergic reactions can occur to those allergic to baker's yeast.

Eye Prophylaxis

Most states mandate **eye prophylaxis** for the newborn although a number of studies suggest that parents can safely choose to refuse this prophylaxis if the mother has had prenatal care and screening for STDs. However, most pediatricians still support prophylaxis. Medications used for prophylaxis include erythromycin eye ointment, tetracycline eye ointment, or 1% silver nitrate drops. **Erythromycin** is usually the drug of choice because it is active against both gonococcal and chlamydial infections. Silver nitrate is rarely used now even though it is effective because it can cause eye irritation. Ointment should be applied to the inside of the lower lids (inner canthus to outer) and the eyes then closed to help to spread the ointment. Excess ointment can be gently wiped from the eyes after 1 minute.

Neonatal Analgesics

Acetaminophen

Acetaminophen (Tylenol®) is used both for control of mild to moderate pain and fever. Acetaminophen can be administered orally and rectally, but absorption is less reliable with the rectal route. Acetaminophen has a half-life of 4 hours, is conjugated in the liver, and is excreted through the kidneys. **Oral dosage** is typically 24 mg/kg as a loading dose and 12 mg/kg every four hours (or 8 hours in infants <32 weeks); **rectal dosage** is 36 mg/kg (loading), followed by 24 mg/kg every 8 hours. Serum levels should be checked if treatment is to continue for >24 hours. Serum levels of 12 to 24 mg/L are required for adequate pain control. Acetaminophen is commonly used for control of pain after **circumcision**, although it is not sufficient for pain control during the procedure.

FENTANYL AND MORPHINE

Fentanyl and morphine are opioid **analgesics/narcotics** that treat moderate to severe pain.

- **Fentanyl** is for painful dressing changes or procedures. Duration of action is 1 to 2 hours and half-life is 2 to 4 hours. *Dosage* is 1 to 4 micrograms/kg every 1 to 2 hours or by continuous infusion. Rapid tolerance develops, requiring higher doses to create the same relief, and increasing the chance of overdose. Fentanyl is metabolized by the liver and excreted by the kidneys. *Side effects* of fentanyl include respiratory depression, peripheral vasodilatation, inhibition of intestinal peristalsis, and chest wall rigidity at higher doses, which compromises ventilation. Fentanyl is less likely to cause hypotension than morphine.
- **Morphine** is for post-operative pain. Duration of action is 3 to 4 hours, and half-life is 2 to 4 hours. Morphine is metabolized by the liver to an inactive metabolite and excreted by the kidneys; 2 to 12% is excreted unchanged in the urine. *Dosage* is 0.02 to 0.1 mg/kg every 1 to 4 hours or by continuous infusion. *Side effects* of morphine include respiratory depression, histamine release, and seizures.

ANTIBIOTICS

Antimicrobials include antibiotics, antifungals, and antivirals. **Antibiotics** may be classified according to their chemical nature, origin, action, or range of effectiveness. **Broad-spectrum antibiotics** are useful against both gram-positive and gram-negative bacteria. **Medium-spectrum antibiotics** are usually effective against gram-positive bacteria, although some may also be effective against gram-negative bacteria **Narrow-spectrum antibiotics** are effective against a small range of bacteria. Antibiotics kill the bacteria by interfering with their biological functions (bacteriocidal) or by preventing reproduction (bacteriostatic). The main classes of antibiotics include the following:

- **Macrolides:** Medium-spectrum antibiotics
- **Penicillins:** Medium-spectrum antibiotics, may be combined with beta-lactamase inhibitors; may cause severe allergic reactions
- **Cephalosporins:** Medium-spectrum antibiotics effective against gram-negative organisms
- **Polymyxins:** Narrow-spectrum antibiotics effective against gram-negative organisms
- **Fluoroquinolones:** Broad-spectrum antibiotics
- **Sulfonamides:** Medium-spectrum antibiotics with action against gram-positive and many gram-negative organisms, as well as Plasmodium and Toxoplasma
- **Tetracyclines:** Broad-spectrum antibiotics (can cause mottling/discoloration of later teeth)
- **Aminoglycosides:** Effective against gram-negative bacteria

GENTAMICIN

Gentamicin is an inexpensive aminoglycosides antibiotic commonly used to treat neonates with gram-negative bacterial infections, like *Staphylococci.* It works by interfering with bacterial protein synthesis, resulting in a defective bacterial cell membrane. Gentamicin is excreted unmetabolized by the kidneys and renal function is directly related to clearance. Clearance is slower in premature neonates secondary to immature kidneys. The peak level (highest concentration in the blood) of gentamicin is measured 30 minutes after infusion is completed and trough level (lowest concentration of the drug in the blood) is measured 30 minutes prior to the next dose. Potential toxicities from elevated gentamicin levels are ototoxicity (ear damage potentiated by concurrent use of furosemide) and nephrotoxicity (kidney damage), so patients with renal failure may only require dosing once every several days. If the pre-dose level falls below 0.5 mg/L and the post dose level falls below 4 mg/L, the gentamicin is sub-therapeutic and will not kill the bacterial infection.

Resuscitation and Stabilization

Providing Warmth

Infants have poor temperature regulation ability, particularly preterm infants who lack brown fat, which is one of the body's tools to regulate body temperature, so **providing warmth** is critical as a component of resuscitation. An infant who is just seconds old and wet will need aggressive measures to keep it warm while any resuscitation efforts are being initiated. Infants lose heat through their head so one of the first steps should be to place a hat on the head. The infant should be placed under a radiant heater and vigorous drying with warmed blankets should begin. Often this stimulation, drying and warming is all that is needed to establish a regular respiration pattern in the neonate. Preterm infants weighing <1500 grams should be placed in a plastic bag (made specifically for this purpose) up to the height of the shoulders to prevent cold shock. A term infant with no apparent distress can be placed on the mother's chest and covered with a warm blanket.

Minimum Neonatal Resuscitation Equipment

Temperature	Thermometer, Warmed drying towels, warmed swaddling blankets, Radiant warmer Phototherapy equipment.
Respiration	Oxygen tank and hood, flow meter, humidifier, heater, tubing, nasal prongs. Bag and mask set-up (assorted sizes). Laryngoscope with size 0 and 1 blades. Endotracheal tubes, sizes 2.5-4. Bulb syringe, suction catheters, sizes 6, 8, and 10 French, suction canister. Cardiorespiratory monitor, oxygen analyzer.
Fluids	IV needles and tubing, infusion pump, umbilical catheters (sizes 2.5 and 5 Fr). Blood pressure monitor, pulse oximeter. Isotonic saline, D10W, sodium bicarbonate. If transfusions are done here, blood drainage system, volume expander, and blood warmer.
Drugs	Epinephrine, Naloxone.
Procedures	Various sterile surgical packs, dressings, chest tubes, scalpels, hemostat. Arterial blood gas equipment and portable x-ray machine.

ABCs of Neonatal Resuscitation

The **ABCs of resuscitation** are a device to help remember in what order to do the steps of the resuscitation process. In this device, the letters stand for the following:

Airway	An airway should be established as the very first thing tended to. If there is no airway, air cannot be moved during resuscitation attempts. This step includes clearing the mouth and nose of secretions and properly positioning the infant in the "sniff" position.
Breathing	This step involves initiating breathing after the airway has been established. This can be done with stimulation, supplemental oxygen, or through artificial ventilation. Oxygen should be initiated at 21% (up to 30% in preterm neonates) and titrated as needed.
Circulation	Once an airway is open and breathing has been established, then circulation is considered. Chest compressions or the administration of volume expanders may be indicated. Epinephrine is only indicated if the heart rate remains <60 despite warming, ventilation and chest compressions.

Establishing Airway and Stimulating Respirations in Neonate

To **establish an airway**, the infant is placed supine with the head slightly extended in the "sniffing" position. A small neck roll may be placed under the shoulders to maintain this position in a very small premature infant. Once the proper position is established, the mouth and nose are suctioned (mouth first, to prevent reflex aspiration of secretions when the nose is suctioned) with a bulb syringe or catheter if necessary. The infant's head can be turned momentarily to the side to allow secretions to pool in the cheek where they can be more easily suctioned and removed to establish the airway. **Stimulating** the newborn is often all that is needed to initiate spontaneous respirations. This tactile stimulation can be accomplished by gently rubbing the infant's back or trunk. Another technique used to provide stimulation is flicking or rubbing the soles of the feet. Slapping neonates as stimulation is no longer practiced and should NOT be used.

Neonatal Chest Compressions

If **chest compressions** are indicated for resuscitation, these steps should be followed.

1. Position the neonate in the "sniffing" position with the neck slightly extended.
2. Make sure there is firm support for the infant's back.
3. Using a two-finger technique, proceed with the compressions on the lower third of the sternum with a depth of one third of the anterior posterior diameter of the chest. The compression rate is 90 compressions per minute and 30 breaths per minute, equaling 120 "events" per minute. One cycle = 3 compressions + 1 breath = 2 seconds.
4. When performing the compressions, the hands should be placed in a circle around the chest to provide support to the infant's back. The ratio of compressions to breaths should be 3 to 1.
5. Check the heart rate again after 30 seconds of compressions—about 45 compressions total.
6. If heart rate is less than 60 beats per minute, continue with another round of compressions, but if the rate is 60 beats per minute or higher, stop compressions.

During chest compressions, oxygen should be delivered at a concentration of 100%.

Administration of Free-Flow Oxygen

If an infant remains cyanotic in the chest area (central cyanosis) after the initial steps of resuscitation have taken place, administering **free-flow oxygen** is the next step to take. Free flow oxygen is administered to the neonate by the use of either a mask hooked up to an oxygen source or by the use of the oxygen tubing itself. If the tubing alone is used, the nurse can hold the tube with a cupped hand helping to direct and concentrate the oxygen at the infant's airway. Free flow oxygen should be administered at a rate of 5 L/minute, initiated at 21% (up to 30% in preterm neonates). If the infant starts to turn pink, the oxygen can be carefully and slowly removed while continuing to closely monitor the infant for returning cyanosis. If the infant remains centrally cyanotic after the administration of free-flow oxygen, bag and mask ventilation must be considered as the next step.

Bag and Mask Ventilation

Ventilation using a **bag and mask** is indicated when one or more of the following occurs and has not responded to other resuscitation attempts:

- Apnea that does not respond to tactile stimulation such as rubbing the chest or back or flicking the soles of the feet.
- Gasping respirations.
- Heart rate of less than 100 beats per minute, determined by auscultation at the apex of the heart or palpation of the base of the umbilical cord.
- Central cyanosis that persists after administering free-flow oxygen, acrocyanosis alone is NOT an indication for the need for further oxygenation or ventilation.

The flowmeter is set at 5-10 L/minute, and opening breath pressures of 30-40 cm H_2O are used for term infants and 20-25 cm H_2O for preterm. Ventilation is done at 40-60 breaths/minute with pressure of 15-20 cm H_2O for normal lungs and 20-50 cm H_2O for immature or compromised lungs.

Flow-Inflating Bag and Mask Ventilation

Bag and mask ventilation is indicated for persistent apnea or gasping respirations, bradycardia (<100 bpm), and persistent cyanosis unrelieved by free-flowing oxygen.

Flow-inflating bag and mask (connected to oxygen flow, which inflates bag) equipment includes:

- Oxygen inlet.
- Flow control valve.
- Pressure manometer attachment.
- Patient outlet for mask attachment.

Advantages: Flow-inflating bag and mask ventilation has the ability to deliver anywhere from 21% (room air) to 100% oxygen; any pressure desired can be set. This type of bag and mask also has the ability to maintain positive end-expiratory pressure (PEEP) and CPAP.

Disadvantages: Because this bag must be connected to a gas (oxygen) source to inflate, it can only be used where a gas supply exists. It requires some experience to deliver the desired quantity of air with each breath. The high pressures possible with this type of equipment make over-inflation of the lungs possible, resulting in pneumothorax. A complete seal is necessary to deliver a tidal volume.

Self-Inflating Bag and Mask Ventilation

Self-inflating bag and mask (does not require gas source) equipment includes:

- Air inlet.
- Oxygen inlet.
- Patient outlet for mask attachment.
- Valve assembly.
- Oxygen reservoir.
- Pop-off valve.
- Pressure manometer attachment.

Advantages: Self-inflating bag and mask ventilation is simple to use and does not require much practice or experience to operate. It can be operated anywhere even if no oxygen source is near and can easily deliver a tidal volume.

Disadvantages: These bags usually have a pop-off valve that will open at a pressure set by the manufacturer to prevent over inflation of the lungs. This valve popping off can prevent the ability to deliver enough pressure to ventilate very noncompliant lungs. Another disadvantage is that if 90% or higher oxygen delivery is desired, this equipment must have a reservoir attached to deliver this concentration. The inability to deliver PEEP is also a disadvantage to the self-inflating bag and mask.

Gastric Suctioning Following Neonatal Resuscitation with a Bag and Mask

When an infant is resuscitated using a bag and mask, air is inadvertently pumped into the stomach as it is being pumped into the lungs, so **gastric suctioning** is necessary. Once respirations have been stabilized, either spontaneously or with mechanical ventilation, the stomach should be aspirated to remove any air pumped into it. If the air is left in the abdomen, it remains distended, causing an upward pressure on the lungs; this compromises lung capacity and breathing effort. Use this procedure.

- Select an orogastric catheter or size 8 Fr. feeding tube.
- Measure the distance from the nose to the earlobe, then to the xiphoid.
- Mark the tube at this distance.
- Advance the tube to the mark.
- Attach a 20 mL syringe to the tube.
- Aspirate the contents of the stomach.
- Leave the tube in place, open to air, taped to the infant's cheek to keep the stomach decompressed.

Epinephrine and Ionotrope

Epinephrine is an endogenous hormone produced by the adrenal glands. It is a sympathomimetic that triggers alpha and beta receptors located in the heart and blood vessels. The effects of epinephrine depend on its dosage and plasma concentration. Low doses of epinephrine have a **positive inotropic effect**, which causes the heart muscle to contract more strongly, and a chronotropic effect, which causes an increase in heart rate and vasoconstricts blood vessels that supply the skin and kidneys. Higher doses of epinephrine cause vasoconstriction in the lungs, viscera, skeletal muscles, brain, and coronary vascular beds. An overdose of epinephrine causes myocardial irritability, arrhythmias, hyperglycemia, and hypokalemia.

Volume Expanders

Volume expanders used in neonatal resuscitation include:

- Normal saline
- Ringer's Lactate
- O- blood, or blood that has been crossmatched with the mother

Prepare 40 mL in a syringe or IV. Give 10 mL/kg over 5-10 minutes. Repeat if necessary. Rapid infusion of a large volume causes intraventricular hemorrhage. (5% albumin in saline is no longer the solution of choice.) Consider volume expanders in instances where neonatal blood loss is suspected, and/or the neonate is showing signs of shock that is not responding to other resuscitative efforts. Blood loss occurs due to trauma of the placenta or umbilical cord, or with neonatal hemolysis. Shock is inadequate tissue and organ perfusion. Signs and symptoms of shock are: Pallor; cold extremities; neurological depression; and weak pulses.

Naloxone Hydrochloride

Naloxone hydrochloride, an opiate antagonist, is not used in the routine resuscitation of an infant but is used in one very specific situation following birth. Naloxone is considered the antidote for narcotics administered to the mother of the infant within 4 hours of birth if the infant shows signs of serious respiratory depression from secondary absorption. If the mother of the infant has narcotics in her system as a result of an addiction to narcotics rather than as treatment for labor pain, however, naloxone cannot be given to this infant. If naloxone is given to an infant born to a narcotic addicted mother, the drug will cause a severe abstinence reaction in the newborn that can result in seizure.

Maternal Postpartum Complications

Hematologic

POSTPARTAL HEMORRHAGE

Postpartum hemorrhage may be early (≤24 hours) or late (≤6 weeks). Normal blood loss with vaginal delivery is about 500 mL and with Caesarean about 1000 mL. ACOG's formal definition of postpartum hemorrhage requires ≥1000mL of blood loss with signs/symptoms of hypovolemia within the first 24 hours after birth, regardless of the mode of delivery. Blood loss is difficult to estimate because it is mixed with amniotic fluid and mucus, and hemorrhage may be internal and not obvious on examination. Usual indications of hemorrhage, such as increased pulse, decreased blood pressure, and decreased output of urine may be delayed until about 2 L of blood loss. A significant drop in hematocrit (10 points) is indicative of hemorrhage. Early hemorrhage poses more risk of mortality than late hemorrhage. When hemorrhage is suspected, such as with steady flow of lochia rubra, then the woman's vital signs should be checked every 5 to 15 minutes and perineal pads weighed (1 mL of blood weighs about 1 g). A soft boggy uterus should be massaged frequently to maintain firmness, with clots expressed. IV access should be maintained. Urinary output <30 mL/hr. should be reported to physician.

Causes of **early postpartal hemorrhage** include:

- **Uterine atony**: most common with multiple gestations, prolonged labor, labor induction, anesthesia, preeclampsia, and placenta previa. Uterine contractions are necessary to occlude blood flow to placenta.
- **Genital lacerations**: may be undetected, or the episiotomy may continue to slowly ooze blood.
- **Hematomas**: resulting from trauma to blood vessels, especially with pudendal anesthesia, forceps or vacuum-assisted delivery, macrosomia, and prolonged second stage of labor.
- **Inversion of the uterus**: rare but may occur with weak uterine muscles, extended labor, anesthesia, use of magnesium sulfate (for preeclampsia), and manual removal of placenta with excess traction.
- **Rupture of uterus**: also rare but can occur with previous C-section, multiparity, and induction with oxytocin.
- Abnormal implantation of placenta.
- **Coagulopathies**: DIC may occur in response to blood loss or may cause blood loss.

Causes of **late postpartal hemorrhage** include:

- **Subinvolution of placental implantation site** (failure of implantation site to shrink and heal) leaves open tissue that may bleed.
- **Retained placental tissue**: Bleeding occurs when it sloughs from implantation site.

POSTPARTAL THROMBOPHLEBITIS

Thrombophlebitis may occur in the postpartal period, with indications of **septic thrombophlebitis** typically evident 3 to 7 days after delivery. **Clot formation** occurs in the vessel walls, leading to occlusion and inflammation. **Fibrinolytic activity** decreases during pregnancy to prevent hemorrhage occurring with delivery; however, this change can promote development of deep vein thrombosis and thrombophlebitis. Additionally, inactivity and bed rest increase risk.

Coagulation usually returns to normal within about 3 days after delivery, so later onset often relates to other factors, such as a history of varicose veins. **Superficial thrombophlebitis** is usually evident by observable symptoms and poses less risk of clots breaking free and migrating than deep vein thrombophlebitis.

- **Femoral**: localized pain and swelling with edema of the leg from impaired circulation, often accompanied by fever and chills.
- **Pelvic**: abdominal pain, fever, and chills as well as generalized lethargy and malaise.

Treatment varies, depending on size and type, but may include heat, anticoagulation, compression (stockings), elevation of affected limb, and limitations on activities.

Postpartal Hematoma

A **hematoma** may form in the perineal area after delivery, especially if an episiotomy is present. Hematomas may form anywhere from the **vulva** to the **upper vagina** because of trauma. Severe vulvar or vaginal pain that is not relieved by usual analgesia may indicate that a hematoma is forming. Hematomas must be monitored carefully. Those <5 cm may resolve over time. Ice packs may help to reduce discomfort. Vital signs should be monitored carefully for signs of hemorrhage. Larger hematomas require surgical excision of the most dependent portion, and drainage. The incision may be closed or left open with drains or packing to prevent recurrence of hematoma. If the hematoma is at the site of the episiotomy, the suture line must be opened to identify the site of bleeding.

HELLP Syndrome

HELLP syndrome occurs in 4 to 12% of those with preeclampsia, most often during weeks 27 to 37, but may develop within 24 hours post-partum, and is characterized by the following:

- **H**—hemolysis
- **EL**—elevated liver enzymes
- **LP**—low platelet count

HELLP syndrome is most common in older multiparous mothers. Hypertension may be less pronounced than in others with preeclampsia. Pain in the right upper quadrant related to liver dysfunction may be misdiagnosed as gastrointestinal upset or gall bladder disease. Mothers often present with flu-like nonspecific symptoms, including headache, nausea and vomiting, and visual disturbances. Prompt diagnosis and treatment are necessary because of high mortality. Platelet transfusions are given if platelet counts <20,000/mm^3 or <50,000 mm^3 with caesarean. The primary treatment is immediate delivery of the fetus as the mother may develop hepatic hemorrhage or permanent liver damage. Both the mother and the fetus are at risk. Neonates are at increased risk and may require mechanical ventilation. Complications include abruptio placentae, DIC, and post-partum hemorrhage.

Pulmonary Embolus

Because hypercoagulation occurs post-partum, coupled with decreased activity, the risk for **pulmonary embolus** increases, especially in the first 24 hours (but risk may persist for 4 to 6 weeks and with Caesarean births). Up to 70% of patients with pulmonary embolus also have DVT, so PE should always be suspected with DVT. Symptoms of PE include dyspnea, chest pain, cough, fever, hemoptysis, tachypnea, tachycardia, and anxiety. Massive PE is characterized by hemodynamic instability and can lead to hypotension, PEA, and death. ECG findings of PE may include right axis deviation and inversion of the T-wave. Most patients will exhibit hypoxemia, but normal blood gas values do not preclude PE. Diagnosis is per chest radiograph, D-dimer, and helical CT-angiography, ventilation-perfusion scanning, or bilateral compression ultrasonography. Treatment may include anticoagulation, thrombolysis, or embolectomy, but all increase the risk of post-partal hemorrhage. Vena cave filters may also be inserted to prevent further clots from entering the lungs. $ECMO_2$ may be used to support the patient if respiratory failure occurs.

DIC

Disseminated intravascular coagulation (DIC), consumption coagulopathy, is a secondary disorder of pregnancy. DIC may be triggered by abruptio placentae, uterine rupture, embolism of amniotic fluid, eclampsia, post-partum hemorrhage, shock (hypovolemic), severe infection with sepsis, and saline/missed abortion. DIC triggers both **coagulation** and **hemorrhage** through a complex series of events that includes trauma causing tissue factor (transmembrane glycoprotein) to enter the circulation and bind with coagulation factors triggering the coagulation cascade. This stimulates thrombin to convert fibrinogen to **fibrin**, causing aggregation and destruction of platelets and forming clots that can be disseminated throughout the intravascular system. These clots increase in size as platelets adhere to the clots, causing blockage of both the microvascular systems and the larger vessels. This can result in **ischemia** and **necrosis**. Clot formation triggers fibrinolysis and plasmin to breakdown fibrin and fibrinogen, causing destruction of clotting factors, resulting in hemorrhage. Both processes, clotting and hemorrhage, continue at the same time, placing the patient at high risk of death, even with treatment.

Symptoms and Treatment

The onset of **symptoms of DIC** may be very rapid, or it may be a slower chronic progression. Those who develop the chronic manifestation of the disease usually have fewer acute symptoms and may slowly develop ecchymosis or bleeding wounds.

The *symptoms* for disseminated intravascular coagulation:

- Bleeding from surgical or venous puncture sites
- Evidence of GI bleeding with distention, bloody diarrhea
- Hypotension and acute symptoms of shock
- Petechiae and purpura with extensive bleeding into the tissues
- Laboratory abnormalities:
    - Prolonged prothrombin and partial prothrombin times
    - Decreased platelet counts and fragmented RBCs
    - Decreased fibrinogen

The *treatment* for disseminated intravascular coagulation:

- Identifying and treating underlying cause
- Replacement blood products, such as platelets and fresh frozen plasma
- Anticoagulation therapy (heparin) to increase clotting time
- Cryoprecipitate to increase fibrinogen levels
- Coagulation inhibitors and coagulation factors

DIC Panel Tests

The disseminated intravascular coagulation (DIC) panel includes a number of tests. Generally, test results will show that measurements of materials needed for clotting are decreased and that clotting times are increased. Typical findings that indicate DIC include:

Activated partial thromboplastin time (aPTT)	**Time increased**
Prothrombin time	Varies from increased time (in 50% of cases) to normal time (25%) to shortened time (25%)
Partial thromboplastin time	Increased time (in 50 to 60%)
Thrombin time	Increased time
D-dimer (a specific polymer that results when fibrin breaks down, giving a marker to indicate the degree of fibrinolysis)	Increased (usually more reliable than FSP)
Fibrinogen	Decreased
Platelets	<100,000.
Fibrin split products (FSP) or Fibrin degradation product (FDP): occur as more clots form and further breakdown of fibrinogen and fibrin occur, interfering with blood coagulation by coating platelets and disrupting thrombin, and attaching to fibrinogen so stable clots can't form.	Increased (in 75 to 100%)
Clotting factor assays (V, VI, VII, X, XIII)	Decreased
Antithrombin III	Decreased (in 90% of cases)

Septic Pelvic Thrombophlebitis

Postpartum **septic pelvic thrombophlebitis** (SPT) is an infection that results from venous stasis of the veins that drain the pelvic organs and the presence of bacteria. The infection can extend along the right (most common) and left ovarian veins resulting in septic thrombosis, which can extend into the vena cava and to the renal vein. This, then, can result in microemboli that migrate through the inferior vena cava to the lungs and other organs. Postpartum SPT is more common after Caesarean than vaginal birth and is associated with postpartum endometriosis/parametritis. Symptoms include chills and fever that is nonresponsive to antibiotics. Patients are otherwise often asymptomatic initially although some may experience pain in one or both of the lower quadrants or uterine tenderness if endometriosis/parametritis is involved. Diagnosis is per CT or MRI and CBC. Treatment is primarily antimicrobial (typically clindamycin, gentamycin and ampicillin). Anticoagulation has not been shown to improve outcomes.

Cardiovascular

Preeclampsia and Eclampsia

Pregnancy-induced hypertension (also called preeclampsia or toxemia) is a disorder that develops in approximately 5% of all pregnancies. Its main features are **new onset elevated blood pressure** with proteinuria OR elevated blood pressure with or without proteinuria with signs of **significant end-organ dysfunction** that develop around 20 weeks of gestation. Proteinuria, while a common feature, is no longer considered a required diagnostic feature of preeclampsia. Initial *treatment* of preeclampsia is magnesium sulfate to prevent seizures in the mother. **Eclampsia** occurs with seizures. Severe cases may require the premature delivery of the infant to relieve the condition. The main detrimental effect on the fetus occurs when longstanding hypertension leads to uteroplacental vascular insufficiency, which impairs the transfer of nutrients and oxygen to the fetus, resulting in intrauterine growth restriction (IUGR). Placental abruption also occurs more frequently. The IUGR is usually asymmetric (fetal head size is normal for gestational age). Infants who are born with IUGR and/or prematurity have increased morbidity and mortality. *Treatment* includes antihypertensive medications, such as thiazide, hydralazine, propranolol, labetalol, nifedipine, and methyldopa, as well as anticonvulsants if seizures occur.

Hypovolemic Shock, Distributive Shock, and Cardiogenic Shock

Shock occurs when the neonate's cardiovascular system is unable to supply organs with adequate perfusion. The three main categories of shock seen in the neonate are:

- **Hypovolemic shock,** where the neonate has inadequate intravascular blood volume because of blood loss from placental abruption, or excessive fluid loss from gastroschisis or omphalocele. Insufficient fluid is available to fill the heart and perfuse tissues adequately.
- **Distributive shock** (also called septic shock) is a type of hypovolemic shock where the capillaries become excessively permeable and fluid moves from the intravascular space into the extracellular spaces. It is often accompanied by vasodilatation, which further exacerbates the decreased intravascular volume.
- **Cardiogenic shock** occurs when the cardiac muscle does not pump with enough strength to maintain tissue perfusion. Cardiogenic shock is caused by myocarditis, hypoxemia, hypoglycemia, acidosis, or cardiac arrhythmias.

Compensated and Uncompensated Shock

Shock occurs when the cardiovascular system is unable to meet the metabolic demands of the neonate. Initially, the neonate **compensates** for inadequate perfusion with these mechanisms to maintain perfusion to vital organs (brain, kidney, liver):

- Vasoconstriction of vessels supplying the skin, skeletal muscle, and gastrointestinal tract, cooling the skin and causing increased capillary refill time.
- Tachycardia.
- Decreased urine output.

When these compensatory mechanisms fail, signs of **uncompensated** shock prevail, including:

- Decreased consciousness, as the brain is inadequately perfused.
- Renal failure, as the kidneys are inadequately perfused.
- Acidosis from anaerobic metabolism, due to hypoxemia and respiratory failure.
- Hypotension as the heart muscle fails in late shock.

Infection

Metritis and Parametritis

Metritis and parametritis are postpartal infections:

- **Metritis** (Endometrial inflammation)
    - May result from C-section, PROM, repeated vaginal examination, fetal scalp electrode, instruments (forceps or vacuum), high-risk behaviors of mother (drug use, smoking, poor nutrition), pre-existing vaginal infection, and aseptic techniques.
    - Indications include foul or scant lochia (depending on organism), uterine tenderness, temperature elevations (sawtooth pattern) 38.3-40 °C, tachycardia, and chills.
- **Parametritis** (Pelvic cellulitis/peritonitis)
    - Infection of connective tissue of broad ligament or all pelvic structures may result from bacterial invasion of cervical laceration or pelvic vein thrombophlebitis. Abscess may form.
    - Indications include chills, high fever (38.9-40 °C), abdominal pain, uterine subinvolution, local and rebound tenderness, tachycardia, abdominal distention, nausea, and vomiting.

Endometritis

Endometritis is an infection of the uterus. It occurs more often after cesarean births than vaginal births. Fever occurs about the third day postpartum, accompanied by abdominal pain, malaise, uterine tenderness, and possibly foul-smelling lochia. Risk factors include cesarean births, prolonged rupture of membranes, protracted labor, invasive procedures during labor and delivery, excess blood loss and anemia, systemic illnesses, diabetes, kidney infections, and smoking. Historically, it has been the most common cause of maternal death after childbirth. Handwashing is the most effective way to prevent it. Many organisms cause endometritis. They reach the uterus from the lower birth canal. Antibiotics are given parenterally and the infection should respond within 48 to 72 hours.

Epinephrine

Epinephrine is a naturally-occurring hormone produced by the adrenal glands. Epinephrine is used to resuscitate both adults and children. It is a sympathomimetic that supports the circulatory system by:

- Increasing heart rate.
- Increasing contraction strength.
- Vasoconstricting vessels in the skin, mucosa, and circulation of the gastrointestinal tract.
- Causing a rise in blood pressure.

If positive pressure ventilation and chest compressions have not caused the neonate's heart rate to rise above 60 beats per minute during resuscitation, then epinephrine is indicated. The recommended IV dose is 0.01-0.03 mg/kg. The usual concentration of epinephrine is 1:10,000 or 0.1mg/ml. Endotracheal administration is no longer recommended, but may be used if no IV access is available. Higher doses are required for endotracheal administration. Prepare 1 mL of epinephrine in a syringe. Dilute epinephrine 1:1 with normal saline if the doctor orders it IT.

Urinary and Wound Infections

Urinary and wound infections in the postpartal period are discussed below:

- **Urinary**
  - May result from birth trauma, urinary retention, and contamination (from a catheter).
  - Indications include dysuria, fever, and urinary retention.
- **Wound**
  - May result from contamination of lacerations, episiotomy, and C-section incisions.
  - Indications include erythema, local pain, purulent discharge, edema, and (rarely) dehiscence.

Postpartal Diabetes Mellitus

Mothers with **diabetes mellitus** require careful evaluation but should be encouraged to be as independent as possible in monitoring their own blood sugars and taking medications, such as insulin. Insulin requirements usually drop by 50 to 75% in the 24 hours after delivery because of the drop in hormone levels, so monitoring **glucose levels** and adjusting **insulin dosage** is important to prevent insulin reactions. The insulin needs should be reestablished over the next few days, taking into consideration diet and exercise. Diabetic mothers should be encouraged to breastfeed. Insulin needs while breastfeeding are often decreased, even with increased caloric intake, so home glucose monitoring and adjustment of insulin doses must continue after discharge. With gestational diabetes, insulin can usually be discontinued after childbirth with monitoring of glucose levels. Oral medications can be used if necessary, although oral antihyperglycemics medications are contraindicated with breastfeeding.

Mood Disorders

Post-Partum Depression

Postpartum major mood disorder, commonly referred to as **postpartum depression,** occurs in >10% of mothers. Onset may occur any time within the first year, but is most common around week 4 postpartum, before the onset of menses. Duration varies but is usually 3 to 14 months (half symptomatic at 6 months). Risk factors include primiparity, history of depression, bipolar disease, or previous postpartum depression, lack of stable and supportive social and family relationships, family history of psychiatric illness, and ambivalence about pregnancy. Symptoms are typical of depression and include sadness, crying, insomnia or excess sleeping, difficulty concentrating or making decisions, phobias, anxiety, lack of interest in activities, and feeling of being out of control or helpless. The mother may be irritable and hostile, especially toward the child. She may also be suicidal. Treatment may include psychotherapy, antidepressants, antipsychotics, and/or lithium. In some cases, the child may need to be cared for by others until the mother's depression lessens.

Postpartum Psychosis

Postpartum psychosis may occur up to 3 months postpartum, but symptoms are usually evident within the first 3 weeks, with sudden onset of **psychotic Criterion A symptoms**, such as delusions, hallucinations, insomnia, anorexia, paranoia, and suicidal and/or homicidal ideation. In 4% of cases, mothers have committed infanticide, sometimes because of voices urging them to do so, so postpartum psychosis is a **medical emergency** that often requires hospitalization. Mothers should be carefully supervised when caring for their children until symptoms have abated, or children may need to be removed from the mother until the mother stabilizes. While postpartum psychosis is most common in mothers with a history of mental illness (such as schizophrenia or bipolar disease), it can occur in mothers with no such history. The cause is unclear but may be a combination of **hormonal imbalance** and **stress/anxiety**. *Treatment* includes psychotherapy, mood stabilizers, antipsychotics, and benzodiazepines. Antidepressants may cause mood cycling if psychosis is associated with bipolar disorder.

Newborn Complications

Cardiovascular

Cyanotic and Acyanotic Congenital Cardiac Defects

Congenital heart disease is one of the leading causes of death in children within the first year of life. There are two main types of congenital heart disease: acyanotic and cyanotic. They may also be classified according to hemodynamics related to the blood flow pattern.

Cyanotic congenital heart disease includes those with decreased pulmonary blood flow and mixed blood flow.

Decreased pulmonary blood flow	Tetralogy of Fallot Tricuspid atresia
Mixed blood flow	Ebstein anomaly Hypoplastic left heart syndrome Total anomalous pulmonary venous return Transposition of great arteries Truncus arteriosus

Acyanotic defects include those with increased pulmonary blood flow or obstructed ventricular blood flow.

Increased pulmonary blood flow	Atrial septal defect Atrioventricular canal defect Patent ductus arteriosus Ventricular septal defect
Obstructed ventricular blood flow	Aortic stenosis Coarctation of aorta Pulmonic stenosis

Tetralogy of Fallot

Tetralogy of Fallot (TOF) is a combination of 4 different defects:

- **Ventricular septal defect** (usually with a large opening).
- **Pulmonic stenosis** with decreased blood flow to lungs.
- **Overriding aorta** (displacement to the right so that it appears to come from both ventricles, usually overriding the ventricular septal defect), resulting in mixing of oxygenated and deoxygenated blood.
- **Right ventricular hypertrophy**.

Infants are often acutely cyanotic immediately after birth while others with less severe defects may have increasing cyanosis over the first year. *Symptoms* include:

- Intolerance to feeding or crying, resulting in increased cyanotic "blue spells" or "tet spells."
- Failure to thrive with poor growth.
- Clubbing of fingers may occur over time.
- Intolerance to activity as child grows.
- Increased risk for emboli, brain attacks, brain abscess, seizures, fainting or sudden death.

Treatment: Total surgical repair at ≤1 year is now the preferred treatment rather than palliative procedures formerly used.

HLHS

Hypoplastic left heart syndrome (HLHS) is underdevelopment of the left ventricle and ascending aortic atresia causing inability of the heart to pump blood, so most blood flows from the left atrium through the foramen ovale to the right atrium and to the lungs with the descending aorta receiving blood through the ductus arteriosus. There may be valvular abnormalities as well. Symptoms may be mild until the ductus arteriosus closes at about 2 weeks causing a marked increase in cyanosis and decreased cardiac output. *Symptoms* include:

- Increasing cyanosis.
- Decreased cardiac output leading to cardiovascular collapse.

Mortality rates are 100% without surgical correction and 25% with correction. *Surgical procedures* include a series of 3 staged operations:

- Norwood procedure connects the main pulmonary artery to the aorta, a shunt for pulmonary blood flow, and creates a large atrial septal defect.
- Glenn procedure.
- Fontan repair procedure.
- Heart transplantation in infancy is preferred in many cases, but the shortage of hearts limits this option.

Transposition of Great Arteries

Transposition of great arteries is the aorta and pulmonary artery arising from the wrong ventricle (aorta from the right ventricle and pulmonary artery from the left), so there is no connection between pulmonary and systemic circulation with deoxygenated blood being pumped back to the body and the oxygenated blood from the lungs is pumped back to the lungs. Septal defects may also occur, allowing some mixing of blood and the ductus arteriosus allows mixing until it closes. *Symptoms* vary depending upon whether there is mixing of blood but may include:

- Mild to severe cyanosis.
- Symptoms of congestive heart failure.
- Cardiomegaly develops in the weeks after birth.
- Heart sounds vary depending upon the severity of the defects.

Treatment may include:

- Prostaglandin to keep the ductus arteriosus and foramen ovale open. Balloon atrial septostomy to increase size of foramen ovale.
- Surgical repair to transpose arteries to the normal position ("arterial switch") as well of repair septal defects and other abnormalities.

CYANOTIC HEART DISEASE

TRICUSPID ATRESIA

Tricuspid atresia is lack of **tricuspid valve** between the right atrium and right ventricle. Blood flows through the foramen ovale or an atrial defect to the left atrium and then through a ventricular wall defect from the left ventricle to the right ventricle and out to the lungs, causing oxygenated and deoxygenated bloods to mix. **Pulmonic obstruction** is common.

Symptoms include:

- Postnatal cyanosis
- Tachycardia and dyspnea
- Increasing hypoxemia and clubbing in older children
- Increased risk for bacterial endocarditis, brain abscess, and stroke

Treatment includes:

- Prostaglandin (alprostadil), to keep the ductus arteriosus and foramen ovale open, if there are no septal defects
- Numerous surgical procedures, including pulmonary artery banding, shunting from the aorta to the pulmonary arteries, Glenn procedure (connecting superior vena cava to pulmonary artery to allow deoxygenated blood to flow to the lungs), atrial septostomy to enlarge the opening between the atria, and Fontan corrective procedure, usually done at 2-4 years after previous stabilizing procedures

TOTAL ANOMALOUS PULMONARY VENOUS RETURN

Total anomalous pulmonary venous return is a defect in which the 4 **pulmonary veins** connect to the right atrium by an anomalous connection to the **systemic venous circulation**, unlike normal pulmonary venous return, which carries oxygenated blood from the lungs to the left atrium where it can then be pumped to the rest of the body. With TAPVR, there is no direct blood flow to the left side of the heart; however, an atrial septal defect is common and allows for the mixed oxygenated and deoxygenated blood to shunt to the left and enter the aorta. There are 4 different types of anomalies, and in some cases pulmonary vein obstruction. If the pulmonary veins are not obstructed, children may initially be asymptomatic.

Symptoms include:

- Heart murmur
- Severe post-natal cyanosis or mild cyanosis
- Dyspnea with grunting and sternal retraction or dyspnea on exertion
- Low oxygen saturation (in the 80s if there is no pulmonary obstruction)
- Cardiomegaly (right-sided hypertrophy)

Surgical repair to attach the pulmonary veins to the left atrium and correction of any other defects may be done immediately after birth or delayed for 1 to 2 months.

Truncus Arteriosus

Truncus arteriosus is the blood from both ventricles flowing into one large artery with one valve, with more blood flowing to the **lower pressure pulmonary arteries** than to the body, resulting in low oxygen saturation and hypoxemia. Usually, there is a **ventricular septal defect** so the blood in the ventricles mixes.

Symptoms include:

- Congestive heart failure with pulmonary edema because of increased blood flow to lungs.
- Typical symptoms of congestive heart failure.
- Cyanosis, especially about the face (mouth and nose).
- Dyspnea, increasing on feeding or exertion.
- Poor feeding and failure to thrive.
- Heart murmur.
- Increased risk for brain abscess and bacterial endocarditis.

Treatment consists of the following:

- Palliative banding of the pulmonary arteries is performed to decrease the flow of blood to the lungs.
- Surgical repair with cardiopulmonary bypass includes closing the ventricular defect, utilizing the existing single artery as the aorta by separating the pulmonary arteries from it, and creating a conduit between the pulmonary arteries and the right ventricle.

Ebstein's Anomaly

Ebstein's anomaly is an abnormality of the **tricuspid valve** separating the right atrium from the right ventricle, with the valve leaflets displaced downward and one adhering to the wall so there is backflow into the atrium when the ventricle contracts. This usually results in enlargement of the **right atrium** and **congestive heart failure**. As pressure increases in the right atrium, it usually forces the **foramen ovale** to stay open, so the blood is shunted to the left atrium, mixing the deoxygenated blood with oxygenated blood that then leaves through the aorta. Symptoms vary widely, depending upon the degree of defect, and range from asymptomatic to life threatening. Ebstein's anomaly may occur with other cardiac defects. Many children are not diagnosed until their teens.

Symptoms include:

- Cyanosis with low oxygen saturation
- Congestive heart failure
- Palpitations, arrhythmias
- Dyspnea on exertion
- Increased risk for bacterial endocarditis

Treatment includes:

- ACE inhibitors, diuretics, and digoxin
- Surgical repair of abnormalities with valve repair or replacement

Acyanotic Heart Disease

Atrial Septal Defect

An **atrial septal defect (ASD)** is an abnormal opening in the **septum** between the right and left atria. Because the left atrium has higher pressure than the right atrium, some of the oxygenated blood returning from the lungs to the left atrium is shunted back to the right atrium, where it is again returned to the lungs, displacing deoxygenated blood.

Symptoms:

- Symptoms may be few, depending upon the degree of the defect but can include Congestive heart failure
- Heart murmur
- Increased risk for dysrhythmias and pulmonary vascular obstructive disease over time
- May be asymptomatic in some infants

Treatment may not be necessary for small defects, but larger defects require closure:

- Open-heart surgical repair
- Heart catheterization and placing of closure device (Amplatz® device) across the atrial septal defect

Atrioventricular Canal Defect

Atrioventricular canal defect is often associated with Down syndrome and involves a number of different defects, including openings between the atria and ventricles as well as abnormalities of the valves. In **partial defects**, there is an opening between the atria and mitral valve regurgitation. In **complete defects**, there is a large central hole in the heart and only one common valve between the atria and ventricles. The blood may flow freely about the heart, usually from left to right. Extra blood flow to the lungs causes enlargement of the heart. Partial defects may go undiagnosed for 20 years. **Symptoms** include:

- Typical congestive heart failure signs
  - Weakness and fatigue
  - Coughing and/or wheezing with production of white or bloody sputum
  - Peripheral edema and ascites
  - Dysrhythmia and tachycardia
- Dyspnea
- Poor appetite
- Failure to thrive; low weight
- Cyanosis of skin and lips

Treatment include:

- Symptom management as indicated
- Open-heart surgery to patch holes in the septum, and valve repair or replacement

PDA

Patent ductus arteriosus (PDA) is failure of the ductus arteriosus that connects the **pulmonary artery and aorta** to close after birth, resulting in left-to-right shunting of blood from the aorta back to the pulmonary artery. This increases the blood flow to the lungs and causes an increase in pulmonary hypertension that can result in damage to the lung tissue.

Symptoms include:

- Essentially asymptomatic in some infants
- Cyanosis
- Congestive heart failure
- Machinery-like murmur
- Frequent respiratory infections and dyspnea, especially on exertion
- Widened pulse pressure
- Bounding pulse
- Atrial fibrillation/ palpitations
- Increased risk for bacterial endocarditis, congestive heart failure, and development of pulmonary vascular obstructive disease

Treatment includes:

- Indomethacin (Indocin®) given within 10 days of birth is successful in closing about 80% of defects.
- Surgical repair can be done with ligation of the patent vessel.

VENTRICULAR SEPTAL DEFECT

Ventricular septal defect is an abnormal opening in the **septum** between the right and left ventricles. If the opening is small, the child may be asymptomatic, but larger openings can result in a left-to-right shunt because of higher pressure in the left ventricle. This shunting increases in the 6 weeks after birth, with symptoms becoming more evident, but the defect may close within a few years. *Symptoms* include:

- Congestive heart failure with peripheral edema
- Tachycardia
- Dyspnea
- Difficulty feeding
- Heart murmur
- Recurrent pulmonary infections
- Increased risk for bacterial endocarditis and pulmonary vascular obstructive disease

Treatment includes:

- Diuretics, such as furosemide (Lasix®), may be used for heart failure.
- ACE inhibitor (Captopril®) decreases pulmonary hypertension.
- Surgery, including pulmonary banding or cardiopulmonary bypass, can be performed to repair the opening with sutures or a patch, depending upon the size.

AORTIC STENOSIS

Aortic stenosis is a stricture (narrowing) of the **aortic valve** that controls the flow of blood from the left ventricle, causing the **left ventricular wall** to thicken as it increases pressure to overcome the valvular resistance, increasing afterload and increasing the need for blood supply from the coronary arteries. This condition may result from a birth defect or childhood rheumatic fever and tends to worsen over the years as the heart grows.

Symptoms include:

- Chest pain on exertion and intolerance of exercise
- Heart murmur
- Hypotension on exertion may be associated with sudden fainting
- Tachycardia with faint pulse
- Poor feeding
- Increased risk for bacterial endocarditis and coronary insufficiency
- Increases mitral regurgitation and secondary pulmonary hypertension
- Sudden death can occur

Treatment in children may be done before symptoms develop, because of the danger of sudden death.

- Balloon valvuloplasty to dilate valve non- surgically
- Surgical repair of valve or replacement of valve, depending upon the extent of stricture

PULMONIC STENOSIS

Pulmonic stenosis is a stricture of the pulmonary blood that controls the flow of blood from the right ventricle to the lungs, resulting in **right ventricular hypertrophy**, as the pressure increases in the right ventricle and pulmonary blood flow decreases. The condition may be symptomatic, asymptomatic, or symptoms may not be evident until the child enters adulthood, depending upon the severity of the defect. Pulmonic stenosis may be associated with a number of other heart defects.

Symptoms include:

- Loud heart murmur
- Congestive heart murmur
- Mild cyanosis
- Cardiomegaly
- Angina
- Dyspnea
- Fainting
- Increased risk of bacterial endocarditis

Treatment includes:

- Balloon valvuloplasty to separate the cusps of the valve for children
- Surgical repair includes the (closed) transventricular valvotomy (Brock) procedure for infants and the cardiopulmonary bypass pulmonary valvotomy for older children

Coarctation of the Aorta

Coarctation of the aorta is a stricture of the aorta, proximal to the ductus arteriosus intersection. The increased blood pressure caused by the heart attempting to pump the blood past the stricture causes the heart to enlarge and also blood pressure to the head and upper extremities while decreasing blood pressure and to the lower body and extremities. With severe stricture, symptoms may not occur until the ductus arteriosus closes, causing sudden loss of blood supply to the lower body. *Symptoms* include:

- Difference in blood pressure between upper and lower extremities.
- Congestive heart failure symptoms in infants.
- Headaches, dizziness, and nosebleeds in older children.
- Increased risk of hypertension, ruptured aorta, aortic aneurysm, bacterial endocarditis, and brain attack.

Treatment includes:

- Prostaglandin (alprostadil), such as Prostin VR Pediatric®, to reopen the ductus arteriosus for infants.
- Balloon angioplasty.
- Surgical resection and anastomosis or graft replacement (usually at 3-5 years of age unless condition is severe). Infants who have surgery may need later repair.

Respiratory

Apnea of Prematurity

Premature infants (especially those <34 weeks) often exhibit **apnea of prematurity (AOP).** AOP begins at birth and is believed to be caused by immaturity of the nervous system, and improves as the brain matures. It may persist for 4 to 8 weeks. There are 3 types of apnea:

- **Central**: no airflow or effort to breathe
- **Obstructive**: no airflow, but effort to breathe
- **Mixed**: both central and obstructive elements (75% of AOP)

Symptoms include:

- Swallowing during apneic periods
- Apnea >20 seconds
- Apnea <20 seconds with bradycardia 30 beats <normal
- Oxygen saturation <85% persisting ≥5 seconds
- Cyanosis

Treatment includes:

- Tactile stimulation (rubbing limbs or thorax or gently slapping bottoms of feet) or gently lifting the jaw to relieve obstruction
- Oxygen or bag/mask ventilation for bradycardia and decreased oxygen saturation
- Continuous positive airway pressure (CPAP) for mixed or obstructive apnea
- Aminophylline/theophylline or caffeine (for central apnea) may increase contractions of diaphragm

Birth Asphyxia

Birth asphyxia is the cause of many problems after birth. Birth asphyxia is defined as an event that alters the exchange of gas (oxygen and carbon dioxide). This interference with gas exchange leads to a decrease in the amount of oxygen delivered to the fetus along with an increase in the level of carbon dioxide the fetus is exposed to. This gas imbalance causes the fetus to switch from normal aerobic metabolism to anaerobic metabolism. Fetal distress results and this distress then leads to increased fetal heart rate, release of meconium into the amniotic fluid, and lowered pH. Infants experiencing birth asphyxia will often present at birth with APGAR scores that are less than 5. Symptoms of birth asphyxia include:

- **Mild:**
  - Overly alert for the first 45 minutes to one hour following birth (infants are normally sleepy after about 15 minutes following birth).
  - The pupils are dilated.
  - The respiratory rate and the heart rate will both be slightly increased.
  - Newborn reflexes and muscle tone are normal.
  - Oxygen may be administered.

- **Moderate:**
  - Hypothermia as evidenced by low body temperature.
  - Hypoglycemia as glucose store are used up trying to supply organs needed energy.
  - Pupils are constricted.
  - Signs of respiratory distress are evident.
  - May experience seizure activity at 12-24 hours of age.
  - Lethargy (floppy infant).
  - Bradycardia.
- **Severe** (requires close monitoring in a NICU):
  - Pale color related to the inability of the heart to perfuse the body.
  - Cerebral edema related to apnea episodes and/or intracranial hemorrhage.

Resuscitation will vary according to the infant's condition, but warming the infant, stabilizing the glucose level, and providing oxygen or EMCO (in severe cases) may be indicated.

TTN

Transient tachypnea of newborn (TTN) occurs when fluid in the lungs is not adequately absorbed after birth. The neonate usually exhibits symptoms within 36 hours of birth, and the condition typically resolves within 3 days. TTN is most common in infants delivered by caesarean section, but premature birth and having a mother who smokes or has diabetes increases risk to infant.

Symptoms include:

- Dyspnea (>60/min)
- Sternal retraction (mild)
- Expiratory grunt
- Nasal flaring
- Poor feeding (because of increased respiratory rate)

Laboratory findings include:

- ABGs: hypoxemia
- Chest radiograph: fluid in lungs

Treatment includes:

- Monitor oxygen saturation levels.
- Provide supplemental oxygen as indicated.
- Provide intravenous fluids or nasogastric feedings if infant is unable to take oral feedings.

Pneumothorax

Pneumothorax is the most common type of air leak syndrome. In infants, increased air pressure caused by the use of mechanical ventilation is the most common cause, but infants may develop spontaneous pneumothorax, especially those infants with fragile lung tissue are at high risk:

- Infants with lung disease, including hyaline membrane disease (HMD).
- Premature infants.
- Infants with meconium aspiration.

Symptoms vary according to the type of pneumothorax (spontaneous, traumatic, or tension) but can include:

- ↑ Respiratory distress with tachypnea and chest wall retractions
- Absence of breath sounds on auscultation.
- Paradoxical chest movement in which the chest contracts during inhalation and expands during exhalation.
- Shift in maximum intensity sounds of heart.
- Bradycardia and cyanosis.

Treatment includes:

- Evacuating air with needle aspiration or chest tubes to water seal drainage.
- Correction of underlying cause.

Chest Tube Insertion/Removal

Chest tubes are inserted in the neonate to treat pneumothorax causing cardiac or respiratory compromise or pleural effusion. **Transillumination** may be used to identify the area of pneumothorax but **chest x-ray** is more accurate. An 8 to 12 Fr. chest tube is placed anteriorly for collections of air and posteriorly/laterally for fluid. The infant is supine with the arm at 90° on the insertion side. The insertion sites are

- **Anterior**: midclavicular line, second or third intercostal space
- **Posterior/lateral**: anterior axillary line, fourth, fifth, or sixth intercostal space

Lidocaine is instilled and an incision made over the rib below the target intercostal space. The tissue is spread and the pleura punctured above the rib with a hemostat, expelling air. The chest tube is inserted 2 to 3cm in preterm and 3 to 4 cm in full-term infants. The purse-string suture is tightened and the chest tube attached to 2 or 3 bottles or a self-contained Pleur-evac underwater seal system. X-ray is taken to confirm placement. Chest tube is removed quickly and pressure dressing applied if there is no bubbling for 24 hours and radiograph is clear.

Needle Aspiration

Neonates receiving bag and mask ventilation or mechanical ventilation risk developing a **pneumothorax**. Signs of pneumothorax include rapid deterioration, poor oxygenation, tachypnea, increased work breathing, impaired circulation, unequal air entry into lungs, displaced apical heartbeat, and increased transillumination on the affected side. If the neonate's clinical status allows it, a chest x-ray will confirm the diagnosis. Air is removed by **needle aspiration.**

The **equipment** for needle aspiration:

- Oral sucrose
- 1% lidocaine
- Fentanyl
- 21-gauge butterfly needle
- 10 mL syringe
- 3-way stopcock attached to the syringe
- 70% isopropyl alcohol swab
- Sterile gloves

The **procedure** for needle aspiration is as follows:

1. Give oral sucrose.
2. Place infant in supine position.
3. Swab second and third intercostal spaces in midclavicular line with alcohol.
4. Infiltrate site with 1% lidocaine 0.5 mL to 1 mL.
5. Drape insertion site.
6. Give 250 mcg fentanyl over 2 to 3 minutes IV.
7. Insert needle directly into second or third intercostal space in mid-clavicular line until air is aspirated into syringe.
8. Expel air through stopcock.

Meconium Aspiration Syndrome

Meconium aspiration syndrome (MAS) occurs when meconium, expelled in the amniotic fluid (occurring in about 20% of pregnancies), is aspirated by the fetus *in utero* or the neonate at first breath. Blood and amniotic fluids may be aspirated as well. Some infants may present with **symptoms** at birth, but sometimes symptoms are delayed for a number of hours:

- Tachypnea.
- Lethargy, depressed state.
- Hypoxemia and hypercapnia.
- Metabolic acidosis may occur.
- Hyperventilation may occur in early stages with hypoventilation in later stages.

Symptoms are similar to transient tachypnea of the newborn (TTN) but they are more severe and the infant appears more compromised. Chest x-rays may show infiltrates, atelectasis, hypoinflated areas as well as hyperinflated areas. Pulmonary hypertension may result. **Treatment** includes:

- Preventive suctioning of the oropharynx as soon as the head is delivered.
- Intubation and suctioning of the trachea for infants with respiratory distress (weak respirations, bradycardia, hypotonia).
- Supplemental oxygen and/or mechanical ventilation as indicated.

Gastrointestinal

Bowel Obstructions

Bowel obstruction occurs when there is a mechanical obstruction of the **passage of intestinal contents** because of constriction of the lumen, occlusion of the lumen, or lack of muscular contractions (paralytic ileus). Obstruction may be caused by congenital or acquired abnormalities/disorders:

Small Bowel Obstructions	Large Bowel Obstructions
Duodenal atresia Malrotation and volvulus Jejunoileal atresia Meconium ileus Meconium peritonitis	Hirschsprung disease Anorectal malformations Meconium plug syndrome

Symptoms include:

- Abdominal pain, distention, and rigidity
- Vomiting and dehydration
- Diminished or no bowel sounds
- Severe constipation (obstipation)
- Respiratory distress from diaphragm pushing against pleural cavity
- Shock, as plasma volume diminishes and electrolytes enter intestines from bloodstream
- Sepsis, as bacteria proliferate in bowel and invade bloodstream

Hypertrophic Pyloric Stenosis

Hypertrophic pyloric stenosis (PS) is obstruction of the pyloric sphincter between the gastric pylorus and small intestine, caused by hypertrophy and hyperplasia of the circular muscle of the pylorus so the enlarged tissue obstructs the sphincter. PS is more common in boys than girls and has a genetic predisposition. Onset of *symptoms* is usually >3weeks:

- Projectile vomiting (1-4 feet) usually shortly after eating but may be delayed for a few hours. Emesis may be blood-tinged but non-bilious.
- Infant is hungry and eats readily, but shows weight loss and signs of dehydration.
- Upper abdominal distention with palpable mass in epigastrium (to right of umbilicus).
- Visible left to right peristaltic waves.

Diagnosis is based on ultrasound. Decreased sodium and potassium levels may not be evident with dehydration.

Treatment includes:

- Intravenous fluids to restore hydration and electrolyte balance.
- Surgical pyloromyotomy: longitudinal incisions through the circular muscle fibers down to the submucosa to release the restriction and allow the muscle to expand.

Intestinal Atresia

When a portion of the bowel comes to a stop and then starts back up again forming a discontinuous or segmented bowel, this is called **intestinal atresia.** This condition usually relates to failures during the 5th to 10th week of fetal development, so it is often associated with other anomalies. The most common site for atresia to occur in the neonate is the duodenum. Atresia can also occur in the ileum, jejunum, colon, and even rarely the stomach. An atresia that occurs anywhere in the intestine except the duodenum is not associated with any other disorders. However, an atresia that occurs in the duodenum (the most common type) is usually (30% of the time) associated with other disorders such as trisomy 21, congenital heart disease, and VACTERL association. The only treatment for intestinal atresia is surgical reconnection of the bowel.

Imperforate Anus

Categories

Imperforate anus (anorectal malfunction) is a congenital abnormality in which the **rectum** is absent, malformed, or displaced from normal position. It may include disorders of the urinary tract. Imperforate anus occurs in 1 in 5000 births, more commonly in males than females. Imperforate anus may include stenosis or atresia of the anus. There are 3 main categories, classified according to the relationship of the rectum to the puborectalis musculature.

- **Low anomalies:** no external opening, but rectum otherwise in normal position through the puborectalis muscle, with normal function and no connection to the genitourinary tract.
- **Intermediate anomalies:** rectum at or below the level of puborectalis muscle, anal dimple evident, and external sphincter in normal position.
- **High anomalies:** rectum ending above the puborectalis muscles, internal sphincter absent often with a rectourethral fistula in males or a rectovaginal fistula in females, and sometimes fistulas to the bladder or perineum.

Diagnosis, Symptoms, and Treatment

Imperforate anus is **diagnosed** by physical examination, digital or endoscopic examination, and contrast radiography with the infant inverted. An opaque marker at the anal dimple will outline the location of a pouch in relation to the normal position of the anus.

Symptoms

Symptoms include:

- Absence of anal opening, no meconium in 24 to 48 hours, abdominal distention, and vomiting
- Rectovaginal fistula or rectourethral fistula (may not be evident at first because stool passes through fistula)
- Fistula between the rectum and the bladder with gas or fecal material possibly expelled through the urethra
- Displacement of the anus, with chronic constipation developing over time

Treatment

Surgery is performed in most cases, type depending upon extent of abnormality:

- With low anomalies, simple excision of anal opening
- Two step or three step procedure for higher anomalies; colostomy first, with later reconstruction of the anus in the proper position, involving anoplasty and pull through procedures
- Manual dilation to treat stenosis

Meconium Plug Syndrome

Meconium plug syndrome (also called functional colonic obstruction) occurs when the first stool obstructs the intestinal tract and no other pathology is present. This will be evident in the first 24 to 48 hours of life, when the infant fails to pass the first meconium stool. Meconium plug syndrome usually occurs in full term infants, infants of diabetic mothers, or infants with hypermagnesemia. The infant may have abdominal distension, poor feeding, and vomiting (often bilious in nature). An x-ray of the abdomen will show dilated loops of bowel. A contrast enema is diagnostic and helps differentiate from other causes of intestinal obstruction. It may also be therapeutic, causing the plug to pass. Infants usually do well after the plug has passed. A small percentage of infants initially identified as having meconium plug syndrome (5 to 10%) have Hirschsprung disease. The cause of meconium plug syndrome is thought to be immaturity of the ganglion cells of the colon.

Congenital Diaphragmatic Hernia

Congenital diaphragmatic hernias (CDH) may cause severe respiratory distress. The primary CDHs that affect infants are **posterolateral** (Bochdalek hernia).

- **Left sided** in 85% of cases. Includes herniation of the large and small intestine and intra-abdominal organs into the thoracic cavity.
- **Right sided** in 13% of cases. May be asymptomatic or involve only the liver and part of the large intestine herniate.

Neonates with left CDH may exhibit **severe respiratory distress** and **cyanosis**. The lungs may be underdeveloped because of pressure exerted from displaced organs during fetal development. There may be a left hemithorax with a mediastinal shift, with the heart pressing on the right lung, which may be hypoplastic. Bowel sounds are heard over the chest area. Pulmonary hypertension and cardiopulmonary failure may occur. *Treatments* include:

- Immediate surgical repair
- HFOV and nitric oxide for pulmonary hypoplasia
- Extracorporeal membrane oxygenation (ECMO) for cardiopulmonary dysfunction

Despite treatment, mortality rates are 50%, and children who survive may have emphysema, with larger volume but inadequate numbers of alveoli.

Hirschsprung's Disease

Hirschsprung's disease (congenital aganglionic megacolon) is failure of **ganglion nerve cells** to migrate to part of the bowel, usually the distal colon, so that part of the bowel lacks enervation and peristalsis, causing stool to accumulate, leading to **distention** and **megacolon**. There is a genetic predisposition to the disease that affects more males than females and is associated with trisomy 21 (Down syndrome).

Symptoms include:

- Failure to pass meconium in 24 to 48 hours
- Poor feeding
- Bilious vomitus
- Abdominal distention

Delayed diagnosis is based on the following:

- Chronic constipation
- Failure to thrive
- Periods of diarrhea and vomiting
- With infection—severe prostration, watery diarrhea, fever, and hypotension

Treatment includes:

- Resection aganglionic section and perform colorectal anastomosis.
- There are a number of procedures—Swenson, Duhamel, and Soave—but recently, minimally invasive laparoscopic or transanal approaches have proven successful.

Short Bowel Syndrome

The neonate's small bowel is approximately 250 cm long. Most absorption of nutrients and vitamins takes place in the first 100 to 150 cm of the jejunum while the ileum absorbs vitamin B_{12} and bile acids. Infants with less than 100 cm of jejunum after surgical removal have significant malabsorption and require aggressive nutritional support. Infants with **short bowel syndrome** (SBS) have diarrhea, steatorrhea, bloating, anemia, electrolyte imbalances, malnutrition, and poor weight gain secondary to decreased absorption of nutrients and vitamins. The severity and exact nature of their symptoms depends on the amount and type of bowel that has been removed. Removal of significant portions of the ileum results in steatorrhea and poor absorption of fat-soluble vitamins (K, A, D, E) and vitamin B_{12}. Removal of significant portions of the jejunum results in poor absorption of calories, proteins, carbohydrates, and fats. Infants require carefully monitoring of serum electrolytes, multivitamins, and a combination of parenteral and enteral nutrition. Over time, the small bowel adapts, increases its absorption, and grows in length.

Cystic Fibrosis and Meconium Ileus

Cystic fibrosis is a congenital disease associated with collection of thick mucus in the **lungs and intestines**. **Meconium ileus** is obstruction of the **ileum** with inspissated (thick) mucilaginous meconium that clings to the side of the narrowed lumen of the intestine and forms hard pellets (usually the first clinical sign of cystic fibrosis). The mucus interferes with absorption of fat, protein, carbohydrates, and other nutrients, leading to malabsorption syndromes. *Diagnosis* is by abdominal x-rays to show air-to- fluid levels and contrast enemas to show obstruction.

Symptoms include:

- *Uncomplicated*: abdominal distention, vomiting, no meconium in first 24 to 48 hours
- *Complicated* (may include volvulus, gangrene, perforations, or bowel atresia): pain, fever, erythema and edema of abdominal wall consistent with peritonitis

Treatment includes:

- Contrast enema with water-soluble contrast (may relieve obstruction by emulsifying fecal material)
- 10 to15cc small volume enemas to flush stool, especially after contrast enema
- Enterotomy, with proximal instillation of wetting agent
- Resection of colon/fecal diversion for perforated or gangrenous bowel
- High protein diet with pancreatic enzyme supplementation

Malrotation/Volvulus

When the intestines return to the abdominal cavity during the tenth to twelfth week of fetal development, they undergo a rotation into their anatomically correct position. Sometimes this rotation fails, and the result is a malrotation. **Malrotation** is a congenital defect in which the intestines are attached to the back of the abdominal wall by one single attachment, rather than a broad band of attachments across the abdomen, essentially suspending the bowels so they can easily twist, resulting in a **volvulus** (twisted bowel), cutting off blood supply. It may untwist, but can lead to **bowel infarction.** Some children with malrotation have **no symptoms**, but most develop some of these *symptoms* by 1 year:

- Cycles of cramping pain about every 15 to 30 minutes
- Abdominal distention
- Diarrhea, bloody stools, or no stools
- Vomiting, occurring soon after crying begins, usually indicating small intestine obstruction; later vomiting usually indicative of large intestine blockage
- Tachycardia and tachypnea
- Decreased urinary output
- Fever

Treatment is by surgical repair.

Gastroschisis

Gastroschisis is extrusion of the non-rotated midgut through the abdominal wall to the right of umbilicus with no protective membrane covering matted, thickened loops of intestine. The abnormality is usually small, but the stomach and almost all of the small and large intestines can protrude. Because the intestines float without protection in amniotic fluid, there may be severe damage to the intestines with bowel atresia and ischemia. Gastroschisis is usually diagnosed with fetal ultrasound and is obvious at birth. These infants lose body temperature, fluids, and electrolytes and receive intravenous fluids. The exposed organs are covered with sterile plastic film for protection and to prevent fluid loss and a naso-gastric feeding tube is inserted. Primary closure is done when infant stabilizes for small abnormalities. Larger abnormalities may require stages with only part of organs returned to cavity and the remaining covered with a Silastic pouch until the abdominal cavity grows and surgical repair can be completed.

Omphalocele

Omphalocele is a congenital herniation of intestines or other organs through the base of the umbilicus with a protecting amniotic membrane but no skin. The sac may contain only a loop or most of bowel and the internal abdominal organs. This sac differentiates gastroschisis from omphalocele. *Diagnosis* is usually with fetal ultrasound.

Symptoms vary widely. Maintaining integrity of tissues by keeping exposed sac or viscera moist and providing intravenous fluids is important. Small omphaloceles are repaired immediately, but more extensive repair is usually delayed until infant is stable if sac is intact. Silvadene® cream toughens the sac, which is usually covered with a silastic (plastic) pouch to protect the tissue. The abdomen may be unusually small, making correction difficult, so surgeons may wait 6-12 months while the abdominal cavity grows. Surgical repair may be done in stages over 8-10 days.

Gastroesophageal Reflux

Gastroesophageal reflux (GER) is involuntary regurgitation of stomach contents into the esophagus, usually caused by decreased tone in the lower esophageal sphincter in neonates, especially preterm.

Symptoms include:

- Frequent non-bilious regurgitation (especially after feeding, usually not associated with respiratory distress).
- Some neonates may have colicky symptoms, and some may cough, choke, wheeze or have periods of apnea.

Treatment includes:

- **Regulating feeding:** Small more frequent amounts, thickened with rice cereal. Continuous gavage rather than bolus may reduce reflux.
- **Positioning:** Prone positioning after feeding/eating reduces regurgitation (although some concern remains about SIDS with neonates). Placing neonate in an upright position (avoiding slumping) after meals or carrying the neonate upright can help but placing in infant seat position may increase intraabdominal pressure.
- **Medications:** Histamine-2 receptor blockers (ranitidine) or proton pump inhibitor (omeprazole), prokinetic agent (metoclopramide) and/or antacids (without aluminum).
- **Surgery:** Considered for severe or life-threatening symptoms.

Neurological

Neonatal Seizures

Causes

Causes of **neonatal seizures** are listed below in order of frequency:

- Hypoxic ischemic encephalopathy after a difficult or traumatic delivery
- Metabolic abnormality:
  - Low levels of glucose, calcium, or magnesium
  - Elevated or low levels of sodium
- Infections:
  - Bacterial meningitis caused by Group B strep, *E. coli, S. pneumoniae*, or Listeria
  - Viral encephalitis caused by herpes simplex, cytomegalovirus, or enterovirus
- Cerebrovascular accidents:
  - Intraventricular hemorrhage
  - Subarachnoid hemorrhage
  - Subdural hematoma
  - Sinus thrombosis
- Seizure syndromes:
  - Epileptic encephalopathies (early myoclonic or early infantile)
  - Benign neonatal seizure syndromes, such as benign familial neonatal convulsions, benign idiopathic neonatal seizures, or benign sleep myoclonus

Types

Seizures indicate an abnormality of the central nervous system and are differentiated by their associated abnormal movements.

- **Subtle seizures** are more common in full term infants, who present with feet pedaling, chewing, apnea, eye movements, or a blank stare.
- **Tonic seizures** are more common in preterm infants, who present with tonic flexion or extension of the limbs, which may be focal (one limb) or generalized.
- **Clonic seizures** occur primarily in full term infants, indicate a focal cerebral injury, and involve slow, clonic movements (1 to 3 movements per second), often in one extremity or on one side of the body.
- **Myoclonic seizures** are rare in neonates, and may be focal, multi-focal, or generalized, with rapid jerking movements of the extremities.

Treatment depends upon identifying underlying cause but may include glucose (if related to hypoglycemia), phenobarbital (drug of choice), fosphenytoin, and phenytoin.

Review Video: Seizures
Visit mometrix.com/academy and enter code: 977061

Initial Management

Seizures in the neonate require immediate treatment to avoid brain injury from hypoxia and hypoglycemia:

- Glucose (10% solution) if indicated for hypoglycemia with bolus 2ml/kg and maintenance ≤8ml/kg.
- Provide supplemental oxygen and ventilation.
- Give a loading dose of Phenobarbital (20 mg/kg IV); if the initial loading dose is ineffective, give an additional 10 to 20 mg/kg IV.
- Draw STAT blood glucose and electrolyte levels.
- Correct electrolyte abnormalities such as low calcium, magnesium, and sodium.
- Give a maintenance dose of 4 mg to 6 mg/kg of Phenobarbital IV every 12 to 24 hours.
- Monitor blood pressure and respiratory status frequently, because large doses of Phenobarbital cause respiratory and cardiac depression.
- Give fosphenytoin, phenytoin, and lorazepam per order if seizures uncontrolled.

Jitteriness

Jitteriness (tremor of chin and extremities) occurs in about half of neonates within the first few days of life and may persist intermittently when the child is excited or crying for ≤2 months. Jitteriness may also be present with drug withdrawal, hypoglycemia, hypocalcemia, and encephalopathy. Jitteriness must be differentiated from seizures, which may have a similar appearance. Characteristics of jitteriness include:

- Lack of ocular deviations or other abnormalities.
- Gentle restraint halts jitteriness.
- Stimulation elicits jitteriness.
- Clonic jerking has both fast and slow elements.
- Autonomic changes involving the heart rate, respirations, and blood pressure are not present.
- EEG is normal.

Jitteriness is distinct from shuddering, a 10-15 second period of fast tremors that may recur ≤100 times daily. Both jitteriness and shuddering are benign conditions that require no treatment.

Subarachnoid Hemorrhage

Subarachnoid hemorrhage is a common injury after trauma and may result from childbirth (one of the most common causes) or from abuse (shaken impact syndrome) along with subdural hematoma. In some cases, no symptoms are evident. The first presenting *symptom* in infants may be seizures, usually on day 2, with the infant appearing normal between episodes of seizures. Seizures are most common in full-term infants, while preterm infants often experience recurrent episodes of apnea. Symptoms will worsen as intracranial pressure rises. *Diagnosis* is per CT scan and lumbar puncture (bloody CSF). Subarachnoid hemorrhage is usually self-limited and requires only supportive care. *Treatment* includes:

- Identifying and treating underlying cause
- Anti-seizure medications
- Antihypertensives
- Surgical repair, if indicated

Epidural Hemorrhage

Hemorrhage is always a concern with head trauma, because even injuries that appear slight can result in vascular rupture, resulting in hemorrhage between the skull and the brain. **Epidural hemorrhage** is bleeding between the dura and the skull, pushing the brain downward and inward. The hemorrhage is usually caused by **arterial tears**, so bleeding is often rapid, leading to severe neurological deficits and respiratory arrest. Initially, the body compensates by rapidly absorbing cerebrospinal fluid and decreasing blood flow, but the compensatory measure is soon overwhelmed. The most common site is the **parietotemporal region**, forcing the medial part of the temporal lobe under the tentorial edge, compressing nerves and vessels. Epidural hemorrhage related to birth trauma is rare, and small hemorrhages may be treated conservatively, but larger hemorrhages require surgical evacuation. *Diagnosis* in neonates is often delayed because of nonspecific symptoms.

Subdural and Subarachnoid Cranial Hemorrhages

Subdural hemorrhage between the dura and the cerebrum, usually from tears in the cortical veins of the subdural space, tends to develop more slowly and can result in a subdural hematoma. If the bleeding is acute and develops within minutes or hours of injury, the prognosis is poor. Subacute hematomas that develop more slowly cause varying degrees of injury. Subdural hemorrhage is a common injury related to birth trauma and child abuse although it can result from coagulopathies or aneurysms. Symptoms of acute injury may occur within 24-48 hours, but subacute bleeding may not be evident for up to 2 weeks after injury. Symptoms may include bradycardia, tachycardia, hypertension, and alterations in consciousness. Subdural taps may suffice for infants, but some infants will require surgical evacuation of the hematoma.

Subarachnoid hemorrhage may result from the childbirth (one of the most common causes) or from shaken impact syndrome. The presenting symptom may be seizures, and other symptoms are similar to those of subdural hematoma. Symptoms worsen as ICP rises.

Intraventricular Hemorrhage

Grading

Intraventricular hemorrhages (IVH) are common in premature neonates less than 32 weeks estimated gestational age. 50% of IVH occur on the first day of life. 90% of cases present within the first three days of life. Depending on the amount and location of bleeding seen on cranial ultrasound, IVH are graded as follows:

	Anatomy	**Severity**
Grade I	The hemorrhage is limited to the germinal matrix (subependymal region).	Mild (5% death rate; 5% motor or cognitive impairment).
Grade II	The hemorrhage extends 10% to 40% into the lateral ventricles on sagittal view, but has not dilated them significantly.	Moderate (10% death rate; 30% to 40% motor or cognitive impairment).
Grade III	The hemorrhage extends 50% or more into the lateral ventricles with significant ventricular dilation.	Severe (27% to 50% death rate; 35% motor or cognitive impairment).
Grade IV	The hemorrhage extends into brain tissue.	Periventricular hemorrhagic infarction (80% death rate; 90% motor or cognitive impairment).

Clinical Presentation in Infants

Intraventricular hemorrhage (IVH) presents within the first 72 hours of life in 90% of affected neonates. 50% of infants less than 35 weeks' gestational age or who weigh less than 1,500 grams have IVH. The rate is declining due to improvements in obstetrical care, nursing management of fluids and respiration.

IVH Category	Signs
Asymptomatic	25%-50% of IVH infants are asymptomatic, or have only a fall in hematocrit and anemia, but ultrasound demonstrates an IVH.
Saltatory	Infants are pale or ashen, and have gradual neurological deterioration (attention, movements, level of consciousness, eye movements).
Catastrophic	Acute onset of decreased level of consciousness, bulging fontanel, cranial nerve abnormalities, decerebrate posturing, and hypotension with drop in hematocrit.

The pediatrician orders with extreme caution: Indocin 0.1 mg/kg/dose IV when the baby is 6 hours old, and 24 hours old, and 48 hours old, **or** Diamox 5 mg/kg/dose PO or IV every 6 hours, which is increased by 25 mg/kg/d (not to exceed 100 mg/kg/d) to suppress CSF production.

Neural Tube Defects

Neural tube defects (NTD) are a spectrum of congenital disorders involving the **meninges** covering the spinal cord. The neural tube is the embryonic structure that eventually forms the brain and spinal cord. Mild forms are asymptomatic. Severe cases are incompatible with life. *Diagnosis* is often made in pregnancy by ultrasound, or by an elevated level of alpha-fetoprotein in the amniotic fluid or in the mother's serum. Causes are multifactorial, with both genetic and environmental components. *Risk factors* for NTD include:

- Diet lacking in folic acid
- Family history of an NTD in a parent or sibling
- Maternal obesity with poorly controlled diabetes
- Maternal use of valproic acid or carbamazepine during pregnancy
- Increasing core temperature 3° to 4 °F (2 °C) through saunas, hot tubs, or fever

Studies have shown that if the mother ingests 400 micrograms of folic acid daily before and during pregnancy, it protects the fetus from developing an NTD.

TYPES

The **neural tube defects**, spina bifida and myelomeningocele, are often used interchangeably, but there is a distinction. Spina bifida is a neural tube defect with an incomplete spinal cord and often missing vertebrae that allow the meninges and spinal cord to protrude through the opening. There are **5 basic types**:

- **Spina bifida***:* Defect in which the vertebral column is not closed with varying degrees of herniation through the opening.
- **Spina bifida occulta***:* Failure of the vertebral column to close, but no herniation through the opening so the defect may not be obvious.
- **Spina bifida cystica**: Defect in closure with external sac-like protrusion with varying degrees of nerve involvement.
- **Meningocele:** Spina bifida cystica with meningeal sac filled with spinal fluid.
- **Myelomeningocele**: Spina bifida cystica with meningeal sac containing spinal fluid and part of the spinal cord and nerves.

MYELOMENINGOCELE

Myelomeningocele, which involves spina bifida cystica with a meningeal sac containing spinal fluid and part of the spinal cord and nerves, comprises about 75% of the total cases of spina bifida. There are numerous physical manifestations.

- **Exposed sac** poses the danger of infection and cerebrospinal fluid leakage; so surgical repair is usually done within the first 48 hours although it may be delayed for a few days, especially if the sac is intact.
- **Chiari type II malformation** comprises hypoplasia of the cerebellum and displacement of the lower brainstem into the upper cervical area, which impairs circulation of spinal fluid. It may result in symptoms of cranial nerve dysfunction (dysphonia, dysphagia) and weakness and lack of coordination of upper extremities.
- **Neurogenic bladder** is common and may require credé massage for infants and later intermittent clean catheterization.
- **Fecal incontinence** is common and is controlled, as the child gets older, with diet and bowel training. (Continued)
- **Musculoskeletal abnormalities** depend upon the level of the myelomeningocele and the degree of impairment but often involve the muscle and joints of the lower extremities and sometimes the upper. Dysfunction often increases with the number of shunts. Scoliosis and lumbar lordosis are common. Hip contractures may cause dislocations.
- **Paralysis/paresis** may vary considerably and be spastic or flaccid. Many children require wheelchairs for mobility although some are fitted with braces for assisted ambulation.
- **Seizures** occur in about a quarter of those affected, sometimes related to shunt malfunction.
- **Hydrocephalus** is present in about 25-35% of infants at birth and 60-70% after surgical repair with ventriculoperitoneal shunt. Untreated, the ventricles will dilate and brain damage can occur.
- **Tethered spinal cord** occurs when the distal end of the spinal cord becomes attached to the bone or site of surgical repair and does not move superiorly with growth, causing increased pain, spasticity, and disability and requiring surgical repair.

ANENCEPHALY

Anencephaly is a neural tube defect in which the **embryological neural tube**, which forms the brain and spinal cord, fails to close at the **cephalic (head) end**, resulting in an infant without most of the brain, skull, or scalp, so that the top of the head is open. The eyes bulge foreword. Because the forebrain is missing, the child has no cognitive ability or sensation of pain. A rudimentary brain stem may be present, supporting reflexive breathing and cardiac function, but the child's condition is not compatible with life. Most are stillborn, and others live a few hours or days. There is no *treatment* possible other than supportive care until death. The condition is often diagnosed with ultrasound. An ethical dilemma exists about the use of these infants' organs for donation with some authorities believing that viable organs should be harvested before brain death.

Encephalocele

Encephalocele is a neural defect that involves a bony defect and herniation of the brain and/or cerebrospinal fluid through part of the skull in a skin-covered sac. In the United States, most commonly the mass is midline in the occipital and occasionally the frontal area. The encephalocele may be as large as the skull or may look like a small nasal polyp. In many cases, other abnormalities may exist, so thorough examination, including angiography and MRI are usually required. Often, the part of the brain that herniates is disorganized, so the condition may be associated with cognitive impairment although in mild cases the child has normal mentation. Surgical repair to place the herniated mass inside the skull and to repair the bony defect is the standard treatment. If the sac is left in place, the skin can erode, resulting in meningitis.

Hematologic

Anemia of Prematurity

Anemia of prematurity (AOP) represents a pathologic exaggeration of the normal decrease in hematocrit that occurs in every newborn. AOP results from a combination of factors:

- **RBC production** decreases because the premature neonate's response to erythropoietin (EPO) has not matured. EPO is the main stimulus for RBC production. The normal progression of EPO production in the fetus is for the liver to initially be the primary site, with transfer to the kidney as the primary site of production in the full-term neonate. The liver is less responsive to hypoxia, and allows for a lower threshold of anemia to progress until EPO production is increased. Lowest Hgb levels are usually at 2-3 months of age.
- **Premature RBCs have a shortened lifespan** when compared to the full-term neonate's because of decreased levels of intracellular ATP and enzyme activity.
- **Frequent blood draws** in premature neonates required for close monitoring deplete the blood supply.

Infants with signs of hypoxemia (poor feeling, tachypnea, tachycardia, pallor) may require transfusions.

Blood-Loss Anemia

Blood loss is the most common cause of **anemia** in the neonate. Anemia is hematocrit or hemoglobin level >2 standard deviations below the mean for age. For a term infant, anemia is a hematocrit <45%. The loss of blood may be internal or external, and may occur in utero, during delivery, or post-delivery. *Treatment* may include packed red blood cell transfusions. Common *causes* of neonatal blood loss include:

Antenatal	Abruptio placentae; Placenta previa Fetomaternal transfusion (passage of fetal blood to the mother) Twin-to-twin transfusion, resulting in one twin with polycythemia and the donor twin with anemia
Perinatal	Trauma to the placenta or umbilical cord Rupture of anomalous cord vessels Fetoplacental transfusion that occurs when the infant is positioned above the level of the placenta after delivery
Postnatal	Internal hemorrhage, such as intracranial hemorrhage or cephalohematoma Damage to internal organs, such as the adrenal gland or liver Iatrogenic blood loss secondary to frequent laboratory sampling, a major cause of anemia in premature infants

Causes of Anemia of Red Blood Cell Destruction

Intrinsic causes – Continued production of abnormal red blood cells that have a decreased survival time because of rare hereditary disorders:

- **RBC enzyme defects,** such as G6PD deficiency, where hemolytic crisis occurs in response to drugs such as sulfonamide antibiotics, or infections.
- **RBC membrane defects,** such as hereditary spherocytosis, where abnormally-shaped red cells are prone to hemolysis.
- **Hemoglobinopathies,** such as thalassemia, which results in the reduced production of one of the protein chains that make up hemoglobin.

Extrinsic causes – Temporary RBC destruction caused by some external stimulus:

- **Immune hemolysis** from transfusion of an incompatible blood product (wrong Rh, ABO, or a minor blood group incompatibility)
- **Acquired hemolysis** from infection, vitamin E deficiency, or poisoning

Vitamin K Deficiency

Vitamin K deficiency in newborns may cause vitamin K deficiency bleeding (VKDB), also called **hemorrhagic disease of the newborn**. Vitamin K is a fat-soluble vitamin produced in the gut. Vitamin K is required by the liver to produce four of the clotting factors—II, VII, IX, and X. At birth, all infants are Vitamin K deficient because of limited transfer of vitamin K across the placenta. Newborns are injected with intramuscular vitamin K just after birth. The injection quickly raises the infant's vitamin K level to normal and maintains the normal level for several months. Infants who do not receive vitamin K prophylaxis at birth will take several weeks (formula fed) to several months (breast fed) to attain normal vitamin K levels. Formula contains higher levels of vitamin K than human milk. VKDB occurs in two forms:

- **Early onset form** occurs within the first 24 hours after birth, and is related to maternal medications that interfere with Vitamin K.
- **Late onset form** occurs after two weeks of age, because of exclusive breastfeeding, diarrhea, hepatitis, cystic fibrosis, alpha 1-antitrypsin disease, or celiac disease.

Hyperbilirubinemia

Hyperbilirubinemia, excess of bilirubin in the blood, is characterized by jaundice. Hyperbilirubinemia is evaluated according to the levels of direct (conjugated) bilirubin and/or indirect (unconjugated) bilirubin:

- **Direct/conjugated bilirubin** levels increase with blockage of bile ducts, hepatitis or other liver damage, including drug reaction.
- **Indirect/unconjugated bilirubin** levels increase with anemias (such as hemolytic disorders) and transfusion reactions.

Four basic types of hyperbilirubinemia and jaundice:

- **Physiologic**: Common in newborns and usually benign, resulting from immature hepatic function and increased RBC hemolysis. Infants have larger red blood cells with a shorter life than adults, leading to more RBC destruction and resulting in an increased load of serum bilirubin, which the liver of the newborn cannot handle. Premature infants have an even greater physiologic jaundice as their RBCs live even shorter lives than the term infant's. Onset is usually within 24-48 hours, peaking in 72 hours for full term or 5 days for preterm infants and declining within a week. Phototherapy is the indicated treatment. (Continued)
- **Hemolytic**: Caused by blood/antigen (Rh) incompatibility with onset in first 24 hours. Preventive treatment is RhoGAM® prenatally or post-natal exchange transfusion. This type of hyperbilirubinemia may also result from ABO incompatibility, but rarely requires treatment other than phototherapy.
- **Breastfeeding associated***:* Relates to inadequate calories during early breastfeeding with onset on 2-3 days. This slows the excretion of stool and allows bilirubin levels to rise. More frequent feeding with caloric supplements is usually sufficient, but phototherapy may be used for bilirubin 18-20 mg/dl.
- **Breast milk jaundice***:* May result from human milk breaking down bilirubin and its being reabsorbed in the gut. Characterized by less frequent stools and onset in 4-5th day, peaking in 10-15 days, but jaundice may persist for a number of weeks. Treatment involves discontinuing breastfeeding for 24 hours.

Indications for Phototherapy and Exchange Transfusion

Phototherapy is often used to treat hyperbilirubinemia to prevent the need for exchange transfusion. For phototherapy, the infant is placed under special lights (15 to 20 cm above the infant) that will decrease the **bilirubin levels** in the blood. Indications include

Weight	Serum bilirubin level
500 to 750 g	5 to 8 mg/dL
751 to 1000 g	6 to 10 mg/dL
1001 to 1250 g	8 to 10 mg/dL
1251 to 1500 g	10 to 12 mg dL

Exchange transfusions may be used for hyperbilirubinemia. Blood <72 hours old is used to maintain potassium levels. Indications include

Weight	Serum bilirubin level
500 to 750 g	12 to 15 mg/dL
751 to 1000 g	>15 mg/dL
1001 to 1250 g	15 to18 mg/dL
1251 to 1500 g	17 to 20 mg/dL

There are many risks associated with exchange transfusions, including vascular complications, such as emboli or thrombosis, often related to umbilical catheters. Cardiac complications include dysrhythmias and overload, leading to arrest. Clotting disorders may result from over-heparinization (reversed with protamine sulfate). Electrolyte and glucose abnormalities as well as infection may occur.

Polycythemia

Risk Factors

Polycythemia occurs in 4% of live born infants. Its etiologies are divided into conditions that cause hypoxia and increased red blood cell (RBC) production and those that cause abnormal transfer of RBCs to the neonate (hypertransfusion):

- **Hypoxia**
  - Disorders that disrupt normal placental function and decrease oxygen delivery to the fetus include preeclampsia, chronic placental abruption, maternal congenital heart disease, postdate pregnancy, and maternal smoking. Many of these are also associated with a growth-restricted neonate (IUGR).
  - Disorders that cause increased oxygen consumption by the fetus include infants of diabetic mothers and those with Beckwith-Wiedemann syndrome. Polycythemia occurs in 30 to 40% of neonates born to mothers with diabetes.
- **Hypertransfusion**
  - Delay in clamping the umbilical cord during delivery allows for increased blood volume to be transferred to the neonate.
  - Twin-twin transfusion creates one twin who is anemic and the second twin with an increased hematocrit in 10% of monozygotic twin pregnancies.

Clinical Signs

Polycythemia is a hematocrit greater than 65%. An elevated hematocrit means that the blood has less plasma and more cellular elements, increasing the viscosity of the blood. Increased blood viscosity results in slowed blood flow and sludging of red blood cells. Small vessels become occluded with microthrombi, resulting in tissue or organ ischemia. Clinical signs of polycythemia include:

- **Dermatologic**: Plethora and increased capillary refill time.
- **CNS**: Lethargy, irritability, abnormal cry, cerebrovascular hemorrhage, and seizures.
- **Pulmonary**: Respiratory distress, cyanosis, apnea, and the development of persistent pulmonary hypertension.
- **Renal**: Hematuria, oliguria, and renal vein thrombosis.
- **Hematological**: Thrombocytopenia secondary to the development of disseminated intravascular coagulation.
- **Gastrointestinal**: Abdominal distension, poor feeding, bloody stools, and necrotizing enterocolitis.
- **Metabolic**: Persistent hypoglycemia and hypocalcemia.

Exchange Transfusions

The infant with polycythemia requires a **partial exchange transfusion** with a plasma substitute in these situations:

- The hematocrit (Hct) is greater than 65%, and the infant is symptomatic.
- The hematocrit is greater than 70%, regardless of symptoms.

Aliquots of the neonate's blood are replaced with isotonic saline to lower the hematocrit to between 50% and 55%. This formula calculates the volume of blood to be exchanged with an equal volume of saline:

$$\text{Exchange vol (mL)} = \frac{\text{initial Hct} - \text{desired Hct}}{\text{initial Hct}} \times \text{weight(kg)} \times 90\,\frac{\text{mL}}{\text{kg}}$$

The procedure is as follows:

- Withdraw no more than 5 mL of blood at a time from the umbilical artery or vein over 2 to 3 minutes.
- Slowly infuse an equal amount of sterile normal saline.
- Repeat the exchange until the desired volume of fluid is swapped.
- Monitor the infant closely during the procedure.
- Measure the hematocrit post procedure.

THROMBOCYTOPENIA

Thrombocytopenia is a platelet count less than 150,000/mcL, caused either by decreased platelet production, increased platelet destruction, or a combination of both. The Hematology lab uses **mean platelet volume (MPV),** a measure of the average platelet size, to differentiate the two. The MPV is normal if the cause is reduced production and elevated if the cause is accelerated destruction. Immature platelets are larger than normal and are released into circulating blood by the bone marrow when mature platelets are being destroyed. The lab may also differentiate the cause by a **retic count** (reticulated platelets are newly-produced platelets). If the retic count is elevated, then platelets are being destroyed, and if it is low, the production of platelets is suppressed. General guidelines for transfusing platelets depend on the clinical stability of the neonate. If the infant is stable, the attending physician considers a transfusion when the count is less than 25,000/mcL. If the infant is unstable, the attending physician considers a transfusion when the count is less than 50,000/mcL.

FETAL ONSET, EARLY ONSET, AND LATE ONSET

Causes of fetal onset include:

- Alloimmune thrombocytopenia: The mother produces antibodies specific to antigens on the neonate's platelets, which cross the placenta, causing thrombocytopenia.
- Autoimmune thrombocytopenia: Mothers with idiopathic thrombocytopenia purpura or lupus produce antibodies against fetal platelets.
- Congenital infection- mediated: CMV, rubella, toxoplasmosis. Neonates with trisomy 13 or 21.

Causes of early onset (<72 hours) are as follows:

- Placental insufficiency occurs in infants who are small for gestational age or with intrauterine growth restriction.
- Perinatal asphyxia.
- Disseminated intravascular coagulation (DIC).

Causes of late onset (>72 hours) include:

- Late onset sepsis.
- Necrotizing enterocolitis.

Jaundice

Jaundice is yellowing of the skin and sclera (eye whites), indicating elevated bilirubin levels (hyperbilirubinemia). **Elevated bilirubin levels** occur normally during the newborn period because of the rapid breakdown of fetal hemoglobin after birth and the immaturity of enzymatic pathways in the newborn's liver, the organ responsible for metabolizing bilirubin. Physiological jaundice describes this normal process, which usually becomes evident on the second or third day of life by yellowing of the face. As bilirubin levels increase, the trunk and extremities become involved and the skin yellows. The baby's eyes are covered, and the baby is placed in under blue lights (phototherapy). For most infants, jaundice is transient and resolves within a few days. Persistent or pronounced jaundice may indicate that further diagnostic testing or intervention is needed.

G6PD Deficiency

Glucose-6-phosphate dehydrogenase (G6PD) deficiency is an X-linked recessive disease and can often present as or similar to hyperbilirubinemia. Because female infants inherit two X chromosomes, it's rare that both are defective, and the normal chromosome compensates, so X-linked recessive disorders affect primarily male children (who get the X chromosome from the mother, not the father) but are passed on by the mother. G6PD is an enzyme utilized to process carbohydrates and to protect red blood cells. G6PD results in premature destruction or red blood cells and hemolytic anemia, which can be triggered by infection, some medications (antimalarial drugs, sulfa, ASAS, NSAIDS, quinidine, quinine, and nitrofurantoin), and eating or inhaling the pollen of fava beans (favism). Infants may be asymptomatic although some may exhibit increased jaundice. In the United States, G6PD is most common in African American males (1 out of 10) and those with Middle Eastern heritage. Treatment includes avoiding triggers, treating infections, and transfusions if necessary.

Infectious Diseases

Neonatal Sepsis

Neonatal sepsis is a particular risk for preterm infants <1000 g and may be associated with a wide range of pathogens, both bacterial and viral. **Early onset** (≤72 hours) is usually related to maternal transmission and **late onset** (4 to 90 days) to invasive devices. Early onset sepsis most often is characterized by pneumonia, and late onset by bacteremia and/or meningitis.

Symptoms vary according to pathogen, onset, and primary site of infection:

- Non-specific signs of respiratory distress, CNS irritation, and metabolic disorders
- Pneumonia: tachypnea, sternal retraction, grunting respirations, cyanosis, and apneic periods.
- Meningitis: stupor, irritability, indications of increasing ICP, bulging anterior fontanel; may be subtle in the neonate
- Decreased cardiac output with pulmonary hypertension; signs of shock
- Hypoglycemia or hyperglycemia; metabolic acidosis
- Jaundice
- DIC
- Necrotizing enterocolitis

Laboratory Findings and Treatment

Laboratory findings (vary):

- Chest radiograph may show pneumonia.
- CT/MRI may show abscesses or obstructive hydrocephalus.
- Ultrasound may show abnormalities of ventricles and brain structures (meningitis).
- Thrombocytopenia is <100,000 μL.
- WBC counts may not be elevated and may not show shift to left, especially initially.
- Immature to total neutrophil ratio is increased.
- Clotting abnormalities may be found (with DIC).
- Culture and sensitivities may not show infection because of small sample size.
- CSF: WBC count and protein level are elevated and positive culture (with meningitis).
- C-reactive protein is increased.

Treatment includes:

- Intravenous antibiotics: aminoglycoside and expanded- spectrum penicillin most commonly; vancomycin or oxacillin, at times, for hospital-acquired infection
- Surgical I &D of abscess
- Ventriculoperitoneal shunt for hydronephrosis related to meningitis
- NPO initially and then enteral feedings or TPN
- Thermoregulation as indicated (radiant warmer, incubator)
- Maintenance of fluid balance and IV fluids as needed
- Intubation/ventilation as needed

Immature-to-total Neutrophil Ration (I:T)

The immature-to-total neutrophil ratio (I:T) is part of the **white blood cell differential**. The ratio of immature neutrophils to the number of total neutrophils can indicate a "left shift" (usually an I:T ratio ≥0.2) and can be used as an early indicator for **neonatal sepsis,** though not absolutely diagnostic. It is especially useful in ruling out sepsis, but according to recent studies, an elevated I:T ratio is not always indicative of infection, and therefore should be interpreted in conjunction with other indicators of sepsis. An I:T ratio of greater than 0.3 suggests the infant may have an infection. The calculation for I:T ratio is:

$$\frac{\text{Immature neutrophils (bands)}}{\text{Total neutrophils (segs and bands)}}$$

The I:T ratio is usually considered along with the **absolute neutrophil count (ANC)** as neutropenia is frequently associated with neonatal sepsis. A normal I:T ratio for the first 12 hours is less than 0.16. This decreases by 24 to 72 hours to less than 0.13. The normal ANC varies from 1800 to 5400 at birth to 7800 to 14,400 at 12 hours, 7200 to 12,600 at 24 hours, and 1800 to 7000 at 72 hours.

Lumbar Puncture Procedure

Lumbar puncture in a neonate is primarily for **sepsis evaluation** and when **CNS infection**, such as meningitis, or **bleeding** is suspected. Resuscitation equipment should be available and cardiorespiratory status and oxygen saturation monitored during the procedure. The infant should receive oral sucrose and/or other analgesia. The nurse places the infant in lateral position with trunk flexed (although excessive flexion must be avoided) or (if term) in sitting position. The lumbar puncture is done with sterile technique. The CSF is usually collected in two tubes with at least 10 drops in each and pressure measured. The specimen should be inspected for signs of pus or blood (which could indicate hemorrhage). Following the procedure, the infant should be kept flat for at least 60 minutes and cardiorespiratory and oxygen saturation continuously monitored during that period. If the infant received narcotic sedation, monitoring should continue for 4 hours and the infant remain NPO for 2 hours. Contraindications include hypotension, respiratory insufficiency, increased intracranial pressure, and abnormalities of spinal column.

Varicella Zoster

Chicken pox, caused by the **varicella zoster virus,** during the first 20 weeks of pregnancy can result in as infant with congenital varicella syndrome, which can cause a number of abnormalities of the skin, extremities, eyes, and central nervous system. Children are often unusually small with distinctive cicatrix scarring on the skin, and chorioretinitis. Brain abnormalities may include microcephaly, hydrocephalus, cortical atrophy, enlargement of the ventricles, and damage to the sympathetic nervous system. The child may suffer intellectual disabilities and developmental delays as well as lack of psychomotor coordination. If the mother is infected at the end of pregnancy and develops a rash from 5 days before to 2 days after delivery, the child may develop neonatal varicella, which poses of high risk to the child with mortality rates of about 30%. Vaccination prior to pregnancy is the best preventive. Premature neonates exposed after birth with ≤28 weeks gestation or ≥28 weeks if mother has no immunity should receive varicella zoster immunoglobulin (VZIG).

Fetal Exposure to Hepatitis

Routine screening of all pregnant women and all newborns helps to identify those infected with **Hepatitis B virus**. Infants are routinely immunized at discharge from hospital, at 2 months and at 6 months of age. In the case of a premature infant, the immunization schedule is started when the infant weighs 2 kg or is 2 months old. If the mother is HVB positive, surface antigen treatment of that infant should include careful bathing (wearing gloves) to remove all maternal blood and body fluids. The infant should also receive an IM injection of the hepatitis B immunoglobulin within 12 hours of birth. This immunoglobulin treatment is up to 95% effective in preventing the development of the disease in the infant.

Hepatitis C is rarely transmitted to the fetus and of those infected about 75% clear the infection by 2 years.

Hepatitis E poses the greatest risk to the mother with a mortality of about 20% during pregnancy and increased risk of fetal complications and death.

Fetal Exposure to Group B Streptococcus

Group B *Streptococcus* (GBS) is the most common neonatal bacterial infection. Many women are asymptomatic carriers. Screening of all pregnant women occurs between 37+0 to 37+6 weeks of gestation followed by antibiotic treatment of the mother during labor can prevent neonatal infection. A mother needs at least 4 hours worth of antibiotic treatment for the infant to benefit. If an infant is born and the mother has not received the recommended treatment, the infant will often be treated with IV ampicillin and gentamicin for 10 to 14 days. If treatment is ineffective or impossible, the infant with a GBS infection that manifests in the first 24 hours after birth may develop pneumonia and/or meningitis, respiratory distress, floppiness, poor feeding, tachycardia, shock and seizures. An infant may be asymptomatic at birth but have late-onset infection occurring at around 7 to 10 days old. Late-onset infections (usually meningitis) are generally more serious than earlier onset, and survivors often have serious damage, such as intellectual disability, quadriplegia, blindness, deafness, uncontrollable seizures, and hydrocephalus.

Bacterial Meningitis

Bacterial meningitis is characterized by inflammation, exudate, WBC accumulation, and brain tissue damage. Predominate pathogens ≤1 month include *E. coli*, Group B streptococci, *Listeria monocytogenes,* and *Neisseria meningitidis*.

- **Early onset:** May exhibit signs of shock within 24 hours of birth with rapid progression of symptoms that include respiratory distress with episodes of apnea, hypotension, thermodysregulation, inconsolable crying, seizures, diarrhea, jaundice, and hepatomegaly.
- **Late onset:** Very nonspecific symptoms can include weight loss, hypo- or hyperthermia, jaundice, irritability, lethargy, irregular respirations with periods of apnea. More specific signs may include increasing signs of illness, difficulty feeding with loss of suck reflex, hypotonia, posturing, weak cry, seizures, and bulging fontanels (may be a late sign). Nuchal rigidity does not usually occur with neonates but may be a late sign.

Treatment includes antibiotic therapy as indicated according to cultures and sensitivities. Initial therapy usually includes ampicillin or penicillin G and an aminoglycoside. Treatment is monitored by examination of CSF with treatment usually for two weeks after CSF becomes sterile. Kernig's sign and Brudzinski's sign are generally absent in neonates.

Neonatal Infections Caused by Maternal STDs

Maternal **sexually-transmitted diseases** can cause infection in the neonate. Common STDs include:

- **Chlamydia**: Infants most commonly exhibit conjunctivitis.
- **Gonorrhea**: Infants exposed to *Neisseria gonorrhoeae* during vaginal delivery most commonly develop bilateral conjunctivitis (ophthalmia neonatorum) if left untreated. In some cases, disseminated gonococcal infection (DGI) can occur in infants.
- **Syphilis**: Infants may be asymptomatic, even with full system infection. Multiple system disorders and abnormalities can occur, including non-viral hepatitis with jaundice, hepatosplenomegaly, pseudoparalysis, pneumonitis, bone marrow failure, myocarditis, meningitis, anemia, edema associated with nephritic syndrome, and a rash on the palms of the hands and soles of the feet
- **Herpes**: Localized lesions may occur at 10-12 days. Disseminated infection may cause pneumonitis, hepatitis, and encephalitis.
- **HIV/AIDS:** Infants are asymptomatic at birth and may test falsely positive.
- **Trichomoniasis**: Infants may be born preterm and with low birth weight (<2500 g).

Sexually Transmitted Diseases

Chlamydia

Chlamydia is the most common sexually transmitted disease in the United States and can be passed on at the time of birth if the infant is delivered vaginally and comes into contact with contaminated vaginal secretions. The organism responsible for this infection is *Chlamydia trachomatis.* Because the mother infected with this organism is usually asymptomatic, preventive care for the newborn is essential. The usual infection site for the newborn is the eye, in the form of conjunctivitis. States now require all newborns be given a prophylactic dose of either erythromycin or tetracycline ointment in the eyes at birth to prevent this infection. While the antibiotic ointment stops the eye infection, a few infants exposed to the pathogen will develop pneumonitis and/or ear infection.

Neisseria Gonorrhoea

Neisseria gonorrhoeae infections are common and may result in recurrent infection, pelvic inflammatory disease (PID), chronic pain, and infertility. Women who become pregnant and have a history of gonorrhea with salpingitis are 7 to 10 times more likely to have an ectopic pregnancy. Signs of infection (dysuria and green foul-smelling discharge from the urethra and the vagina) may occur 3 to 5 days after contact. However, many women are asymptomatic, especially on initial infection, and may be unaware they have the infection while pregnant. Vaginal delivery increases risk to the neonate, but infection can occur with caesarean. Newborns usually develop conjunctivitis 2 to 5 days after birth. Infants exhibit bilateral purulent ocular discharge, edema of the eyelids, and chemosis (edema of conjunctiva). Without treatment, the infection can progress and may result in rupture of the globe and blindness. In rare cases, the neonate may develop sepsis or meningitis from untreated infection. However, routine prophylaxis (usually erythromycin ointment) to the neonate's eyes is an effective treatment.

Cytomegalovirus

Cytomegalovirus, a member of the herpes simplex virus group, can cause asymptomatic infection in women. Over 50% of women are seropositive and may have chronic infections that persist for years. Cytomegalovirus is the most common intrauterine viral infection. Cytomegalovirus can be transmitted placentally or cervically during delivery (infecting ≤2.5% of neonates) and can put the fetus at high risk with death rates of 20-30% among infants born with symptoms. About 90% of survivors have neurological disorders, such as microcephaly, hydrocephalus, cerebral palsy, and/or intellectual disability. In less severe infections, symptoms (intellectual disability, hearing deficits, learning disabilities) may be delayed. Commonly, the neonate is small for gestational age (SGA). The brain and liver are commonly affected, but all organs can be infected. Multiple blood abnormalities can occur: anemia, hyperbilirubinemia, thrombocytopenia, and hepatosplenomegaly.

Herpes Simplex Virus

Most pregnant women infected with **herpes simplex virus** (HSV) are asymptomatic and unaware of infection. Most vertical transmissions occur when the neonate travels through a colonized birth canal. The risk of transmitting HSV during the birth process varies greatly, depending if the infection is a new infection (primary) or a secondary outbreak. The transmission rate from women with a primary HSV infection is approximately 50%, while the transmission rate is 1-2% if the infection is a recurrence of HSV. Signs of a neonatal infection with HSV include:

- Skin, eye, and mucous membrane blistering at 10-12 days of life.
- Disseminated disease may spread to multiple organs, leading to pneumonitis, hepatitis, and intravascular coagulation.
- Encephalitis may be the only presentation, with signs of lethargy, irritability, poor feeding, and seizures.

A mother with active herpes should deliver by cesarean section within 4-6 hours after membranes rupture. An infant is inadvertently exposed to an active lesion should be treated with acyclovir.

Fetal Exposure to Syphilis

An infant can be exposed to the **syphilis** organism, *Treponema pallidum,* during gestation and become infected *in utero* starting with the 10th-15th week of gestation. Many infected fetuses abort spontaneously or are stillborn. The infant born infected with syphilis can be asymptomatic at birth or can have a full multi-system infection. An infant who is symptomatic may have non-viral hepatitis with jaundice, hepatosplenomegaly, pseudoparalysis, pneumonitis, bone marrow failure, myocarditis, meningitis, anemia, edema associated with nephritic syndrome, and a rash on the palms of the hands and soles of the feet. Other symptoms, such as interstitial keratitis and dental and facial abnormalities may occur as the child develops. Treatment involves an aggressive regimen of penicillin administration with frequent follow-up until blood tests are negative.

Treatment for Mothers with HIV/AIDS to Prevent/Reduce Transmission

Optimal **treatment for mothers infected with HIV/AIDS** reduces the perinatal transmission rate to as low as 1 to 2%.

- **Antiviral therapy during the pregnancy**: A reduced viral load in the mother lessens the likelihood of prenatal transmission.
- **Elective caesarian section before the amniotic membranes rupture**: Emergency caesarian, rupture of membranes longer than 4 hours, and the need for an episiotomy all increase the likelihood of infection during delivery.
- **Antiviral medications for the neonate for the first 6 weeks of life**: The first dose should be given within the first 6 to 12 hours after delivery.
- **Avoiding breastfeeding**: The risk of HIV transmission with breastfeeding is 0.7% per month of breastfeeding.

Fetal Exposure to AIDS/HIV

Most children infected with **AIDS/HIV** acquire the infection from their mothers (vertical transmission). The perinatal transmission rate is 30% in untreated HIV positive mothers, usually acquired during delivery. Neonates are usually asymptomatic but are at risk for prematurity, low birth weight, and small for gestational age (SGA). Infants may show failure to thrive, hepatomegaly, interstitial lymphocytic pneumonia, recurrent infections, and CNS abnormalities. Optimal treatment reduces the perinatal transmission rate to as low as 1-2%:

- Antiviral therapy during the pregnancy: A reduced viral load in the mother lessens the likelihood of prenatal transmission.
- Elective caesarian section before the amniotic membranes rupture is especially recommended for women with a viral load >1000 copies/mL and is associated with reduced rates of vertical transmission. Emergency caesarian, rupture of membranes longer than 4 hours, and the need for an episiotomy all increase the likelihood of infection during delivery.
- Antiviral medications for the neonate for the first 6 weeks of life. The first dose should be given within the first 6-12 hours after delivery.
- Avoiding breastfeeding: The risk of HIV transmission with breastfeeding is 0.7% per month of breastfeeding.

Immunologic Clinical Laboratory Tests for HIV

The **immunological** status of infants with **HIV** positive mothers is assessed in a series of tests performed over the first two years in order to institute treatment and decrease transmission to ≥2%:

- Birth (≥24 hours): ELISA and rapid tests are used to identify those neonates who test positive at birth. Confirmatory testing is done with the neonate's blood (not cord blood due to possibility of maternal contamination), usually using DNA PCR, which is about 99% sensitive by 1 month, but does NOT detect very recent infection (for instance, infection acquired during the birth). RNA PCR may be used for some subtypes of HIV infection.

In the United States, testing is based on identifying mothers with HIV. If the mother's status is not known, then some states require mandatory testing of the infant, but laws vary. Based on positive findings, treatment is begun within 24 hours without waiting for confirmatory test results. Breastfeeding is avoided. Subsequent testing is done at 2, 4, 12, and 18 months.

Genetic, Metabolic and Endocrine

Hypoglycemia

Hypoglycemia is low blood sugar of 30 mg/dL or less during the first day after birth, or below 45 mg/dL thereafter. One neonate in every 25,000 experiences persistent hypoglycemia. Half of hypoglycemic neonates develop brain damage. The hypoglycemic patient may be asymptomatic, or may have these symptoms: Apnea; tachypnea; respiratory distress; vomiting; diminished oral intake; tachycardia; bradycardia; jitteriness; lethargy; brisk Moro reflex; seizures; coma; and temperature instability. Suspect hypoglycemia in these circumstances:

- Elevated insulin levels in the infant with a brittle diabetic mother.
- Premature or SGA baby.
- KATP-HI diffuse or focal disease, GDH-HI, or GK-HI genetic disorders.
- Septic shock.
- Hyperthyroidism.
- Inadequate glucose stores in malnourished infants and poor feeders.
- Hypoxemia or ischemia.
- Ingestion of alcohol, beta blockers, or salicylates.

Treatment is 5 mg/kg/day-20 mg/kg/day oral diazoxide, two or three times per day. The doctor may also order hydrochlorothiazide, nifedipine, octreotide, and glucagon. Partial pancreatectomy is required if drugs are ineffective.

Glucose-Bolus-Associated Hypoglycemia

A **glucose-bolus-associated occurrence of acute hypoglycemia** can arise if a glucose bolus is given and not followed up with a **continuous infusion**, because the body will produce more insulin to cover the bolus, which will then start to use glucose stores as soon as the bolus stops. To prevent this, a steady infusion should be continued for a sufficient time period for the infant's insulin production to stabilize. Most infants with hypoglycemia are asymptomatic. *Symptoms* of hypoglycemia stem from central nervous system excitation (jitteriness, high-pitched cry, exaggerated Moro reflex, and seizure) or depression (lethargy, apnea, poor feeding, and temperature instability). Bedside tests for hypoglycemia with reagent sticks may overestimate hypoglycemia and should be confirmed with a serum level. Hypoglycemic infants are treated with either oral or IV infusion of glucose while awaiting results from the laboratory. If the infant is truly hypoglycemic, the blood glucose test is repeated frequently until the infant displays a stable blood glucose level.

Causes and Risk Factors

The following are common causes of hypoglycemia in the neonate along with their risk factors:

- **Decreased glucose availability** - Risk factors include preterm birth, glycogen storage diseases, intrauterine growth restriction, and prolonged fasting.
- **Increased glucose utilization** - Risk factors include cold stress and hypothermia, sepsis, labored breathing, perinatal asphyxia, Rh incompatibility, persistent neonatal hyperinsulinism, and maternal tocolytic drugs. An umbilical artery catheter placed with the tip right above the pancreas delivers glucose directly to the pancreas and can stimulate too much insulin production.
- **Elevated insulin levels** - Risk factors include infant of diabetic mother (elevated glucose levels trigger increased insulin production), islet cell hyperplasia, abrupt cessation of IV glucose, exchange transfusion, and Beckwith-Wiedemann syndrome.

SODIUM, HYPONATREMIA, AND HYPERNATREMIA

Sodium (Na) regulates fluid volume, osmolality, acid-base balance, and activity in the muscles, nerves and myocardium. It is the primary cation (positive ion) in ECF, necessary to maintain ECF levels needed for tissue perfusion:

- Normal neonatal value: 133-146 mEq/L.
- Hyponatremia: <133 mEq/L. (Critical value <120).
- Hypernatremia: >146 mEq/L. (Critical value >160).

Hyponatremia develops with excessive water gain or excessive sodium loss. Late symptoms include apnea, irritability, twitching, and seizures when serum sodium drops below 120 mEq/L, but infants are often asymptomatic. In the first days after birth, hyponatremia is usually secondary to excessive water gain (dilutional hyponatremia), reflected in a weight gain or absence of expected weight loss. Conditions causing dilutional hyponatremia include syndrome of inappropriate antidiuretic hormone (SIADH), renal dysfunction with decreased urine output, and overhydration. Treatment involves identifying and treating underlying cause, restricting fluid, and replacing sodium if necessary. **Hypernatremia** is caused by dehydration, excess use of sodium containing solutions, and diabetes insipidus. Late symptoms include seizures. Underlying cause must be identified and treated.

HYPOCALCEMIA

The ionized form of **serum calcium** is the only biologically available form in the body.

- Cord: 8.2 to 11.2 mg/dL
- 0 to 10 days: 7.6 to 10.4 mg/dL
- 11 days to 1 yr: 9.0 to 11.0 mg/dL
- Critical value for hypocalcemia: <7 mg/dL

Signs of **hypocalcemia** include jitteriness, irritability, stridor, tetany, high-pitched cry, seizures, and decreased myocardial contractility, with decreased cardiac output. An electrocardiogram may show a prolonged QT interval and a flattened T-wave. Early onset hypocalcemia usually presents in the first 3 days of life and is associated with prematurity, birth asphyxia, and infants of diabetic mothers. Late onset hypocalcemia presents after the first week of life and is associated with DiGeorge syndrome, hyperphosphatemia, vitamin D deficiency, magnesium deficiency, diuretic therapy, and hypoparathyroidism. Hypocalcemia is treated with a slow infusion of calcium gluconate. Rapid infusion may cause bradycardia. Tissue infiltration with calcium causes necrosis, so the administration site must be monitored.

HYPERCALCEMIA

Hypercalcemia (>12 mg/dL) is rare, occurring less often than hypocalcemia. Signs of hypercalcemia include: Vomiting; constipation; hypertension; hypotonia; lethargy and seizures. Possible causes of hypercalcemia include: Congenital hyperparathyroidism; maternal hypoparathyroidism; hypervitaminosis D; hyperthyroidism; hypophosphatasia; subcutaneous fat necrosis; Williams syndrome; and adrenal insufficiency. Idiopathic hypercalcemia is diagnosed when no other cause can be found. Iatrogenic hypercalcemia occurs because of excess administration of calcium or vitamin D, or phosphate deprivation. Treatment depends on the exact cause, but may include:

- Correction of the underlying cause.
- Furosemide (Lasix) after adequate hydration to increase calcium excretion.
- Glucocorticoids to inhibit intestinal absorption of calcium.
- Use of low calcium and low vitamin D formulas.

Magnesium, Hypermagnesemia, and Hypomagnesemia

Magnesium is the second most abundant intercellular cation:

- Neonate: 1.5-2.2 mg/dL.
- Critical values: <1.2 mg/dL and >3 mg/dL (neonates)

Hypermagnesemia most commonly results from maternal administration of magnesium prior to delivery. Maternal serum chemistries are reflected in newborn blood values. Magnesium is used in the pregnant woman as a tocolytic agent to stop pre-term labor, and also for treatment of pre-eclampsia. Signs of hypermagnesemia in an infant include hypotonia, hyporeflexia, constipation, low blood pressure, apnea, and marked flushing secondary to vasodilatation. Elevated magnesium blocks neurosynaptic transmission by interfering with the release of acetylcholine. Treatment is usually supportive, as the elevated serum magnesium will be cleared by the infant's kidneys. In severe cases the infant may require respiratory and/or blood pressure support.

Hypomagnesemia in neonates occurs with preterm birth, respiratory distress syndrome, and neonatal hepatitis. *Symptoms* include:

- Neuromuscular excitability/ tetany.
- Seizure and coma.
- Tachycardia with ventricular arrhythmias.
- Respiratory depression.

Treatment includes diagnosing underlying cause and magnesium replacement.

Serum Potassium Changes After Birth

Electrolyte levels in the newborn reflect those of the mother at birth. Shortly after birth, within the first 24 to 72 hours, **serum potassium** concentrations are expected to rise without exogenous potassium delivery and with normal renal function, resulting from a shift of potassium from the intracellular space to the extracellular space. **Potassium shift** is more extreme in premature infants and can result in life- threatening hyperkalemia. Over the next several days, the potassium level will fall to normal in an infant with normally functioning kidneys. Preterm infants' serum electrolytes, including potassium, should be carefully monitored in the first 48 hours of life and until values have stabilized.

- Normal neonatal values: 3.7 to 5.9 mEq/L
- Hyperkalemia: >6 mEq/L; critical value: >6.5 mEq/L
- Hypokalemia: <3.5 mEq/L; critical value: <2.5 mEq/L

HYPERKALEMIA

Hyperkalemia is a serum potassium level greater than 6 mEq/L in a non-hemolyzed blood sample. Squeezing the infant's heel too hard during blood collection can cause the sample to hemolyze and give an artificially elevated laboratory value. Causes of hyperkalemia in the newborn fall into 3 categories:

- Excessive potassium supplementation.
- Transcellular shift, where potassium concentrated inside cells moves outside cells, due to low pH, cellular damage, intraventricular hemorrhage or trauma.
- Decreased potassium secretion by the kidneys, due to congenital adrenal hyperplasia with elevated secretion of aldosterone or renal failure.

Cardiac manifestations of hyperkalemia include potentially fatal arrhythmias like bradycardia, tachycardia, supraventricular fibrillation, and ventricular fibrillation. EKG shows peaked T waves (earliest sign), and a widened QRS complex.

TREATMENT

Hyperkalemia must be treated promptly because it may develop into a lethal cardiac arrhythmia, especially if the blood potassium value is >7 mEq/L and the infant's electrocardiogram shows abnormalities. Follow these steps to lower potassium levels:

- Discontinue all potassium administration.
- Elevate the blood pH by inducing hyperventilation.
- Give sodium bicarbonate to shift extracellular potassium back inside cells.
- Administer insulin and/or inhaled albuterol to enhance the shift of extracellular potassium back inside cells. *Monitor glucose levels closely.*
- Increase excretion of potassium by giving furosemide (Lasix) or sodium polystyrene sulfonate (Kayexalate).
- Give calcium gluconate concurrently to help stabilize the myocardium and lessen the chance of the infant developing an arrhythmia.
- In extreme cases, consider dialysis or exchange transfusion.

HYPOKALEMIA

Hypokalemia is a serum potassium level less than 3.5 mEq/L. Common causes of hypokalemia are chronic diuretic use and excessive nasogastric drainage. Alkalosis accentuates hypokalemia by triggering the sequestration of potassium from the extracellular fluid to inside the cell. Electrocardiograph manifestations of hypokalemia include a flattened T wave (earliest manifestation), ST segment depression, and appearance of U waves (second recovery wave following the T wave). These changes are identical to those seen with hypomagnesemia. Hypokalemia is usually not of concern until the level drops below 3.0 mEq/L. Signs of hypokalemia include cardiac arrhythmias, ileus, and lethargy. *Treatment* is with Slow-K and can be intravenous or oral. Rapid administration of potassium is associated with possible life-threatening cardiac dysfunction.

Metabolic and Respiratory Acidosis

Pathophysiology

- Metabolic acidosis
  - Increase in fixed acid and inability to excrete acid, or loss of base, with compensatory increase of CO_2 excretion by lungs.
- Respiratory acidosis
  - Hypoventilation and CO_2 retention, with renal compensatory retention of bicarbonate (HCO_3) and increased excretion of hydrogen.

Laboratory

- Metabolic acidosis
  - Decreased serum pH and PCO_2 normal if uncompensated and decreased if compensated.
  - Decreased HCO_3.
  - Urine pH <6 if compensated.
- Respiratory acidosis
  - Increased serum pH and increased PCO_2.
  - Increased HCO_3 if compensated and normal if uncompensated.
  - Urine pH >6 if compensated.

Causes

- Metabolic acidosis
  - DKA, lactic acidosis, diarrhea, starvation, renal failure, shock, renal tubular acidosis, starvation.
- Respiratory acidosis
  - COPD, overdose of sedative or barbiturate, obesity, severe pneumonia/atelectasis, muscle weakness (Guillain-Barré), mechanical hypoventilation

Symptoms

- Metabolic acidosis
  - Neuro/muscular: drowsiness, confusion, headache, coma
  - Cardiac: decreased BP, arrhythmias, flushed skin
  - GI: nausea, vomiting, abdominal pain, diarrhea
  - Respiratory: deep inspired tachypnea
- Respiratory acidosis
  - Neuro/muscular: drowsiness, dizziness, headache, coma, disorientation, seizures
  - Cardiac: flushed skin, VF, ↓BP
  - GI: absent
  - Respiratory: hypoventilation with hypoxia

METABOLIC AND RESPIRATORY ALKALOSIS

PATHOPHYSIOLOGY

- Metabolic alkalosis
    - Decreased strong acid or increased base, with compensatory CO_2 retention by lungs.
- Respiratory alkalosis
    - Hyperventilation and increased excretion of CO_2, with compensatory HCO_3 excretion by kidneys

LABORATORY

- Metabolic alkalosis
    - Increased serum pH
    - PCO_2 normal if uncompensated and increased if compensated
    - Increased HCO_3
    - Urine pH >6 if compensated
- Respiratory alkalosis
    - Increased serum pH
    - Decreased PCO_2
    - HCO_3 normal if uncompensated and decreased if compensated
    - Urine pH >6 if compensated

CAUSES

- Metabolic alkalosis
    - Excessive vomiting, gastric suctioning, diuretics, potassium deficit, excessive mineralocorticoids and $NaHCO_3$ intake
- Respiratory alkalosis
    - Hyperventilation associated with hypoxia, pulmonary embolus, exercise, anxiety, pain, and fever
    - Encephalopathy, septicemia, brain injury, salicylate overdose, mechanical hyperventilation

SYMPTOMS

- Metabolic alkalosis
    - Neuromuscular: dizziness, confusion, nervousness, anxiety, tremors, muscle cramping, tetany, tingling, seizures
    - Cardiac: tachycardia and arrhythmias
    - GI: nausea, vomiting, anorexia
    - Respiratory: compensatory hypoventilation
- Respiratory alkalosis
    - Neuro/muscular: light-headedness, confusion, lethargy
    - Cardiac: tachycardia and arrhythmias.
    - GI: epigastric pain, nausea, and vomiting
    - Respiratory: hyperventilation

Inborn Error of Metabolism

Phenylketonuria

Phenylketonuria (PKU) is an inborn error of metabolism that results from a deficiency of the liver enzyme that changes phenylalanine to tyrosine (phenylalanine is a product that results when protein is digested). These infants are unable to digest protein. The symptoms of this disorder will show up sometime before 3 months if not caught in a screening. The first symptoms will be vomiting, poor feeding effort, and irritability. Later, if not treated, the infant will develop eczema and will have urine that smells musty. Once this condition is diagnosed, the infant must be put on a strict diet that restricts phenylalanine. Extensive family training must take place to educate the family about the diet. If the infant does not follow this diet restriction, intellectual disability will result. PKU screening within 7 days of birth is required in all 50 states.

Galactosemia

Galactosemia, an autosomal recessive disorder, is the most common inborn error of metabolism. In this disorder, the infant is lacking the enzyme that converts galactose to glucose. Because lactose is made up of galactose and glucose, the infant who cannot convert the galactose in lactose to glucose cannot tolerate lactose. Usually the neonate is asymptomatic but develops symptoms rapidly. The clinical manifestations seen with galactosemia include jaundice, vomiting, diarrhea, inability to gain weight and hypoglycemia. An infant with this condition that does not receive treatment can contract a serious gram negative infection related to damage to the intestinal lining, and death may occur at 1-2 weeks. This condition must be treated by removing all lactose products and replacing the formula with soy or lactose free formula. If left untreated, severe intellectual disability can result.

Cystic Fibrosis

Cystic fibrosis (mucoviscidosis or CF) is a progressive congenital disease that particularly affects the pancreas and lungs causing digestive and respiratory problems. It is caused by a genetic defect that affects sodium chloride movement in cells, including mucosal cells that line the lungs, causing the production of thick mucus that clogs the lungs and provides a rich medium for bacteria. While most patients with cystic fibrosis at one time died in childhood, the life expectancy is now about 30 years. About 15% to 20% of neonates with CF have meconium ileus (obstruction of small intestine with meconium) at birth. Other infants have no symptoms at first but show failure to thrive in the first 4-6 weeks and may develop a cough and wheezing. Cystic fibrosis patients usually suffer from recurrent respiratory infections of the lower respiratory tract. The most common infective agents are *Pseudomonas aeruginosa* and *Burkholderia cepacia* complex. The screening test for CF is IRT/DNA. If the IRT/DNA is positive, the infant is scheduled for a sweat test and buccal swab.

Multifactorial Inheritance

Complex or multifactorial inheritance relates to an interaction of many different genes as well as the environment and life style choices. Thus, a genetic disorder may depend upon genes inherited from both parents as well as unidentified environmental factors (smoking, drug use, diet) interacting in such a way as to produce an abnormality. This type of inheritance pattern is much less predictable than the others. Neural tube defects, for example, are caused by multifactorial inheritance. In some cases, an infant may inherit only a tendency toward a disease, such as diabetes type 2, but development of the disease may depend up weight, diet, smoking, and other factors as the child matures. Complex diseases include such things as asthma, heart disease, and osteoarthritis. Multifactorial traits often run in families, with risk 50% in first-degree relatives (parents), 25% in second degree (grandparents, aunts, uncles), and 12.5% in 3rd degree (cousins).

AUTOSOMAL INHERITANCE PATTERNS

Autosomal inheritance patterns involve genetic abnormalities in chromosome pairs 1-22:

- **Autosomal recessive***:* This occurs when two parents (without active disease) each have a copy of the same abnormal recessive gene and both pass the abnormal copy to offspring. The *recurrence risk* (the chance to have affected offspring) for two carrier parents with the same abnormal gene mutation is 25% for each pregnancy and 50% chance the child will become a carrier. Autosomal recessive disorders, such as cystic fibrosis, Tay Sachs, and sickle cell anemia, are seen more frequently among certain ethnic groups and in offspring of related parents.
- **Autosomal dominant***:* This means that only one abnormal dominant gene needs to be inherited to cause the condition. Autosomal dominant diseases include Huntington's disease and Marfan syndrome. The *recurrence risk* for an affected parent to pass the disease to a child is 50% with each pregnancy, but there is no carrier state.

SEX-LINKED INHERITANCE

Sex-linked inheritance involves the sex chromosomes (chromosome 23). Y-linked disorders such as Klinefelter syndrome are rare, but they will be passed from the father to all male children. X-linked diseases, such as hemophilia and Duchenne muscular dystrophy, usually occur in males because males have only one X chromosome, so a single recessive gene on that X chromosome causes the disease. Females have two X chromosomes, so the normal gene on an unaffected X chromosome can usually compensate. Although the Y chromosome is the other half of the XY chromosome pair in the male, the Y chromosome is much smaller than the X chromosome and doesn't contain most of the genes of the X chromosome—it's not a complete match—so there is no compensating gene to protect the male. Thus, females carry the disease and males inherit the disease. A man with an X-linked recessive disorder will not pass the disease to his sons (because they don't inherit his X chromosome), but his daughters will inherit the mutated gene, so they have one abnormal X (from the father) and one normal (from the mother). These daughters then have a 50% chance of having sons who are affected and a 50% chance of having daughters who carry one copy of the mutated gene. X-linked dominant inheritance also differs depending upon whether the mother or father carries the defective gene. There is no carrier state with X-linked dominant disorders. If the father has the disease, such as Rett's syndrome, all daughters will inherit. If the mother has the disease, each child, regardless of gender, has a 50% chance of inheriting.

Infant of Diabetic Mother

Infants of diabetic mother (IDM) often present with:

- Birth trauma secondary to cephalopelvic disproportion, including shoulder dislocation.
- Hypoglycemia from sudden withdrawal of maternal glucose and elevated insulin in the infant.
- Respiratory distress syndrome because elevated insulin inhibits surfactant production.
- Polycythemia (excessive red blood cell production) and hyperviscosity because of elevated insulin and glucose increase the metabolic rate and oxygen consumption.
- Iron deficiency because polycythemia leaches iron from the heart and brain.
- Hyperbilirubinemia because of increased red blood cell destruction after birth.
- Cardiovascular malformations, such as intraventricular hypertrophy with outflow tract obstruction, transposition of the great arteries, ventral septal defects, and coarctation of the aorta.
- Congenital malformations, such as anencephaly, spina bifida, renal agenesis, and duodenal atresia.
- Electrolyte abnormalities, including hypocalcemia and hypomagnesemia.

Complications

There are several **complications resulting from IDM,** including:

- **Seizure activity***:* This can occur in some of these infants due to the lack of sufficient fuel for the brain when the infant becomes hypoglycemic. Glucose is the fuel the brain needs to function properly and when it is in short supply, the brain is essentially starved.
- **Shoulder dystocia***:* This is a condition that is directly related to an infant that is large for gestational age (LGA) because of diabetes. Large babies will often experience shoulder dislocation at birth as they try to fit through the birth canal.
- **Thrombosis** sometimes forms in the kidneys (venous or arterial) as a result of a high hematocrit and increased viscosity of blood.
- **Increased diabetic risk:** 2% of female and 6% of male IDMs will go on to develop juvenile type one diabetes.

Hypoglycemia

Infants of diabetic mothers (IDM) are exposed to elevated levels of **glucose** during their intrauterine development, as glucose freely crosses the placenta; the blood glucose level of the developing fetus mirrors that of the mother. The fetus increases production of insulin at around 20 weeks gestation, in response to the mother's elevated blood glucose. When the umbilical cord is cut, it abruptly disrupts the neonate's supply of glucose. The infant's greatest risk for **hypoglycemia** occurs between 30 and 90 minutes after delivery. Because insulin levels are elevated in the fetus, the newborn may have an increased glucose need for several days to prevent hypoglycemia—as high as 10 to 15 mg/kg/min. Glucose is given as a continuous infusion to prevent the newborn from developing rebound hypoglycemia after a bolus of glucose. IDM infants show fewer symptoms of hypoglycemia when compared to other neonates and may also suffer from hypocalcemia, hypomagnesemia, and hyperbilirubinemia. Hypoglycemia is an easily treatable condition that, when left untreated, causes long-term neurological damage.

Fetal Exposure to Heroin

Heroin is a highly addictive, opioid narcotic that is a common drug of abuse. Heroin users are at increased risk of poor nutrition, iron deficiency anemia and preeclampsia-eclampsia, all negatively affecting the fetus. Infants with prenatal heroin exposure display symmetric intrauterine growth restriction (IUGR) and are often born prematurely. About 60-80% of these infants will undergo neonatal abstinence syndrome (NAS). Heroin has a relatively short half-life and symptoms of NAR typically begin 48-72 hours after delivery. Several different body systems are affected by NAS and include:

CNS Dysfunction	GI Dysfunction	Miscellaneous Signs
High-pitched cry hyperactive. Reflexes increased muscle. Irritability. Tremors.	Poor feeding. Periods of frantic sucking or rooting. Vomiting. Loose or watery stools. Vomiting.	Frequent yawning. Sneezing multiple times. Sweating. Fever. Tachypnea.

Withdrawal Symptoms in Neonate

Fetal exposure to drugs, such as opioids, methadone, cocaine, crack, and other recreational drugs, causes **withdrawal symptoms** in about 60% of infants. There are many variables, which include the type of drug and the extent and duration of maternal drug use. For example, children may have withdrawal symptoms within 48 hours for cocaine, heroin, and methamphetamine exposure, but there may be delays of up to 2 or 3 weeks for methadone. Short hospital stays after birth make it imperative that children who are at risk are identified so they can receive supportive treatment, particularly since they often feed poorly and can quickly become dehydrated and undernourished. Polydrug use makes it difficult to describe a typical profile of **symptoms**, but they usually include:

- Tremors
- Irritability
- Hypertonicity
- High-pitched crying
- Diarrhea
- Dry skin
- Seizures (in severe cases)

Treatment is supportive. Infants with opiate exposure may be given decreasing doses of opiates, such as morphine elixir, with close monitoring until the child is weaned off of the medication.

Managing Symptoms of Intrauterine Drug Exposure

High-Pitched Crying and Inability to Sleep

Interventions for high-pitched crying are as follows:

- Keep room quiet with low light.
- Swaddle the infant securely in a flexed position with the arms close to the body.
- Hold infant close to body.
- Rock swaddled infant slowly and rhythmically.
- Walk with swaddled infant held close.
- Offer pacifier, possibly with sugar solution, if acceptable.
- Give a warm bath.
- Play soft music.
- Placing the infant in a dark room with no stimulation at all for a period of time may be effective if other methods fail.

Interventions for inability to sleep are as follows:

- Decrease environmental stimuli and maintain quiet.
- Waterbed or sheepskin.
- Feed frequently in small amounts.

Nasal Stuffiness

Interventions for nasal stuffiness/sneezing are as follows:

- Aspirate nasopharynx as needed.
- Feed slowly and give time for rest between sucking.
- Monitor respirations.

Poor Feeding

Interventions for poor feeding and frantic sucking of fingers/fist are as follows:

- Feed small frequent amounts with enteral feedings if necessary.
- Weigh daily.
- Provide nonnutritive sucking with pacifier to relieve frantic sucking.

Regurgitation

Interventions for regurgitation are as follows:

- Weigh frequently and monitor fluids and electrolytes.
- Observe for dehydration and provide IV fluids as needed.
- Place supine with head elevated after feedings.

Hypertonicity

Interventions for hypertonicity are as follows:

- Monitor temperature and decrease environmental temperature if infant's temperature >37.6 °C.
- Change infant's position frequently to avoid pressure sores.
- Place on sheepskin or waterbed to prevent pressure.

Diarrhea

Interventions for diarrhea are as follows:

- Change diaper frequently and cleanse skin with mild soap and water. Apply skin barrier as needed.
- Expose irritated skin to air.

Tremor/Seizures

Interventions for tremor/seizures are as follows:

- Decrease environmental stimuli and handling.
- Change position frequently.
- Observe for scratches, blistering, or abrasions.
- Place on sheepskin or waterbed to reduce friction and pressure.
- Maintain patent airway and observe for apnea.
- Monitor for hyperthermia.

Fetal Alcohol Syndrome

Fetal alcohol syndrome (FAS) is a syndrome of birth defects that develop as the result of maternal ingestion of alcohol. Fetal alcohol spectrum disorders (FASD) is an umbrella diagnosis that includes FAS along with infants impacted by alcohol in utero that do not meet the full FAS criteria. Despite campaigns to inform the public, women continue to drink during pregnancy, but no safe amount of alcohol ingestion has been determined. FAS includes:

- **Facial abnormalities**: Hypoplastic (underdeveloped) maxilla, micrognathia (undersized jaw), hypoplastic philtrum (groove beneath the nose), short palpebral fissures (eye slits between upper and lower lids).
- **Neurological deficits**: May include microcephaly, intellectual disability, and motor delay, hearing deficits. Learning disorders may include problems with visual-spatial and verbal learning, attention disorders, delayed reaction times.
- **Growth restriction**: Prenatal growth deficit persists with slow growth after birth.
- **Behavioral problems**: Irritability and hyperactivity. Poor judgment in behavior may relate to deficit in executive functions.

Indication of brain damage without the associated physical abnormalities is referred to as alcohol-related neurodevelopmental disorder (ARND).

Screening of the Newborn

Screening of the newborn to detect genetic diseases varies somewhat from one state to another. Because about 1 in 200 newborns has chromosomal abnormalities, screening is an important tool, although many birth defects, such as defects caused by maternal alcohol abuse or vitamin deficiency, are not genetic in origin. Screening tests for these genetic diseases are available:

- Biotinidase deficiency (autosomal recessive).
- Congenital adrenal hyperplasia (autosomal recessive).
- Congenital hearing loss (autosomal recessive, autosomal dominant, or mitochondrial).
- Congenital hypothyroidism (autosomal recessive or autosomal dominant).
- Cystic fibrosis (autosomal recessive).
- Galactosemia (autosomal recessive).
- Homocystinuria (autosomal recessive).
- Maple syrup urine disease (autosomal recessive).
- Medium-chain Acyl-CoA dehydrogenase (autosomal recessive).
- Phenylketonuria (autosomal recessive).
- Sickle cell disease (autosomal recessive).
- Tyrosemia (Two types are autosomal recessive; a third type is unclear).

Congenital Adrenal Hyperplasia

Congenital adrenal hyperplasia (CAH) is an autosomal recessive defect that results in a cortisol deficiency, and is often accompanied by an aldosterone deficiency. 90 to 95% of CAH cases are due to a deficiency in 21-hydroxylase, the enzyme responsible for catalyzing two reactions in the adrenal glands:

- 17-Hydroxyprogestorne → 11-deoxycortisol → cortisol
- Progesterone → deoxycorticosterone → aldosterone

The cortisol deficiency results in shock, hypoglycemia, and circulatory collapse. The infant becomes dehydrated when CAH is accompanied by aldosterone deficiency (salt wasting), because of excessive loss of urinary sodium. Symptoms do not usually occur until the infant is 2 to 4 weeks old. Metabolic abnormalities of hyperkalemia, hyponatremia, hypoglycemia, and metabolic acidosis are present shortly after birth. Some infants have milder forms of CAH and are not diagnosed until later in life. Elevated levels of ACTH cause hypertrophy of the adrenal glands and increased production of androgens. Elevated androgens *in utero* virilize the female infant, so she has ovaries and uterus but external genitalia are often ambiguous.

Maternal Newborn Practice Test

1. Correct statements about breastfeeding and formula-feeding include which of the following?

a. there is a faster return to pre-pregnancy weight in mothers of formula-fed infants
b. there is a lower incidence of milk-protein allergy in formula-fed infants
c. there is an improved immunity in breastfed infants

2. The dark red uterine discharge expelled in the first 2-3 days postpartum is

a. lochia rubra
b. lochia serosa
c. lochia alba

3. The fetal/neonatal lung substance that improves pulmonary compliance by decreasing alveolar surface tension is

a. meconium
b. prostaglandin
c. surfactant

4. Obesity during pregnancy is associated with an increased risk of

a. fetuses that are small-for-gestational age
b. cesarean birth
c. rapid postpartum weight loss

5. Immediately after an uncomplicated delivery without meconium, a full-term newborn is warmed, dried, suctioned, and positioned appropriately but has a heart rate of 80 beats/min. According to neonatal resuscitation guidelines, the next step in managing this infant is

a. positive-pressure ventilation
b. chest compression
c. epinephrine administration

6. Clinical practice that is consistent with established recommendations or standards is best characterized by

a. standards that are used primarily to minimize providers' legal liability
b. recommendations that are used to standardize patient care based on evidence-based guidelines
c. standards that are based on methods that have proven effective over a substantial period of time

7. All of the following are elements of the postpartum breast assessment EXCEPT:

a. firmness, tenderness and redness
b. engorgement and nipple soreness/cracking
c. lumps indicating possible cancerous growths

8. Vitamin K is administered to newborn infants to prevent

a. bleeding
b. neonatal jaundice
c. gonococcal conjunctivitis

9. Perineal pain in the first 4-6 hours after vaginal delivery are initially managed with

a. oral analgesic medications
b. ice packs to the perineum
c. frequent perineal pad changes

10. The biophysical profile evaluates fetal wellbeing by combining fetal heart rate monitoring with

a. ultrasonographic examination of established fetal parameters
b. fetal movement counting ("kick counts")
c. external monitoring of uterine contractions

11. The least expensive type of infant formula is

a. formula concentrate
b. ready-to-feed formula
c. powdered formula

12. Six to twelve hours after the vaginal delivery of a single infant and placenta, the uterine fundus should be palpable at or below the level of the

a. pubic symphysis
b. umbilicus
c. epigastrium

13. Infants delivered by elective cesarean section are at increased risk for

a. neonatal jaundice
b. low birth weight
c. neonatal respiratory distress

14. In caring for a family who has experienced a perinatal fetal death, it is helpful to

a. share personal stories of recovery that have been witnessed in the past
b. maximize consistency in assigned nursing staff
c. guide the family to a bereavement room as soon as possible, to allow privacy in mourning

15. Ineffective or shallow infant latch with breastfeeding may lead to increased

a. reflux in the infant
b. milk let-down
c. nipple pain

16. Reddish-orange crystals noted in the urine of a 48-hour-old newborn are

a. a sign of congenital renal disease
b. a sign of vitamin K deficiency
c. a normal finding

17. Which of the following statements about the nurse's medical record documentation is correct?

a. it provides an accurate account of patient status and response to care
b. it consists of both objective and subjective notes regarding the patient and care provided
c. the physician's medical record documentation is more important than the nurse's medical record documentation in legal proceeding

18. Breastfeeding in the immediate postpartum period can improve uterine contractions because of the release of

a. prolactin
b. oxytocin
c. human chorionic gonadotropin

19. Gas exchange in utero in the fetus is performed by the

a. fetal heart
b. fetal lungs
c. placenta

20. An early sign of magnesium sulfate toxicity is

a. seizure activity
b. loss of deep tendon reflexes
c. flushed skin and nausea

21. Breastfeeding is usually contraindicated if the mother has

a. a history of treated breast cancer
b. human immunodeficiency virus
c. latent tuberculosis

22. A method of heat production unique to newborn infants is the metabolism of

a. bilirubin
b. brown fat
c. prostaglandin

23. If the postpartum uterine fundus is boggy on palpation, the nurse does which of the following?

a. notifies the physician immediately
b. massages the uterus until it feels firm
c. re-examines the fundus in 15-20 minutes

24. A sign of impaired attachment between the postpartum mother and her infant is

a. decreasing maternal interaction with the infant over time
b. maternal request to rest and refuse visitors
c. maternal encouragement for family members to hold the infant

25. An Rh-negative mother who has given birth to an Rh-positive infant and has no evidence of sensitization (i.e., maternal indirect Coombs test negative) should be administered

a. Rh immune globulin (Rhogam) within 72 hours of delivery
b. no additional medication
c. cross-matched packed red blood cells within 4 hours of delivery

26. A common complication in the newborn infant of a diabetic mother is

a. hyperglycemia
b. anemia
c. hypoglycemia

27. Hindmilk (milk that flows later in a feeding) has a higher concentration of which of the following substances than foremilk?

a. fat
b. protein
c. colostrum

28. The postpartum patient who has undergone a forceps-assisted vaginal delivery is at increased risk for

a. postpartum hemorrhage
b. eclampsia
c. postpartum depression

29. Early decelerations with a normal fetal heart rate variability during labor have which of the following indications?

a. they often indicate fetal congenital heart disease
b. they do not indicate fetal hypoxia
c. they may indicate fetal acidemia

30. A cephalohematoma in the newborn infant has which of the following characteristics?

a. it does not cross suture lines
b. it typically resolves within 12 hours of birth
c. it is more common after a cesarean birth

31. Infectious mastitis in the breastfeeding mother has which of the following characteristics?

a. it is treated by cessation of breastfeeding
b. it usually occurs within 48 hours of delivery
c. it can often be prevented with proper breastfeeding technique

32. Neonatal jaundice that is present in the first 24 hours of life is considered

a. physiologic
b. pathologic
c. unconjugated

33. A common cause of neonatal sepsis is

a. *neisseria gonorrhoeae*
b. group B *Streptococcus*
c. *Gardnerella vaginalis*

34. All of the following clinical features would be expected with "postpartum blues" (adjustment reaction with depressed mood) EXCEPT

a. frequent tearfulness
b. irritability
c. suicidal ideation

35. The newborn's sensory capacity to attend to and fixate on a visual stimulus (e.g., caregiver's face) is known as

a. habituation
b. orientation
c. self-quieting

36. To prevent contamination and encourage drying of the umbilical cord stump, caregivers should be advised to

a. give the newborn daily tub baths
b. pull on the cord stump daily
c. fold diapers down to avoid covering the cord stump

37. Compared to infants delivered in occiput anterior vertex presentation, infants delivered vaginally in a breech presentation have which of the following risks?

a. a higher risk of birth trauma
b. a lower risk of fetal asphyxia
c. a lower risk of umbilical cord prolapse

38. Treatment of engorgement in the breastfeeding mother includes

a. application of warm compresses before breastfeeding
b. less frequent breastfeeding
c. antibiotics and cold therapy

39. Pregnancy in the breastfeeding postpartum mother is at the lowest likelihood

a. within one month of delivery
b. throughout the duration of breastfeeding
c. when menstruation resumes

40. The sign most concerning for congenital heart disease in the newborn infant is

a. fever
b. central cyanosis
c. acrocyanosis

41. The expected physiologic weight loss in the term newborn's first week of life is

a. up to 20% of birth weight
b. no weight loss
c. up to 10% of birth weight

42. A mother who gives birth by cesarean delivery is encouraged to

a. ambulate as soon as possible after delivery
b. delay seeing her infant until she is no longer requiring pain medications
c. take shallow, purse-lip breaths to minimize pain

43. In a patient with preeclampsia, the development of eclampsia is characterized by

a. elevated liver enzymes
b. hypertension
c. seizures

44. A gestational age assessment in the preterm newborn is likely to demonstrate

a. hyperflexion of the upper and lower extremities in the infant's resting posture
b. minimal breast bud tissue
c. highly developed ear cartilage

45. The drug-exposed infant is most likely to have symptoms of withdrawal in the newborn period after chronic intrauterine exposure to

a. caffeine
b. marijuana
c. oxycodone

46. In caring for a newborn male's recently circumcised penis (non-Plastibell technique), the infant's caregivers are advised to

a. apply a small amount of petroleum ointment to the glans with diaper changes
b. avoid cleaning the penis with warm water
c. pull off the thin, yellowish film that forms on the glans

47. A respiratory pattern characterized by 10-15 seconds of shallow rapid breathing followed by a 5-10 second respiratory pause with spontaneous return of breathing and no associated distress or color change is called

a. periodic breathing
b. central apnea
c. transient tachypnea of the newborn

48. Sticky, greenish black stool is considered characteristic of

a. a newborn infant
b. a breastfed infant
c. a formula fed infant

49. A newborn infant opens her mouth and turns her head to the right when her right cheek is touched, which is consistent with which of the following reflexes?

a. rooting reflex
b. moro reflex
c. tonic neck reflex ("fencing" reflex)

50. Parents of newborn infants are instructed to place infants on their back to sleep to decrease the risk of

a. gastroesophageal reflux (GERD)
b. sudden infant death syndrome (SIDS)
c. bronchiolitis

51. Characteristics of jitteriness include

a. ocular deviations
b. clonic jerking with fast and slow elements
c. increased heart rate

52. After using a breast pump, the woman should

a. rinse removable parts in cold water, then wash with warm soapy water
b. immediately sterilize the removable parts in boiling water
c. wash removable parts in very hot soapy water

53. The most common neonatal bacterial infection is

a. *Staphylococcus aureus*
b. Pseudomonas aeruginosa
c. Group B *Streptococcus*

54. The neonate usually passes meconium within

a. 6 to 8 hours
b. 8 to 24 hours
c. 48 to 72 hours

55. A few weeks after delivery, if a woman complains that she cannot sleep, has little appetite and has begun having anxiety attacks and fears that she cannot take adequate care of her neonate, the most likely cause is

a. postpartum depression
b. postpartum blues
c. postpartum psychosis

56. If a neonate's hemoglobin is 19.3 shortly after birth, a typical value at 7 days is

a. 22.4 g/dL
b. 19.3 g/dL
c. 17.4 g/dL

57. HELLP syndrome is characterized by (H) hemolysis, (EL) elevated liver enzymes, and (LP)

a. lateral pain
b. low (blood) pressure
c. low platelet count

58. The vaccination that should be routinely administered to all newborns within 24 hours of birth is

a. hepatitis A.
b. hepatitis B.
c. rotavirus.

59. If a quad screen shows high AFT, and normal hCG, uE^3 and INH-A, this indicates

a. neural tube defect
b. trisomy 21
c. multiple gestation

60. The infantile form of Tay-Sachs disease is classified as a

a. chromosomal abnormality
b. blood disorder
c. metabolic defect

61. The nutritional supplement given to women to prevent neural tube defects is

a. folic acid
b. magnesium
c. iron

62. If a woman complains that she is exhausted because the neonate nurses so frequently during the night that the woman cannot get any sleep, the nurse should advise the woman to

a. give bottle feedings during the night so the neonate will sleep longer
b. nurse the infant on a strict 3- to 4-hour schedule
c. sleep when the baby sleeps, day and night

63. The CARE principles applied to the care of a pregnant woman refer to (C) communication, (A) advocate, (R) respect, and (E)

a. enable
b. educate
c. engage

64. The recreational drug that most increases the risk of spontaneous abortion is

a. marijuana
b. methamphetamine
c. MDMA

65. By about the sixth day after birth, over a 24-hour period, most infants urinate approximately

a. 12 to 14 times
b. 8 to 12 times
c. 6 to 8 times

66. The neural tube defect that is most likely to result in hydrocephalus is

a. spina bifida occulta
b. myelomeningocele
c. meningocele

67. When using the BUBBLE-HE mnemonic to remember the steps to a comprehensive postpartal assessment, the initial BUB refers to

a. breasts, uterus, bladder
b. bowels, urine, and breasts
c. bowels, uterus, and bonding

68. Human milk can be kept frozen in the freezer section of a side-by-side refrigerator-freezer for

a. 2 weeks
b. 3 to 4 months
c. 6 months

69. If a pregnant woman at 38-weeks of gestation complains of dizziness when lying flat, the most likely cause is

a. hyperventilation and shortness of breath
b. nutritional imbalance
c. supine hypotensive syndrome

70. If a woman's pregnancy classification is G4, T2, P1, A1, L3, the number of total pregnancies is

a. 3
b. 4
c. 6

71. If the fundal height is halfway between the woman's symphysis pubic and umbilicus, the approximate weeks of gestation are

a. 8
b. 12
c. 16

72. The cell free fetal DNA test assesses for

a. chromosomal disorders
b. neural tube defects
c. fetal alcohol syndrome

73. How much weight is a woman with a pre-pregnancy BMI of 22.0 is expected to gain during pregnancy?

a. 15 to 20 pounds
b. 25 to 35 pounds
c. 28 to 40 pounds

74. The presence of bilirubin in amniotic fluid usually indicates

a. chromosomal abnormalities
b. infection
c. Rh-sensitized pregnancy

75. Severe post-dural puncture (spinal) headache is best treated with

a. epidural blood patch
b. opioid analgesia
c. caffeinated beverages

76. If bottle-feeding a neonate with cleft lip and cleft palate, the nipple should be

a. shorter than normal size
b. normal size for gestation
c. longer than normal size

77. Ultrasonography can be used to estimate fetal age with crown-rump length (CRL) at approximately

a. 6 to 8 weeks
b. 7 to 12 weeks
c. 13 to 14 weeks

78. When palpating the uterus after delivery, it is necessary to

a. support the lower uterine segment
b. support the upper uterine segment
c. press down firmly with both hands

79. Asymmetric intrauterine growth restriction is caused by problems that occur during the

a. first trimester
b. second trimester
c. third trimester

80. If a woman in labor is receiving a benzodiazepine to relieve anxiety, nausea, and pain, the medication that should also be available on the unit is

a. flumazenil
b. naloxone
c. N-acetylcysteine

81. A patient who experienced placenta previa is at increased risk of hemorrhage during the postpartal period because

a. the placenta was smaller than normal
b. the area of implantation does not contract effectively
c. the placenta implanted very high in the uterus

82. Following spontaneous rupture of the membranes during labor, if the fetal heart rate becomes markedly bradycardic with variable decelerations, this likely indicates

a. cord prolapse
b. placenta previa
c. fetal head compression

83. During the process of lactation, the breasts usually begin filling and feel firm and warm by the

a. first day
b. second day
c. third day

84. The most common cause of subinvolution is

a. uterine atony
b. retained placental fragments
c. hematoma

85. If shoulder dystocia occurred during delivery, the newborn should be examined for

a. fractured clavicle and Erb's palsy
b. skull fracture and cerebral palsy
c. spinal cord injury and paralysis

86. Labor and delivery is defined as precipitate if labor lasts less than

a. one hour
b. three hours
c. five hours

87. Ensuring that a woman has given informed consent and understands her rights and all of the risks and benefits of a procedure or treatment supports the ethical principal of

a. beneficence
b. nonmaleficence
c. autonomy

88. If a woman complains of persistent constipation in the postpartal period, the best treatment approach is usually a(n)

a. increase in fluid intake
b. high fiber diet
c. stool softener

89. When conducting a review of the literature as part of evidence-based research, the level of evidence that is based on a quasi-experimental study, such as a matched case-control study, would be categorized as

a. Level I
b. Level II
c. Level III

90. In the postpartal period, the uterine fundus should no longer be palpable after

a. 14 days
b. 10 days
c. 7 days

91. The antibiotic agent that should be avoided for long-term use while a woman is breastfeeding is

a. tetracyclines
b. erythromycin
c. cephalosporins

92. If a nurse administers the wrong drug to a patient but the patient suffers no ill effects, the elements of malpractice that are missing are

a. Duty to use care and breach of duty
b. Duty to use care and damages
c. Damages and causation

93. Necrotizing enterocolitis in a preterm infant is usually caused by

a. ischemic bowel
b. severe constipation
c. generalized infection

94. If, on palpating the uterus in the postpartal period, the nurse finds the fundus is displaced superior to the umbilicus and to the right, the nurse should suspect that the cause is

a. uterine atony
b. bladder distention
c. uterine hemorrhage

95. Methylergonovine (Methergine®) may be administered to a woman after delivery in order to

a. promote uterine contractions
b. relieve pain and discomfort
c. reduce maternal hypertension

96. A woman who is breastfeeding and needs to take smoking cessation medication in order to stop smoking should avoid

a. nicotine patches
b. nicotine gum
c. varenicline

97. A woman who has taken methadone during pregnancy and wants to breastfeed should

a. take the lowest dose of methadone
b. continue the same dose of methadone
c. stop taking methadone

98. If a neonate's skin is dry and peeling with no vernix and loss of subcutaneous fat, the likely gestational age is

a. 42 to 44 weeks
b. 35 to 40 weeks
c. 24 to 26 weeks

99. In the immediate postpartal period, a woman's gastric motility is generally

a. within normal limits
b. increased
c. decreased

100. If a woman's white blood cell count was 20,000 after delivery and increased to 40,000 by the second day, this likely indicates

a. normal postpartal elevation
b. acute infection
c. chronic infection

101. If testing after birth shows that a neonate has inherited galactosemia, an inborn error of metabolism, the neonate should be fed

a. human milk
b. whey-based formula
c. soy-based formula

102. If a breastfeeding woman shows a nonimmune rubella titer prior to discharge, the woman should be

a. given the MMR vaccine and continue breastfeeding
b. given the MMR vaccine and stop breastfeeding for a few days
c. told to take the MMR vaccine in 3 to 6 months

103. The breastfeeding position that is good to relieve plugged milk ducts and engorged breasts is

a. cradle hold
b. football hold
c. side-lying hold

104. When assisting with the lumbar puncture of a preterm neonate, the correct position for the neonate is

a. lateral with trunk flexed
b. lateral with trunk in neutral position
c. sitting with head supported

105. If a new mother presents with irritation of the nipple and verbalizes discomfort during breastfeeding, it is most likely that the infant is

a. latching to both the nipple and the areola
b. latching only to the nipple, with the nipple ending at the infant's soft palate
c. latching only to the nipple, with the nipple ending at the infant's hard palate

106. If a neonate exhibits neck rigidity after birth, this may indicate injury to the

a. sternocleidomastoid muscle
b. levator scapula muscle
c. platysma muscle

107. B. A demarcated unraised red-purple lesion caused by capillaries below the skin on a child's face is a

a. nevus vasculosus (strawberry mark)
b. nevus flammeus (port-wine stain)
c. erythema toxicum

108. If a woman with flat nipples has started using a nipple shield while breastfeeding but the infant is not gaining adequate weight, the nurse should advise the woman to

a. provide supplemental bottle feedings
b. use the nipple shield for only 1 or 2 minutes
c. stop breastfeeding

109. If a nursing neonate has a 5:1 suck/swallow ratio, this indicates

a. non-nutritive suckling
b. fast but adequate suckling
c. normal suckling

110. If a new mother asks about bottle-feeding human milk so the father can experience feeding the infant, she should be advised to wait for at least

a. 24 to 48 hours
b. one week
c. 4 weeks

111. Until a neonate regains body weight, the neonate should be nursed at least every

a. 2 hours
b. 3 hours
c. 4 hours

112. A normal percentage of weight loss for a neonate in the first few days of life is

a. 5%
b. 8%
c. 10%

113. When expressing milk from the breast, a woman should

a. alternate between the C and the U hold in fixed positions
b. start with the C hold but move about the breast clockwise
c. use the C hold and hold the hand in a fixed position

114. Women may experience exacerbation of autoimmune disorders, such as lupus erythematosus, after labor and delivery because

a. the woman's immune system is no longer suppressed
b. the woman is in a weakened condition
c. the woman is experiencing increased stress and anxiety

115. If, on the first post-partum day, the woman's fundus is firm and lochia appears normal but the woman complains of perineal discomfort and BP falls to 88/50 and pulse increases to 112, the nurse should suspect a(n)

a. uterine hemorrhage
b. vaginal laceration
c. hematoma

116. If a neonate's cardiac status appeared normal at birth but 48 hours later the neonate experiences a precipitous drop in circulation to the lower body, the likely congenital heart defect is

a. ventricular septal defect
b. aortic stenosis
c. coarctation of the aorta

117. Following delivery, if the fundus feels contracted and in the right position but free flow of bright red blood is evident vaginally, this is likely due to

a. vaginal or cervical laceration
b. normal post-delivery lochia
c. uterine hemorrhage

118. The hormone that stimulates the alveoli to produce milk is

a. oxytocin
b. estrogen
c. prolactin

119. If a woman reports that her neonate cries frantically when hungry, this likely means that

a. there the possibility of an underlying disease process that must be investigated
b. the woman is missing signs of hunger
c. the woman is not breastfeeding correctly

120. Following an unmedicated delivery, a neonate should ideally begin breastfeeding during the first

a. 10 to 20 minutes
b. 1 to 2 hours
c. 3 to 4 hours

121. A woman who develops postpartal DVT should be carefully monitored for signs of

a. pulmonary embolus
b. infection
c. hemorrhage

122. During stage two of milk production (the postpartum period), hormonal changes include

a. increased progesterone and decreased prolactin
b. increased progesterone and decreased estrogen
c. decreased progesterone and increased prolactin

123. In order to prevent post-dural puncture (spinal) headache, the woman should

a. be administered ibuprofen
b. lie flat for several hours
c. increase hydration

124. During the "claiming" part of parent-neonate attachment, the parent usually first compares the child to other family members by noticing how the neonate is

a. similar
b. unique
c. different

125. After delivery, a woman is likely to exhibit signs and symptoms of hypovolemic shock with blood loss greater than

a. 500 mL
b. 1000 mL
c. 1500 mL

126. The phase of maternal role transition during which the woman begins to feel like a mother is

a. taking in
b. taking hold
c. letting go

127. If a neonate's chest circumference is 34 cm, the head circumference would normally be about

a. 32 cm
b. 36 cm
c. 38 cm

128. An indication that the woman may not be bonding with her neonate is when the mother

a. exhibits disgust when the infant urinates and refuses to change the diaper
b. points out that the neonate looks like a paternal grandparent
c. asks that the infant be placed in the nursery during the night

129. Paternal-neonate bonding includes three stages: Commitment, attachment, and

a. knowledge
b. preparation
c. acceptance

130. If a woman admitted in labor plans to relinquish her infant for adoption, the nurse should

a. avoid any mention of adoption
b. acknowledge the adoption plans
c. ask the woman if she has changed her mind

131. To prevent contamination, reconstituted formula for bottle feeding should not be stored in the refrigerator for more than

a. 6 hours
b. 12 hours
c. 24 hours

132. To facilitate bonding between the woman and her neonate if the woman chooses to bottle feed, the nurse should encourage the woman to

a. maintain eye contact with the neonate
b. hold the infant with the head higher than the body
c. swaddle the infant tightly in a blanket

133. The neonate of a diabetic mother whose blood glucose levels were elevated above 145 mg/dL during labor is likely to experience

a. hyperglycemia and hypercalcemia
b. hypoglycemia and hypocalcemia
c. hypoglycemia and hypercalcemia

134. The primary risk factor for metritis (uterine infection) is

a. hematoma
b. vaginal birth
c. caesarean birth

135. A woman with gestational diabetes is at risk of delivering a neonate with

a. microsomia
b. macrosomia
c. congenital defects

136. If a woman with a history of bipolar disease develops marked hyperactivity about two weeks after delivery with signs of postpartum psychosis, including confusion and anger toward the infant, the first intervention should be to

a. remove the neonate from the home
b. urge the woman to seek treatment
c. immediately refer services to help the mother care for the infant during this period

137. If a neonate is born with gastroschisis, the exposed organs should be

a. pushed back into place and covered with dry dressing
b. irrigated and covered with wet dressings
c. covered with moist gauze and wrapped in plastic

138. Following delivery, the best preventive measure to reduce the risk of developing deep vein thrombosis (DVT) is

a. ASA prophylaxis
b. early ambulation
c. adequate hydration

139. A first-line treatment for gestational hypertensive disorders is

a. nifedipine
b. hydrochlorothiazide
c. furosemide

140. A woman should be encouraged to room-in with her neonate during hospitalization in order to

a. reduce maternal anxiety
b. initiate maternal responsibility
c. facilitate bonding

141. On the day of delivery, a diabetic woman who has been receiving insulin for type 1 diabetes will probably require

a. the same dosage
b. a higher dosage
c. a lower dosage

142. If a neonate has a hematocrit of 67%, this likely indicates

a. polycythemia
b. anemia
c. hypovolemia

143. If a Haitian woman states she does not want to name her baby girl, the nurse should assume

a. the woman is not bonding with the neonate
b. delayed naming is a cultural norm
c. the woman is unhappy with the child's gender

144. Following delivery, postpartum blues typically subsides within about

a. 4 days
b. 10 days
c. 16 days

145. X-linked disorders affect

a. male offspring primarily
b. female offspring primarily
c. male and female offspring equally

146. If a woman expresses concern that her 3-year-old child does not seem to love the neonate, the nurse should advise the woman that

a. the child may need professional help to develop a bond
b. the mother should pay less attention to the neonate
c. young children develop affection over time

147. A woman who is nursing her neonate usually needs to increase fluid intake by about

a. 500 mL day
b. 1000 mL day
c. 2000 mL day

148. An antidepressant that is generally considered reasonably safe to continue during pregnancy for women with a history of severe depression is

a. paroxetine (Paxil®)
b. tranylcypromine (Parnate®)
c. citalopram (Celexa®)

149. A neonate exposed to or infected with herpes simplex is treated with

a. cephalosporin
b. acyclovir
c. corticosteroid

150. Conditions associated with oligohydramnios include

a. urinary tract anomalies
b. chromosomal abnormalities, such as trisomy 21
c. obstructional lesions of GI tract

151. Laboratory abnormalities associated with disseminated intravascular coagulation include

a. increased platelet counts
b. increased fibrinogen
c. prolonged prothrombin

152. When assisting a patient to take a sitz bath to relieve swelling and discomfort of hemorrhoids, the nurse should assure that the water temperature does not exceed

a. 100 °F (38 °C)
b. 105 °F (41 °C)
c. 110 °F (43 °C)

153. If a normal speaking voice is 50 to 60 decibels, the noise levels in the nursery and NICU should be maintained at

a. ≤45 decibels
b. ≤50 decibels
c. ≤60 decibels

154. With kangaroo care, the neonate in minimal clothing is placed

a. in a swaddling blanket and held
b. between the mother's bare breasts
c. in a sling across the mother's breasts

155. If a neonate has a patent ductus arteriosus, the usual initial treatment is

a. captopril
b. prostaglandin
c. indomethacin

156. In the neonate, the nurse should immediately report any periods of apnea that last for more than

a. 10 seconds
b. 20 seconds
c. 30 seconds

157. The wet neonate's temperature falls rapidly after birth if not promptly dried and warmed because of

a. evaporation
b. convection
c. radiation

158. Following birth, damage to the neonate's upper brachial plexus (C5 to C7) is likely to result in

a. Ipsilateral Horner syndrome
b. Klumpke's palsy
c. Erb's palsy

159. The purpose of administering vitamin K to a neonate is to

a. facilitate clotting
b. prevent clotting
c. treat anemia

160. According to Safe Sleep guidelines, parents should be taught to place a neonate on the back

a. when the neonate is sleeping and unattended
b. during the night
c. during the first two weeks

161. Starting immediately after hospital discharge, the neonate should have "tummy time"

a. 2 to 3 times a day
b. whenever the neonate is awake
c. 4 to 6 times a day

162. The normal position for the neonate's ears is with the insertion point of the top of the ear parallel to the

a. eyebrow
b. outer canthus of the eye
c. nostrils

163. When placing a newborn in a safety car seat, the seat should be rear-facing and

a. reclined 30-45 degrees
b. upright
c. flat

164. If a neonate must undergo a medical procedure, sucrose analgesia (SweetEase™) should be given to the infant

a. when the procedure starts
b. 10 minutes before the procedure
c. 2 minutes before the procedure

165. According to the Silverman-Anderson Index, a neonate exhibiting see-saw movement of the chest/abdomen, pronounced intercostal and xiphoid retraction, nasal flaring, and audible grunt would receive a score of

a. 2
b. 6
c. 10

166. The neonatal hearing test that measures the integrity of the middle and inner ear and the outer hair cells of the cochlea is the

a. auditory brainstem response
b. otoacoustic emissions test
c. bone-conduction test

167. The eye prophylaxis for neonates that is generally the drug of choice is

a. erythromycin
b. silver nitrate
c. tetracycline

168. If air becomes trapped in the alveoli because of meconium aspiration during labor and delivery, the neonate is at risk for

a. pulmonary embolism
b. air embolism
c. pneumothorax

169. ABO incompatibility can occur if

a. the mother is B and the fetus is A
b. the mother is O and the fetus is B
c. the mother is A and the fetus is C

170. If a neonate with Down syndrome has skin that appears mottled at times (pale in some areas and flushed in others), especially if the neonate is exposed to cool air, the most likely cause is

a. acrocyanosis
b. erythema toxicum
c. cutis marmorata

171. In order for a child to be born with cystic fibrosis, an autosomal recessive disorder,

a. both parents must carry the defective gene
b. either parent must carry the defective gene
c. the mother must carry the defective gene

172. If a neonate is born to an HIV infected mother, the neonate should begin antiretroviral medications within

a. 6 weeks
b. 24 to 48 hours
c. 6 to 12 hours

173. In order to prevent intracranial hemorrhage, a neonate with thrombocytopenia generally requires a platelet count of at least

a. 100,000
b. 50,000
c. 30,000

174. If a neonate's mother was addicted to methamphetamine use during her pregnancy, the neonate in withdrawal will likely exhibit

a. hyporeflexia
b. high-pitched crying
c. inability to sleep

175. Neonates who are bottle fed need to be burped

a. every 2 to 3 ounces
b. if appears uncomfortable
c. at the end of feeding, regardless of volume

Answer Key and Explanations

1. C: Whenever possible, breastfeeding is the nutritional method of choice for the newborn infant and has many advantages for both the infant and the postpartum mother. The nutritional composition of human milk is ideal for the newborn infant and cannot be entirely replicated in formula. Breastfed infants have improved immunity relative to formula-fed infants, including a decreased risk for respiratory and gastrointestinal infections, serious bacterial infections, and allergic disease, including milk-protein allergy. Advantages for the breastfeeding mother include faster postpartum weight loss and a lower risk of breast and ovarian cancer later in life.

2. A: The uterine discharge expelled in the postpartum period is called lochia and consists of blood cells, epithelial cells, uterine debris, and the superficial layer of the endometrial decidua basalis. Lochia rubra is expelled in the first 2-3 days of the postpartum period; it is dark red in color and may include expulsion of small clots, usually as a result of pooling of the lochia rubra in the upper vagina. Lochia serosa is a pink-colored discharge and is expelled on days 4-10 postpartum. Lochia alba is a white-yellow discharge that is seen for 1-2 weeks following the lochia serosa. Variations in volume and duration are common, but the overall trend with lochia should be a lighter color and volume as time elapses. Assessment of lochia volume and character is important in the postpartum period to monitor for excessive postpartum bleeding.

3. C: Surfactant is a lipoprotein that is produced in the lung alveoli beginning at 24 weeks' gestation. Surfactant reduces the surface tension of the alveoli by coating their inner surface. This results in a decreased tendency for the alveoli to collapse. Surfactant deficiency leads to progressive respiratory distress as a result of impaired lung compliance, ultimately leading to hypoxia, respiratory failure, and metabolic acidosis, all of which further impair surfactant production. Respiratory distress due to surfactant deficiency is called respiratory distress syndrome (RDS) and is most commonly seen in preterm infants. The morbidity and mortality of RDS are markedly reduced with the early assessment of fetal lung maturity, identification of high-risk infants, and the endotracheal administration of surfactant replacement therapy.

4. B: Maternal nutritional status is an important determinant of both maternal and fetal wellbeing. Women with a normal body mass index whose pregnancy weight gain is within the recommended range have the lowest risk for complications in pregnancy and delivery. Poor weight gain during pregnancy is associated with an increased risk of preterm delivery and low birth weight. Obesity and pregnancy weight gain above the recommended range are associated with an increased risk of gestational diabetes, cesarean delivery, fetal macrosomia, fetal demise, postpartum hemorrhage, fetal neural tube defects, and difficulty with postpartum weight loss.

5. A: Neonatal resuscitation guidelines allow for all care providers managing newborn infants to proceed along a standardized algorithm to stabilize the infant as soon as possible after delivery. Initial steps may vary with deliveries involving meconium-stained amniotic fluid in an attempt to avoid worsening meconium aspiration. In the newborn without meconium-stained amniotic fluid, the infant is warmed, dried, suctioned (if necessary), and placed in a position that allows for unobstructed breathing. Heart rate, respiratory effort, and color are then evaluated. If the infant has poor respiratory effort or rate or the heart rate is lower than 100 beats/min, positive-pressure ventilation is provided. If positive-pressure ventilation does not improve the heart rate to 100 beats/min, then chest compression and epinephrine administration are indicated.

6. B: Medical care providers need to stay up-to-date with current recommendations and care guidelines to ensure that they are providing quality, evidence-based care to patients, while protecting themselves from allegations of medical mismanagement. While methods that have proven effective over a substantial period of time may continue to do so, it is important that clinical practice incorporate recent research and best practices into their standardized methods. When situations arise in clinical practice that require deviation from established standards of practice, thorough documentation in the medical record, detailing the provider's medical decision-making process is particularly important. Medical care that is consistent with established guidelines can minimize a provider's legal liability. The primary purpose of following professionally established standards, however, is providing safe, high-quality, evidence-based care to the patient.

7. C: Assessment of the breasts is an important component of the comprehensive nurse assessment in the postpartum period. During pregnancy, elevated estrogen and progesterone levels cause the breasts to enlarge and become more glandular. The postpartum patient should have her breasts assessed for firmness, tenderness, redness, and engorgement in addition to nipple soreness or cracking. In the breastfeeding patient, a crucial part of the nurse assessment is evaluation of infant latch and removal from the breast. In the non-breastfeeding patient, techniques for lactation suppression and pain management can be reviewed and demonstrated. The postpartum mother should be reminded of the importance of self-breast examinations for lumps indicative of malignancy, but the immediate postpartum period will prove difficult to identify lumps upon assessment due to the number of changes the breasts are going through at this time.

8. A: Newborns are vitamin K-deficient as a result of poor transfer of vitamin K across the placenta and low capability of the liver to store vitamin K in the newborn period. Several clotting factors depend on the presence of adequate vitamin K for proper function. As a result, vitamin K deficiency leads to an increased risk of serious bleeding. Newborns at increased risk for vitamin K deficiency include breastfed infants, as there are low levels of vitamin K in human milk, and infants born to mothers taking anticonvulsant medication. Bleeding as a result of a vitamin K deficiency often presents as bleeding of the umbilicus, gastrointestinal tract, circumcision or venipuncture sites, or rarely, intracranium. Vitamin K administered routinely after delivery prevents most cases of bleeding in the neonate that results from a vitamin K deficiency.

9. B: Perineal pain is present in virtually all postpartum patients after vaginal delivery. Ice pack application, sitz baths, and careful cleaning after voiding (e.g., using a "peri-bottle" to squirt water onto the perineum) are helpful supportive care measures to reduce and manage postpartum perineal pain. Topical anesthetics or soothing agents (e.g., witch hazel) may also be applied. Analgesics are not typically first line treatment for perineal pain. Changing the "peri-pad" frequently can reduce the risk of contamination of perineal wounds but is not typically helpful for reducing pain. Perineal lacerations need to be monitored for signs of poor healing or infection, such as erythema, marked swelling, and discharge or wound dehiscence.

10. A: There are multiple methods for the evaluation and monitoring of fetal wellbeing. In high-risk pregnancies (e.g., maternal hypertension, multiple gestation) or in cases where there are other concerns for fetal wellbeing (e.g., decreased fetal movement, previous fetal demise), antepartum fetal monitoring is generally indicated. Fetal movement counting (e.g., maternal perception of fetal movement) is considered normal if the mother perceives ten distinct movements over a 2-hour period (after 32-34 weeks' gestation). The nonstress test involves fetal heart rate (FHR) monitoring and is considered reassuring ("reactive") if there are at least two fetal heart rate accelerations (>15 beats/min above baseline, lasting >15 seconds) in a 20-minute period. The biophysical profile combines FHR monitoring with ultrasonographic evaluation of fetal tone, fetal movement, amniotic fluid volume, and fetal respiratory movements.

11. C: Powdered formula is the least expensive form of commercially available infant formula, but it must be reconstituted, using water. Proper mixing (60 mL water for each scoop of powdered formula) is crucial to avoid medical complications in the infant because of inappropriately concentrated or dilute formula. Among the three forms available, powdered formula preparation has the highest risk for contamination. Formula concentrate is mixed with water to its appropriate concentration, while ready-to-feed formula is given without any mixing required. Although ready-to-feed formula is the easiest to use, its cost is significant. Whichever type of formula is used, proper mixing and storage guidelines must be reviewed with postpartum families.

12. B: Immediately after vaginal delivery of the placenta, the normal uterus contracts to grapefruit-size, and the fundus is palpable between the umbilicus and the pubic symphysis. During the first 6-12 hours after delivery, the ligaments and muscles supporting the uterus relax somewhat, and the fundus is palpable at or below the umbilicus. Beginning approximately 24 hours after delivery, the shrinking uterus descends about 1 cm/d into the pelvis, reaching pre-pregnancy size and location by 6 weeks' postpartum. Excessive blood loss, infection, and retained placental fragments can lead to an interruption of the normal postpartum uterine contractions, leading to uterine atony. A common cause of uterine atony and displacement of the uterine fundus after delivery is bladder distention.

13. C: Approximately one-third of infants in the United States are delivered by cesarean section. Cesarean delivery may be performed for maternal indications, fetal indications, or both. Examples of common indications for cesarean birth include placenta previa, breech presentation, placental abruption, congenital anomalies, fetal distress, maternal infection, and previous delivery by cesarean section. Women who deliver by cesarean section are at increased risk for infection, thromboembolic events, and anesthesia complications. Infants delivered by cesarean section are at increased risk for respiratory complications, physical injury (e.g., laceration, fracture), early breastfeeding difficulties, and admission to a neonatal intensive care unit.

14. B: Facilitating and assisting with the family's grief process after a perinatal death is an important nursing intervention and is best accomplished with consistency in the nursing staff. This allows for establishment of a therapeutic relationship between the nurse and the grieving family. Ideally, the nurse assists the family in expressing their feelings about the loss, participating in decision-making about the birth and postpartum period (including seeing the deceased infant), and becoming aware of the resources available for ongoing support during the journey through the grieving process. Sharing personal stories may appear as an effort to normalize an extremely unique and private experience for the family, and should be avoided. Although not all parents choose to see or spend time with the deceased infant, it can be very helpful in assisting the family to accept the loss of the infant, therefore utilizing a bereavement room should not be rushed.

15. C: Establishing successful and satisfying breastfeeding for both the mother and infant depends on proper teaching of multiple factors, including signs of infant hunger, ways to wake the sleepy infant, breast and nipple care, proper positioning of mother and infant, and proper infant latch on the breast. The infant's mouth should be attached not just to the nipple but far back onto the areola. A shallow latch on the nipple is painful for the mother, and milk let-down is often inhibited. The infant's lower lip should be out and the infant's nose should be close to (but not compressed against) the breast. Establishing the proper latch can be time-consuming and frustrating initially, but most infants and mothers ultimately accomplish the proper latch with teaching and support.

16. C: Uric acid crystals appear reddish-orange in color ("brick dust") and are often mistaken for blood in the infant's diaper. Urate crystals form most commonly when an infant is dehydrated and are, therefore, quite common in the neonatal period, particularly in the breastfed infant. The crystals themselves are not harmful or dangerous and require no further intervention aside from an assessment of the infant's hydration status. True hematuria in the neonatal period is not a normal finding and requires further evaluation of the genitourinary tract.

17. A: Timely and accurate medical record documentation is a critical skill of all patient care providers. The bedside nurse is the care provider who most often assesses the patient, and his or her documentation is often the best representation of the patient's clinical status. Although the nurse's priority is providing excellent direct patient care, thorough documentation is important. The maternal/newborn nurse's documentation should include objective data about maternal/fetal status (e.g., vital signs, fetal heart rate monitoring); recognition of problems or complications; nursing actions in response to changes in the patient's status; communication with other providers, including their responses; communication with the patient and family members; and details of the patient's response to interventions. In legal cases alleging medical mismanagement, the medical record is often the most critical document available to a provider who must defend his or her actions.

18. B: Breast stimulation from infant sucking or a breast pump leads to prolactin release from the anterior pituitary and oxytocin release from the posterior pituitary. Milk production is stimulated by prolactin release, while milk secretion is stimulated by oxytocin release. Oxytocin also stimulates uterine contractions. Initiation of breastfeeding in the postpartum period can, therefore, lead to improved uterine contractions and a decreased risk of postpartum hemorrhage as a result of uterine atony. Human chorionic gonadotropin is an important hormone of early pregnancy for maintenance of the corpus luteum.

19. C: One of the most critical physiologic adaptations of the newborn infant is the use of the lungs as the primary organs of gas exchange. In utero, oxygen from maternal blood flows through the placenta into the umbilical vein. From the umbilical vein, it travels to the right side of the fetal heart and is then diverted across the foramen ovale or ductus arteriosus to the fetal body. In the fetal circulation, pulmonary vascular resistance is high, and there is relatively little pulmonary blood flow. Fetal waste and carbon dioxide flow through the umbilical arteries into the placenta and are eliminated through the maternal circulation. When the newborn infant takes a breath after birth, the inhaled oxygen stimulates dilation of the pulmonary vessels, and blood flow to the lungs increases as pulmonary vascular resistance falls. This process is crucial for a smooth transition to extrauterine life.

20. B: Magnesium sulfate is administered in the obstetrical setting for the treatment of preterm labor because it relaxes smooth muscle and for the treatment of preeclampsia and eclampsia because it depresses the central nervous system. Magnesium sulfate is usually administered as a continuous intravenous drip, and side effects are dose-related. Common side effects include nausea, generalized weakness, lethargy, flushing, headache, and blurry vision. Patients need to be monitored closely for signs of magnesium sulfate toxicity to avoid life-threatening complications of magnesium administration. Loss of deep tendon reflexes (typically assessed with the patellar tendon reflex) is often the first sign of toxicity. Other signs of toxicity include a significantly depressed level of consciousness, hypotension, and respiratory depression. If magnesium sulfate toxicity is not recognized and promptly treated, the patient may experience total respiratory or cardiovascular collapse. Calcium gluconate is the antidote for magnesium sulfate toxicity and should be readily available for patients receiving magnesium sulfate.

21. B: Human milk and breastfeeding provide such great benefit to both the breastfeeding mother and infant that true contraindications to breastfeeding are relatively few and should be evaluated on a case-by-case basis. Generally accepted contraindications to breastfeeding (in most cases) include HIV infection, human T-lymphotropic virus 1 infection, active tuberculosis, active herpes breast lesions, illicit substance abuse or dependence, and chemotherapy or radiation therapy in the breastfeeding mother. Galactosemia in the infant is also a contraindication to breastfeeding. Recently diagnosed breast cancer may interfere with breastfeeding so that the mother can initiate treatment, but treated breast cancer is not a contraindication. Similarly, treated or latent tuberculosis is not a contraindication to breastfeeding, in contrast to active, untreated tuberculosis.

22. B: Newborn infants are at risk for significant heat loss because of their large skin surface area relative to body mass, small amount of subcutaneous fat, and limited ability to shiver as a means of generating heat. Brown fat is produced from 26 weeks gestation until 1 month after birth and is metabolized in response to cold stress. Metabolism of brown fat requires oxygen and glucose and produces acids as a byproduct of the process. Brown fat metabolism ("nonshivering thermogenesis") is one of the few means by which the newborn infant produces heat. Cold stress in the newborn infant can lead to hypoglycemia, metabolic acidosis, and increased caloric requirements. Environmental interventions, such as use of a radiant warmer, drying, hats, and blankets, are crucial to prevent cold stress in the newborn infant.

23. B: Periodic assessment of the uterine fundus is a crucial part of postpartum care. The postpartum fundus should feel firm to palpation once the placenta has been delivered. A boggy fundus is a sign of uterine atony or relaxed uterine muscles. Uterine atony is a common cause of postpartum hemorrhage and should be recognized and treated promptly. Many postpartum patients can lose a large amount of blood within the uterine cavity before becoming symptomatic of serious blood loss. The first step in treating uterine atony is external fundal massage to stimulate the uterine muscles to contract. Bladder distention may lead to uterine atony and results in the fundus being displaced laterally. If bladder distention is suspected, the patient is encouraged to void. Should these interventions not be effective, the physician should be notified.

24. A: The postpartum nurse is in an excellent position to observe and support early attachment between the postpartum patient and her infant. Early opportunities for the mother to hold, interact with, and feed the infant as soon as possible after delivery can encourage mother-infant bonding. Important components to assess include the frequency and type of contact between the mother and infant (e.g., eye contact, close touch/hold), sensitivity to the infant's needs, responsiveness to the infant's needs, and the mother's interpretation of the infant's behaviors. Decreasing maternal interaction with the infant over time indicates impaired attachment, while maternal requests for rest or for family members to hold the infant are healthy and supported actions. Factors that may interfere with mother-infant bonding include maternal or infant medical complications, inadequate postpartum pain management, negative past pregnancy or postpartum experiences, and inadequate family or partner support. All patients, but particularly the first-time mother, benefit from education and positive reinforcement for appropriate infant care behaviors in the postpartum period.

25. A: If an Rh-negative woman is pregnant with an Rh-positive fetus and fetal red blood cells enter the maternal circulation, Rh antibodies form in the maternal circulation. This process is referred to as "sensitization." A subsequent pregnancy with a Rh-positive fetus in the sensitized Rh-negative mother leads to hemolysis of fetal red blood cells as maternal anti-Rh antibodies cross the placenta, leading to severe fetal anemia. Rh immune globulin (Rhogam) confers passive antibody protection against Rh antigens, preventing maternal Rh-antigen antibody protection. The indirect Coombs test detects Rh-positive antibodies in the maternal circulation and is, therefore, the test of choice for maternal sensitization screening. If a Rh-negative mother delivers a Rh-positive infant and there is no evidence of maternal sensitization, Rhogam is administered within 72 hours of delivery. Rhogam is also administered after abortion, antepartum hemorrhage, amniocentesis, chorionic villus sampling, trauma, or any procedure or incident where there is a reasonable likelihood of maternal exposure to Rh-positive fetal blood.

26. C: Infants born to a diabetic mother (IDM) are at increased risk for multiple complications in the newborn period. Maternal hyperglycemia causes fetal hyperglycemia as glucose freely crosses the placenta. Fetal hyperglycemia leads to increased fetal insulin production, which exerts a growth hormone-like effect (causing macrosomia). After birth (when the infant is no longer exposed to maternal hyperglycemia), the newborn's elevated insulin level causes a rapid fall in serum glucose, typically within 1-6 hours after birth. Symptoms of neonatal hypoglycemia include temperature instability, tremors, and poor feeding. Other complications in the newborn period of the IDM include hyperbilirubinemia, birth trauma, polycythemia, and respiratory distress syndrome.

27. A: The composition of mature human milk varies significantly as a single feeding progresses. The milk that flows at the beginning of a feeding is called foremilk. The milk that flows beginning at let-down (milk-ejection reflex) is called hindmilk. Foremilk is high in protein and low in fat, while hindmilk is high in fat (and calories) but with a low protein content. The let-down reflex typically occurs 1-2 minutes after the infant begins sucking. Hindmilk is released from the breast alveoli into the ducts in response to oxytocin release. Colostrum is the milk that is present immediately after birth and until the mother's mature milk "comes in." Colostrum is a thick, yellow fluid with large amounts of immunoglobulin and protein and is relatively low in fat compared with mature milk.

28. A: A significant amount of blood loss can occur in the postpartum period before it becomes clinically apparent. As a result, the postpartum nurse needs to be aware of risk factors for postpartum hemorrhage and early signs of significant blood loss. Early postpartum hemorrhage (within 24 hours of delivery) may be caused by a combination of factors. Uterine atony (inappropriate relaxation of the uterine musculature) is a common cause of early postpartum hemorrhage. Risk factors for uterine atony include uterine distention (e.g., multiple gestation, macrosomic infant), preeclampsia, retained placental fragments, bladder distention, medication (e.g., magnesium sulfate), and instrumented delivery (e.g., forceps and vacuum extraction). Genital lacerations (e.g., perineum, cervix, vagina) can also cause significant postpartum blood loss. Risk factors for genital lacerations include instrumented delivery, macrosomic infant, nulliparous mother, and precipitous vaginal delivery. Retained placental fragments, vulvar or pelvic hematomas, and uterine inversion are additional causes of early postpartum hemorrhage.

29. B: Intrapartum fetal heart rate monitoring requires documentation and interpretation of five variables: baseline fetal heart rate, baseline heart rate variability, presence or absence of fetal heart rate accelerations, fetal heart rate decelerations, and changes in the fetal heart rate pattern as labor progresses. Interpretation of fetal heart rate monitoring can be complex and challenging but is an important component of intrapartum fetal monitoring. In general, when fetal heart rate monitoring demonstrates a normal baseline rate with accelerations, moderate variability, and no late or variable decelerations, the fetus is neither hypoxemic nor acidotic. Early decelerations with normal variability are associated with uterine contractions; fetal head compression, which occurs with the uterine contraction, leads to stimulation of the vagus nerve, leading to a decrease in fetal heart rate, which resolves as the contraction subsides. Early decelerations are not associated with fetal hypoxia and require no intervention.

30. A: Cephalohematoma may occur in up to 2% of births and is far more common in vertex vaginal delivery than cesarean births. Blood vessels between the cranial bone and the periosteal layer rupture, leading to the formation of a hematoma in the subperiosteal space, which is limited in its extension by cranial suture lines. Cephalohematoma typically becomes clinically apparent in the first 1-2 days after birth and may take weeks to months to resolve. This is in contrast to a caput succedaneum, a subcutaneous collection of edematous fluid, which crosses suture lines, is typically present at birth, and resolves within hours to days after birth.

31. C: Mastitis is an infection of the connective tissue of the breast that occurs almost exclusively in lactating women. Mastitis is unusual in the immediate postpartum period, and is typically seen beginning 2-3 weeks after delivery in the breastfeeding patient. Human milk is an excellent medium for bacterial (and fungal) growth and typically becomes infected when bacteria from the infant's mouth or maternal skin ascend through a traumatized nipple. Mastitis typically presents with focal, unilateral breast pain and may be accompanied by fever and flu-like symptoms. The affected breast region is typically warm, red, and tender. Treatment of mastitis includes frequent breastfeeding, warm packs, pain relievers, and systemic antibiotics. Increased breast-emptying by frequent nursing or pumping leads to a rapid resolution of symptoms and a decreased risk of progression to breast abscess. Because nipple trauma and milk stasis are major contributing causes of mastitis, proper nipple care and breastfeeding technique can prevent many cases of mastitis. The postpartum patient who is breastfeeding her newborn should be instructed in proper infant latch, nipple care, and positioning techniques, which enhance complete emptying of both breasts.

32. B: Jaundice is common in the neonatal period, occurring in up to 50% of full-term newborns and 80% of preterm infants. Prenatally, fetal unconjugated bilirubin crosses the placenta to be conjugated and excreted. Postnatally, unconjugated bilirubin is converted in the liver to its water-soluble form and then excreted in the infant's urine and stool. The infant is physiologically vulnerable to hyperbilirubinemia in the first several weeks of life for several reasons: there are low levels of hepatic enzymes necessary to convert bilirubin to its water-soluble form; there is a large unconjugated bilirubin load as a result of an increased rate of red blood cell destruction (in the newborn), and there is an increased reabsorption of bilirubin from the immature gastrointestinal tract. Physiologic jaundice as a result of these expected factors does not become clinically apparent until after 24 hours of life. Jaundice that is present in the first 24 hours after birth is considered pathologic and may result from abnormal hemolysis (e.g., ABO incompatibility) or underlying liver disease.

33. B: Group B *Streptococcus* (GBS) remains a common cause of neonatal sepsis and may lead to early-onset illness (within 1 week of birth) or late-onset illness. Infants with early-onset GBS disease are seriously ill and may present with pneumonia, apnea, and shock. Meningitis is more common in late-onset GBS disease. Approximately 20-25% of pregnant woman are colonized by GBS in their lower gastrointestinal or urinary tracts and can transmit the infection to the infant during vaginal delivery. Intrapartum antibiotic administration in pregnant women with positive GBS cultures (or other risk factors) at least 4 hours before delivery significantly reduces the incidence of early-onset GBS disease in newborns. *Gardnerella vaginalis* is the etiologic agent in bacterial vaginosis and is not a cause of neonatal sepsis. *Neisseria gonorrhoeae* may cause neonatal conjunctivitis but is not a cause of neonatal sepsis.

34. C: Postpartum "blues" (or adjustment reaction with depressed mood) occurs in more than half of postpartum mothers and is characterized by mild depressive symptoms in addition to happier periods. Postpartum "blues" typically occurs within a few days of delivery and lasts approximately 1-2 weeks. The postpartum "blues" are thought to be caused by rapid swings in prolactin, estrogen, and progesterone levels after delivery. Typical features include frequent tearfulness, fatigue, anxiety, irritability, and feelings of being overwhelmed. Signs of major depression (e.g., suicidal ideation) or psychosis are not features of the postpartum "blues."

35. B: The newborn infant is equipped with multiple behavioral and sensory mechanisms for interacting with his or her environment. Orientation describes the newborn's ability to notice, follow, and fixate on appealing visual and auditory inputs. The infant's ability to orient in this way encourages parent-infant bonding as the infant responds to caregivers' faces and voices. The newborn's ability to decrease his or her response to a repetitive stimulus (e.g., ambient noise, flashing lights) is habituation. Self-quieting refers to the infant's ability to calm him- or herself (e.g., with hand-sucking) when distressed. The degree to which an infant can habituate or self-quiet is often a large component of parental perception of the infant's temperament.

36. C: Proper care of the umbilical cord is important to prevent infection. Hospitals and families differ in the specifics of umbilical cord care, depending on tradition and cultural beliefs. Some medical providers advocate daily use of alcohol or antibacterial ointments, although there is no definitive data supporting their use. In general, the umbilical cord stump should be kept dry and either exposed to air or covered loosely with clean dressings or clothing. The base of the cord stump and the skin around the umbilicus can be cleaned several times daily with water and a cotton swab. Baths involving submersion of the abdomen in water should be avoided until the stump has fallen off. Pulling the cord stump is not recommended.

37. A: Infants in breech presentation at the time of delivery have a markedly increased incidence of perinatal injury and death, regardless of whether delivery is vaginal or surgical. Breech presentation occurs in 3-4% of all deliveries and is more common with congenital fetal anomalies, preterm deliveries, uterine or placental malformations, and multiple gestation. Risks to the fetus or newborn with breech presentation include increased risk of umbilical cord prolapse, fetal asphyxia/nonreassuring fetal status, spinal cord/brachial plexus injuries, dystocia, and perinatal death. Most infants in breech presentation at the time of delivery are delivered by cesarean section.

38. A: Breast engorgement differs from the normal feeling of fullness that the breastfeeding mother experiences when milk first "comes in." Engorgement is characterized by firm, warm, and painful breasts. Engorged breasts often appear taut and shiny and may be accompanied by axillary swelling and low-grade fever. The infant often has difficulty latching onto the engorged breast. Treatment of breast engorgement in the breastfeeding mother includes more frequent feedings at least 10-15 minutes on each breast to allow adequate emptying of both breasts, warm (or cold) compress application to stimulate let-down and soften the breasts, and pain relievers as needed for further relief. Supportive nursing bras may help with discomfort between feedings. Antibiotics are only indicated in the case on infection, such as mastitis.

39. A: Postpartum patients vary a great deal in the timing of their return to sexual activity. Because pregnancy can occur with the first ovulation after pregnancy (before first menstruation occurs), contraception and family planning issues should be discussed with all postpartum patients before discharge. Women who are not breastfeeding generally have a faster return of ovulation and menstruation compared with women who are breastfeeding. Breastfeeding is a fairly effective contraceptive method in the postpartum period (lactational amenorrhea method) provided that the mother is fully breastfeeding (day and night), is amenorrhoeic, and less than 6 months postpartum. A decrease in breastfeeding leads to an increased likelihood of ovulation and, therefore, an increased risk of pregnancy. Therefore, it is possible to get pregnant while breastfeeding. Other forms of postpartum contraception include progestin-only oral contraceptives, combined estrogen/progestin oral contraceptive, intrauterine devices, sterilization, and barrier methods. Depending on whether the patient is breastfeeding, recommended timing for each method varies.

40. B: Cyanosis limited to the distal extremities and perioral regions is known as acrocyanosis and is a common and normal finding in newborn infants. Central cyanosis (lips and tongue in addition to the trunk and extremities) in the newborn infant is not a normal finding. Central cyanosis in the neonate that persists after appropriate immediate post-delivery resuscitation is usually a sign of serious pulmonary disease (e.g., persistent pulmonary hypertension, respiratory distress syndrome), congenital heart disease (e.g., transposition of the great vessels, total anomalous pulmonary venous return), and sepsis. Fever may be present in the infant with sepsis/neonatal infection, but is not a finding that is highly specific for congenital heart disease.

41. C: The full-term healthy newborn infant can be expected to lose 5-10% of birth weight in the first 5-7 days of life as a result of fluid shifts and adjustment to feeding. Infants who are exclusively breastfed generally lose more weight than formula-fed infants as a result of the wait for maternal milk production to begin. Preterm infants and infants who are large-for-gestational age may have increased weight loss after birth as well. If an infant is having difficulty with feedings or is losing more weight than would be expected, close monitoring is warranted with feeding evaluation and support and frequent weight checks. Most healthy infants should return to their birth weight by 2 weeks of age.

42. A: Care of the postpartum patient after a cesarean delivery involves the usual postpartum care, in addition to close attention to the conditions unique to the mother who has undergone abdominal surgery. Postsurgical patients have an increased need for analgesic medications and other pain-relieving techniques after delivery. Early contact with her infant and early breastfeeding help with mother-infant bonding. Patients should be encouraged to take deep breaths regularly after cesarean delivery to minimize the risk of pulmonary infections. Leg exercises and early ambulation after cesarean delivery decrease the risk of venous thrombosis and speed the return of normal gastrointestinal motility.

43. C: Preeclampsia is a disease unique to pregnancy and typically presents anytime from late pregnancy to the postpartum period. Preeclampsia is characterized clinically by new onset hypertension with or without proteinuria, and edema. Preeclampsia is more common in first pregnancies. Preeclampsia leads to decreased organ perfusion, including the uterus and placenta. A form of preeclampsia with severe features is known as the HELLP syndrome in which lab findings include: hemolysis (H), elevated liver enzymes (EL), and low platelets (LP). Eclampsia is characterized by the onset of seizures or coma in women with preeclampsia, assuming the absence of alternate etiologies of seizure or coma.

44. B: Estimation of gestational age in the stable newborn infant is an important component of newborn assessment. Complications in the neonatal period more commonly occur in association with gestational age rather than birth weight. In other words, a small-for-gestational-age infant born at 35 weeks' gestation has a less complicated newborn course than a large-for-gestational-age infant born at 31 weeks' gestation. There are multiple tools available for estimation of gestational age, all of which combine evaluation of both external physical characteristics and neuromuscular development. Preterm infants tend to have decreased muscle tone, resulting in a less flexed resting posture. Preterm infants also have more lanugo, thinner skin, fewer plantar foot creases, less developed ear cartilage, and less breast bud tissue than term infants. Tests for neuromuscular development include assessment of the angle of the wrist, assessment of the popliteal, hip, and ankle flexion, and observation of the infant's resting posture.

45. C: Chronic maternal narcotic use during pregnancy leads to neonatal withdrawal symptoms within 72 hours of birth. Symptoms of drug withdrawal include high-pitched cry, vomiting, irritability, seizures, diarrhea, and sneezing. Maternal alcohol use can lead to fetal alcohol syndrome, which is characterized by specific facial features, developmental disability and feeding or growth problems. Fetal exposure to cocaine may lead to abnormal brain development, behavioral disturbances, and an increased risk for sudden infant death syndrome. Heavy maternal marijuana use may be associated with mild neonatal withdrawal symptoms, but a link between isolated marijuana use and neonatal withdrawal symptoms has not been definitively established. Heavy maternal caffeine ingestion may lead to symptomatic withdrawal in the exposed infant but is less likely to cause neonatal withdrawal syndrome.

46. A: Although circumcision rates in the United States have been dropping in recent years, at least half of newborn males are circumcised. There are multiple clamp devices used for neonatal circumcision, as well as the Plastibell. Home care of the penis recently circumcised with one of the clamp devices should involve gentle warm water cleaning with diaper changes, petroleum ointment application, and monitoring for bleeding or infection. A thin, yellow layer of granulation tissue is an expected finding on the recently circumcised penis and should not be removed. If a Plastibell is in place, no ointment should be applied until the Plastibell has fallen off (usually by 7 days after circumcision).

47. A: Periodic breathing is a normal respiratory pattern in the newborn infant and is observed more commonly in preterm infants. As opposed to true apnea, periodic breathing is not associated with any cardiorespiratory compromise and resolves without intervention or stimulation. A pause in respiration that is prolonged (>15-20 seconds) or of any duration with associated with signs of cardiorespiratory compromise is not consistent with periodic breathing. Periodic breathing most commonly occurs during sleep. Transient tachypnea of the newborn is due to retention of excess lung fluid during delivery and is characterized by 12-72 hours of tachypnea with variable degrees of hypoxia and respiratory distress. Central apnea is due to an abnormality in brain control of respiratory stimulation and effort.

48. A: The newborn infant's first bowel movement (meconium) is a sticky, greenish black substance made up of bile salts and intestinal debris. Meconium may be passed during birth as a response to perinatal stress and can lead to respiratory distress and meconium aspiration syndrome if inhaled before or during delivery. Most healthy infants pass their first meconium stool by 24 hours of life. Delayed passage of meconium beyond 48 hours of life can indicate underlying disease, such as cystic fibrosis or Hirschsprung disease. Once feeding has been established, the stools transition to normal breastfed or formula-fed stools typical in infants. Breastfed stools are mustardy yellow in color with a cottage cheese consistency, while formula fed stools are slightly darker orange/tan, and slightly thicker in consistency (similar to peanut butter).

49. A: There are several reflexes found in the healthy term newborn. The rooting reflex occurs when the infant's cheek is touched, causing the infant to turn the head toward the side of contact with their mouth (to "find" the site for feeding). The Moro reflex is demonstrated when the infant is startled by sudden noise or movement and consists of the infant extending the arms suddenly and then slowly pulling them back to the body, often accompanied by a brief cry. The tonic neck reflex ("fencing" reflex) describes the extension of the infant's arm or leg on the side toward which the head is turned with associated flexion of the contralateral extremities. Other normal newborn reflexes include the grasping, sucking, and stepping reflexes.

50. B: Sudden infant death syndrome (SIDS) is the leading cause of death in 1-12-month-old infants. Rates of SIDS have declined by more than 50% since the initiation of the Back to Sleep campaign, which educates parents about the risks of placing infants on their stomachs to sleep. Other important recommendations that decrease the risk of SIDS include placing the infant on a firm surface to sleep, minimizing or eliminating second-hand cigarette smoke exposure, and using a pacifier during sleep. Gastroesophageal reflux symptoms may be more prominent in the supine position. The incidence of bronchiolitis is not affected by the infant sleep position.

51. B: Characteristics of jitteriness include:

- Clonic jerking with both fast and slow elements.
- Halted by gentle restraints.
- Elicited by stimulation.
- Lack of ocular deviation.
- Absence of autonomic response (increased heart rate, respirations, blood pressure).

Jitteriness is tremors of the chin and extremities, and is common in infants within a few days and may persist for up to months. Jitteriness is a benign condition but may indicate drug withdrawal, hypoglycemia, hypocalcemia, and encephalopathy.

52. A: After using a breast pump, the woman should rinse the equipment in cold water and then wash it in warm soapy water. If this isn't possible (such as when a woman is away from home), the woman should at least rinse the removable parts and then place them in a plastic bag so they can be washed later. The removable parts should be boiled for 20 minutes to sterilize or run through a dishwashing cycle once every 24 hours.

53. C: The most common neonatal bacterial infection is Group B *Streptococcus* (GBS) because most woman are carriers but asymptomatic. For this reason, women should be screened at 37+0 to 37+6 weeks of gestation and those who are positive administered antibiotics during labor. The woman needs at least 4 hours of antibiotics to provide adequate protection of the neonate from infection. Signs of infection in the neonate usually occur about 24 hours after birth although some infants have delayed symptoms 10 to 14 days after birth.

54. B: The neonate usually passes meconium within 8 to 24 hours although it may be delayed as long as 48 hours. First meconium is thick, dark, and tarry. Transitional stools for the next few days are usually brown to green, after which the child should pass normal stools. Stools of breastfed babies are usually yellow-gold and mushy, while bottle-fed are pale yellow and pasty in color. Bowel sounds can usually be heard within 30 to 60 minutes of birth as air begins to move down the GI tract (first to the stomach) as the child breathes.

55. A: If a few weeks after delivery, a woman complains that she cannot sleep, has little appetite and has begun having anxiety attacks and fears that she cannot take adequate care of her neonate, the most likely cause is postpartum depression. Onset may occur within the first 6 months but is not usually present initially, unlike postpartum blues. Symptoms of postpartum psychosis are much more severe and may include paranoia, hallucinations, and disorientation.

56. C: If a neonate's hemoglobin is 19.3 g/dL at birth, a typical value at 7 days is 17.4 g/dL. Hemoglobin is high immediately after birth because the placental environment is relatively hypoxic, but the hemoglobin begins to fall after birth with exposure to the higher oxygen content of ambient air and with an increase in adult hemoglobin. By 3 months, the hemoglobin usually ranges from 9.3 to 13.3 g/dL.

57. C: HELLP syndrome is characterized by (H) hemolysis, (EL) elevated liver enzymes, and (LP) low platelet count. HELLP syndrome is most common in multiparous women during weeks 27 to 37 but may occur within 24 hours after delivery. Pain in the right upper quadrant related to liver dysfunction may be misdiagnosed as gastrointestinal upset or gall bladder disease. Initial symptoms are often flu-like, including headache, nausea and vomiting and visual disturbances. Mortality rates are high without prompt diagnosis and treatment.

58. B: The vaccination that should be routinely administered to all newborns within 24 hours of birth is hepatitis B. The second dose should be given within the first to second month and the third dose between 6 and 18 months. If the neonate's mother is hepatitis B positive, then the neonate should receive the vaccination within 12 hours of birth and 0.5 mL of hepatitis B immune globulin (HBIG). If the mother's status is unknown, the neonate should also receive the vaccination within 12 hours of birth and the mother tested.

59. A: The Quad Screen includes: (1) Alpha-fetoprotein (AFP), (2) Human chorionic gonadotropin (hCG), (3) Estriol (uE^3), and (4) Inhibin A (INH-A).

Disorder	AFP	hCG	uE^3	INH-A
Neural tube defects	High	Normal	Normal	Normal
Trisomy 21	Low	High	Low	High
Trisomy 18	Low	Low	Low	Low
Multiple gestation	High	High	Normal	Normal

60. C: The infantile form of Tay-Sachs disease is classified as a metabolic defect. The infant lacks an enzyme necessary to metabolize fatty substances, so these build up in the body and damage the brain and nerve cells. Symptoms are usually evident by about 6 months, but there is currently no treatment. The child progressively loses control of muscles and becomes blind and paralyzed. Life expectancy ranges from 4 to 5 years.

61. A: The nutritional supplement given to women to prevent neural tube defects is folic acid. Folic acid deficiency causes megaloblastic anemia in which immature red blood cells enlarge rather than divide, so there are fewer red blood cells. However, because cells need to duplicate during pregnancy as the fetus grows, adequate folic acid is critical. Women should receive 0.4mg folic acid daily and, for deficiency, 1mg folic acid and iron supplements (because folic acid deficiency is associated with iron deficiency anemia).

62. C: If a woman complains that she is exhausted because the neonate nurses so frequently during the night that the woman cannot get any sleep, the nurse should advise the woman to sleep when the baby sleeps, day and night. Over time, the baby will establish a more regular nursing schedule, but initially neonates often want to nurse very frequently, especially in the evening, and irregularly. Bottle-fed babies usually go longer between feedings than babies that are nursed.

63. A: The CARE principles applied to the care of a pregnant woman refer to

- (C) Communication: Sharing information through speaking, writing, signs, or other means. Exhibiting mutual understanding and sympathy.
- (A) Advocate: Speaking for the person and the person's rights.
- (R) Respect: Paying attention, showing consideration, and respecting another.
- (E) Enable: Empowering the person through information, resources, and support.

64. B: The recreational drug that most increases the risk of spontaneous abortion is methamphetamine (commonly referred to as "meth" or "crank"). Methamphetamine is a stimulant drug that can be snorted or smoked. Methamphetamine has been associated with increased placental abruption and premature delivery. Infants may go through a form of withdrawal and exhibit tremors and poor muscle tone at birth. They may also have congenital abnormalities and may develop neurobehavioral problems.

65. C: While infants vary, by about the sixth day after birth, over a 24-hour period, most infants urinate approximately 6 to 8 times, having increased steadily from one diaper on the first day and two on the second day. The neonate's output depends on the intake, so if urinary output is inadequate, the patient may not be getting enough milk. Urine should be pale yellow in color. If the baby is jaundiced, the infant may excrete dark urine.

66. B: The neural tube defect that is most likely to result in hydrocephalus is myelomeningocele, which is a condition in which there is an opening in the spine through which the meninges and spinal cord protrude, in an exterior sac. Myelomeningocele is also associated with weakness or paralysis of the lower extremities and poor or no control of bowels and bladder. Surgery is done to close the defect and prevent CSF infection. Some require a ventriculoatrial shunt.

67. A: The mnemonic BUBBLE-HE is used to remember the steps to a comprehensive postpartal assessment:

- B: breasts—inspect carefully for firmness, color, temperature, abnormalities.
- U: uterus—check fundal location and tone.
- B: bladder—determine time of last urination and palpate bladder.
- B: bowels—determine last BM and presence of flatus.
- L: lochia—assess color, amount, presence of clots, signs of bleeding (free flow of blood).
- E: episiotomy (incision)—use REEDA assessment.
- H: Homan's signs (legs)—check for pain, swelling, redness, warmth in calves and pulses and sensation in legs and feet.
- E: Emotions: Assess level of exhaustion/fatigue and affect.

68. B: Human milk can be kept frozen in the freezer section of a side-by-side (separate door) refrigerator-freezer for 3 to 4 months. If the freezer compartment is inside the refrigerator (at the top) the milk should not be kept for more than 2 weeks because the temperature varies as the refrigerator is opened and closed. Deep freezers with a temperature of 0° C/32° F maintain temperature the best, so human milk can be frozen and stored for up to 6 months. Human milk is safe to use for up to 4 hours if stored at room temperature and up to 7 days if refrigerated.

69. C: If a pregnant woman at 38-weeks of gestation complains of dizziness when lying flat, the most likely cause is supine hypotensive syndrome. This drop in blood pressure and associated dizziness results when the enlarged uterus and growing fetus cause pressure on the inferior vena cava, resulting in decreased cardiac output. Similar symptoms may occur with anemia, hypoglycemia, and dehydration, but if these are ruled out, the woman should be advised to lie on the side rather than flat and to take deep breaths and raise herself slowly from lying to sitting position.

70. B: If a woman's pregnancy classification is G4, T2, P1, A1, L3, the number of total pregnancies is 4. The woman has been pregnant 4 times with 2 pregnancies carried to term, 1 premature birth, 1 abortion, and 3 living children. This classification system is in general use do describe a woman's reproductive history:

- G: Gravida refers to the number of times that a woman has been pregnant.
- T: Term pregnancies, the number of pregnancies carried to term.
- P: Preterm delivery, the number of preterm deliveries.
- A: Abortions, may be spontaneous or induced.
- L: Living births, the number of infants born living.

71. C: If the fundal height is halfway between the woman's symphysis pubis and umbilicus, the approximate weeks of gestation are 16. The fundal heights directly correlate to the weeks of gestation from week 22, but the weeks of gestation can be estimated by the fundal position:

- Symphysis pubis: 12 weeks.
- Halfway between symphysis pubis and umbilicus: 16 weeks.
- At umbilicus: 22 weeks.
- One-third of distance between umbilicus and xyphoid process: 28-30.
- Two-thirds of distance between umbilicus and xyphoid process: 32 weeks.
- At xyphoid process: 36 weeks. Then begins to drop again at 38 to 40 weeks as the head engages.

72. A: The cell free fetal DNA test assesses for chromosomal disorders. Testing typically covers 3 common chromosomal disorders: trisomy 21 (Down syndrome), trisomy 18 (Edwards syndrome), and trisomy 13 (Patau syndrome). The DNA testing may also test for other rarer disorders, especially if there is a family history indicating increased risk. The cell free fetal DNA test, which can be done during or following week 10 of gestation, is presently still considered a screening test and must be verified by further testing, such as chorionic villus sampling or amniocentesis.

73. B: During pregnancy, a woman with BMI of 22.0 (which is classified as a normal weight for the mother) is expected to gain 25 to 35 pounds. Weight gains are recommended according to the woman's BMI:

BMI	Classified	Recommended weight gain
<18.5	Underweight	28 to 40 pounds
18.5 to 24.9	Normal weight	25 to 35 pounds
25 to 29.9	Overweight	15 to 25 pounds
30+	Obese	11 to 20 pounds

Women pregnant with twins should generally gain about 15 to 25 pounds more than women with singletons.

74. C: The presence of bilirubin in amniotic fluid usually indicates Rh-sensitized pregnancy and fetal hemolytic syndrome. Bilirubin may be monitored routinely beginning at 25-weeks of gestation to evaluate the severity of the syndrome in the developing fetus. Rh incompatibility occurs if the mother is Rh- and the father is Rh+, putting their infant at risk for hemolytic disease of the newborn (HDN) or Rh disease, (erythroblastosis fetalis). Sensitization can occur during abortion, placental abruption, amniocentesis, cesarean section, chorionic villus sampling, cordocentesis, delivery, ectopic pregnancy, and toxemia.

75. A: Severe post-dural puncture (spinal) headache is best treated with an epidural blood patch, which seals the cerebrospinal leak that causes the headache. Caffeinated beverages or medication with caffeine may provide temporary relief of the headache, and hydration is important, but usually not adequate alone. With the woman lying prone, the physician takes 20 to 25 mL of venous blood from a vein and then slowly injects it into the epidural space. The patient may feel some initial pressure, but this should prevent further leakage and resolve the headache within a few hours.

76. C: If bottle feeding a neonate with cleft lip and cleft palate, the nipple should be longer than normal size so the milk is delivered to the back of the throat, past the open cleft. The neonate should be fed in upright position to prevent aspiration. The mother should be encouraged to breast feed the neonate as breastfeeding is often successful with cleft lip and cleft palate although the mother must be sure to keep the infant upright.

77. B: Ultrasonography can be used to estimate fetal age with crown-rump length (CRL) at approximately 7 to 12 weeks. The heart rate can be assessed at 6 to 7 weeks gestation. Other measurements used to estimate fetal age include gestational sac dimensions at about 8 weeks and biparietal diameter (BPD) and femur length after 12 weeks. Ultrasonography can be used throughout pregnancy to estimate gestational age, to confirm the viability of the fetus, to identify gender, and to identify fetal abnormalities.

78. A: When palpating the uterus after delivery, it is necessary support the lower uterine segment with one hand while palpating with the other. Applying pressure to the fundus without properly supporting the lower uterine segment may result in increased bleeding, hemorrhage, and/or uterine inversion. The lower segment is supported by placing one hand directly above the symphysis pubis firmly (but avoiding distal pressure) while placing the other hand at the umbilicus and pressing inward and downward until the fundus is palpated.

79. C: Asymmetric intrauterine growth restriction is caused by problems that occur during the third trimester and typically result from problems with the function of the uterus and placenta and/or nutritional deficiency. Usually the brain and heart have normal development and the neonate has normal length but is in less than the 10th percentile for weight. The abdominal organs may be underdeveloped. The neonate will usually develop normally with adequate nutrition after birth.

80. A: If a woman is labor is receiving a benzodiazepine to relieve anxiety, nausea, and pain, the medication that should also be available on the unit is flumazenil. Flumazenil is an antagonist for benzodiazepines and may be necessary to reverse the effects if excessive sedation occurs. Benzodiazepines may result in some degree of amnesia, so some women may want to avoid their use. Naloxone should also be available for patients receiving narcotic analgesia. N-acetylcysteine is a reversal agent for acetaminophen overdoses.

81. B: A patient who experienced placenta previa is at increased risk of hemorrhage during the postpartal period because the area of implantation does not contract effectively. With placenta previa, the placenta implants very low in the uterus or over the cervical os. Additionally, the blood supply in the lower segment of the uterus is less than in the upper segment, so the placenta tends to grow to a larger size to compensate. This leaves a greater denuded area that can bleed after expulsion of the placenta.

82. A: Following spontaneous rupture of the membranes during labor, if the fetal heart rate becomes markedly bradycardic with variable decelerations, this likely indicates cord prolapse, which occurs when part of the cord is below the presenting part of the fetus, blocking blood flow. While prolapse may be occult and occur at any time during labor, it is most common after rupture of the membranes because the pressure literally washes the cord downward. Risk increases with an exceptionally long cord, mal-presentations, multiple gestations, hydramnios, and preterm birth.

83. C: During the process of lactation, the breasts usually being filling and feel firm and warm by the third day. The breasts are usually soft during the first two days but produce colostrum in small amounts, as the neonate's stomach capacity is very small immediately after birth. By the fourth day, the breasts will feel full before the neonate nurses and then should feel soft if the emptying of the breast was adequate. If the mother's breasts remain very firm and uncomfortable after nursing, a breastfeeding specialist should review breastfeeding techniques with the mother to ensure the neonate is latching and nursing effectively.

84. B: The most common cause of subinvolution is retained placental fragments and infection. Subinvolution is a restricting of the rate at which the uterus returns to nonpregnant size. Indications of subinvolution include prolonged lochia, pelvic pain or discomfort, intermittent bleeding or hemorrhage, backache, and lethargy and malaise. An unpleasant or foul vaginal odor is usually present with infection. Treatment requires identifying and treating the cause. Methylergonovine (Methergine®) is often given to promote contractions and antibiotics for infection.

85. A: If shoulder dystocia (difficult delivery of the shoulders) occurred during delivery, the newborn should be examined for fractured clavicle and Erb's palsy. The anterior or posterior (less common) shoulder becomes literally stuck behind the pubis. Shoulder dystocia poses risks to both the mother and fetus and may result in death of the fetus or severe impairment because the cord becomes compressed and the lungs cannot expand because the fetus is lodged in the birth canal. Risk factors for shoulder dystocia include macrosomia, diabetic mother, obese mother, abnormal anatomy of pelvis, prolonged pregnancy, older maternal age, and induced labor.

86. B: Labor and delivery is defined as precipitate if labor lasts less than three hours. Women who are multiparous are at greatest risk because of loss of muscle tone. They may experience dilation of 10 cm within an hour while nulliparous women may experience dilation of 5 cm an hour. In some cases, the mother may have experienced little pain prior to delivery. Precipitate labor may also occur with hypertonic uterine contractions. If there is inadequate relaxation of the uterine muscle between contractions, the fetus may suffer hypoxia.

87. C: Autonomy is the ethical principle that the individual has the right to make decisions about her own care, based on informed consent and understanding of risks and benefits. Beneficence is an ethical principle that involves performing actions that are for the purpose of benefitting another person. Nonmaleficence is an ethical principle that means healthcare workers should provide care in a manner that does not cause direct intentional harm to the patient.

88. C: If a woman complains of persistent constipation in the postpartal period, the best treatment approach is usually a stool softener, such as docusate sodium or Bisacodyl, both of which can be taken while the woman is breastfeeding. While the woman should be encouraged to drink ample fluids and to include fiber in the diet, constipation is common because hormonal changes decrease bowel motility. Also, if the woman had an episiotomy or tearing, the woman may avoid bearing down because of pain.

89. C: When conducting a review of the literature as part of evidence-based research, the level of evidence based on a quasi-experimental study, such as a matched case-control study, would be categorized as level III:

- Level I: Meta-analysis, randomized controlled studies.
- Level II: One or more well-designed study, may or not be randomized.
- Level III: As above.
- Level IV: Comparative non-experimental studies.
- Level V: Case reports and clinical examples but without empirical evidence.

90. B: In the postpartal period, the uterine fundus should no longer be palpable after 10 days. Immediately after delivery, the fundus should be palpable at about the midline point between the umbilicus and the symphysis pubis, and it should continue to descend at about the rate of 1 cm per day. It's important that the woman urinate prior to assessment of the fundus because a full bladder may displace the fundus. The nurse should note the position of the fundus vertically as well as any lateral deviation.

91. A: The antibiotic agent that should be avoided for long-term use (>14 days) when a woman is breastfeeding is tetracyclines. While some studies indicate that short-term use may be acceptable, tetracycline is usually avoided because it may result in permanent tooth staining and enamel defects in the infant's developing teeth. Tetracycline should also be avoided during pregnancy because it may restrict skeletal growth in the fetus and cause the same dental problems. Cephalosporins and erythromycin are safe to use while breastfeeding.

92. C: If a nurse administers the wrong drug to a patient but the patient suffers no ill effects, the elements of malpractice that are missing are damages (because the patient suffered no ill effects) and causation (because there must be damages before there can be causation). The four elements necessary for malpractice are: duty to use care, breach of duty, damages, and causation. In order to prove malpractice, evidence must show that all 4 elements are present.

93. A: Necrotizing enterocolitis in a preterm infant is usually caused by ischemic bowel. If the neonate has episodes of hypoxia, oxygen is shunted to the heart and lungs and other organs, such as the intestines, may become hypoxic. If oxygenation is inadequate, areas of necrosis occur, and this interferes with peristalsis, so stool begins to build up. Sepsis may also occur, putting the neonate at grave risk.

94. B: If, on palpating the uterus in the postpartal period, the nurse finds the fundus is displaced superior to the umbilicus and to the right, the nurse should suspect that the cause is bladder distention. The nurse should ensure the bladder is empty prior to uterine palpation. Spontaneous urination usually occurs within 6 to 8 hours. The woman should urinate an average of 150 mL per hour to prevent bladder distention. The postpartal period is one of diuresis up to 3000 mL a day for the first few days, and the bladder can easily become distended because of decreased bladder tone.

95. A: Methylergonovine (Methergine®) may be administered to a woman after delivery in order to promote uterine contractions. Uterine atony or subinvolution may result in postpartal hemorrhage if not treated. Methylergonovine is usually administered at 200 mcg IV at 2- to 4-hour intervals after delivery or at 200 to 400 mcg PO every 6 to 12 hours for 2 to 7 days. Blood pressure must be carefully monitored, and methylergonovine should be used with care in hypertensive patients.

96. C: A woman who is breastfeeding and needs to take smoking cessation medication in order to stop smoking should avoid varenicline. Low dose nicotine patches (14-mg or 7-mg) decrease exposure to nicotine and other chemicals compared to smoking. Blood levels of nicotine vary considerably with nicotine gum, depending on how fast and frequently the gum is chewed, so women should be advised to avoid using the gum for 2 to 3 hours before breastfeeding.

97. B: A woman who has taken methadone during pregnancy and wants to breastfeed should continue the same dose of methadone. The danger to the infant is greater if the mother reduces the doses or stops the methadone and returns to substance abuse. However, the infant should be monitored for excessive drowsiness. The drug's peak occurs 4 to 5 hours after the woman takes an oral dose, so the mother should try to avoid breastfeeding at that time. When breastfeeding, the infant receives about 2 to 3% of the maternal dose.

98. A: If a neonate's skin is dry and peeling with no vernix and loss of subcutaneous fat, the likely gestational age is 42 to 44 weeks. Post-term infants may weigh >4000 g. Other indications include long and thin body, long fingernails (meconium staining may be evident), long hair, and hypothermia. The neonate may suffer from cold stress because of decreased brown fat, and may have hypoglycemia. Post-term infants are at increased risk of meconium aspiration and seizures resulting from hypoxia.

99. C: In the immediate postpartum period, a woman's gastric motility is generally decreased because of both hormonal effects and the lack of adequate abdominal muscle tone. Because of this, the postpartal woman often experiences abdominal distention from gas and constipation. Spontaneous bowel movements usually occur by the second or third day after delivery, but the woman may benefit from increased fluids and fiber and stool softeners, especially if the stool is hard and the woman must strain to defecate.

100. B: If a woman's white blood cell count was 20,000 after delivery and increased to 40,000 by the second day, this likely indicates an acute infection. The WBC count is commonly between 20,000 and 30,000 after delivery but it should start to fall and return to normal levels within 3-7 days. A sudden marked increase is always cause for concern and further tests and should be carried out to determine the cause of the increase.

101. C: If testing after birth shows that a neonate has inherited galactosemia, an inborn error of metabolism, the neonate should be fed soy-based formula. Because the child cannot metabolize galactose, which is derived from metabolism of lactose, the infant can never have any product that contains either, and this eliminates all milk products, including human milk. Failure to diagnose and treat can result in organ damage (liver, kidneys), intellectual disabilities, cataracts, and death.

102. A: If a breastfeeding woman shows a nonimmune rubella titer prior to discharge, the woman should be given and MMR vaccine and continue breastfeeding. The MMR vaccination should not be taken by the woman during pregnancy or the month prior to becoming pregnant because the live virus used in the vaccine poses a risk to the developing fetus. The varicella vaccination should also be avoided. Safe vaccinations include tetanus and diphtheria toxoids, hepatitis B, influenza, rabies, and meningococcal.

103. B: The breastfeeding position that is good to relive plugged milk ducts and engorged breasts is the football hold. The baby's legs are tucked under the arm on the side the child is nursing. This position is often used with twins if the woman wants to nurse both infants at the same time. The football hold is also a good position for women who have had a Caesarean and have abdominal tenderness.

104. A: When assisting with the lumbar puncture of a preterm neonate, the correct position for the neonate is lateral with the trunk flexed (being careful to avoid over-flexion). If the neonate is term, this position or sitting position with the head supported may be used. Following the procedure, the infant should be kept flat for at least 60 minutes and cardiorespiratory and oxygen saturation continuously monitored during that period. If the infant received narcotic sedation for the procedure, monitoring should continue for 4 hours and the infant should remain NPO for 2 hours.

105. C: When an infant latches only to the nipple, the nipple is not able to extend as deeply into the infant's mouth as required for effective breastfeeding. The nipple must extend into the infant's mouth to the soft palate because if it ends at the hard palate, the suckling movements will result in irritation and discomfort. If, when a new mother is trying to breastfeed, the neonate latches on to just the nipple, the nurse should advise the woman to insert a finger at the side of the infant's mouth to break the suction and to start over. Appropriate latching (to both the nipple and areola) typically does not cause discomfort or irritation.

106. A: If a neonate exhibits neck rigidity after birth, this may indicate injury to the sternocleidomastoid muscle. The neonate should be able to hold the head up slightly when lying prone, but the head lags because of weakness of the neck muscles when lifted from supine position. The sternocleidomastoid muscle, one of the largest in the neck, allows the head to turn from right to left and the neck to flex. Because the muscle originates in the clavicle and sternum, clavicular injuries can damage the muscle.

107. B: A demarcated unraised red-purple lesion caused by capillaries below the skin on a child's face is a nevus flammeus (port-wine stain). Nevus vasculosus (strawberry mark) is a capillary hemangioma and is a raised, demarcated dark red lesion. Erythema toxicum is a transient rash characterized by perifollicular lesions (1-3 mm), white or yellow with pustules, which appears suddenly over all of the body (except the palms and soles). The cause of erythema toxicum is not known.

108. B: If a woman with flat nipples has started using a nipple shield while breastfeeding but the infant is not gaining adequate weight, the nurse should advise the woman to use the nipple shield for only 1 to 2 minutes and then remove it for the rest of the nursing period as the nipple usually elongates enough for the infant to latch on within this time. The breast stimulation is inadequate with a nipple shield, and the infant must work harder to nurse.

109. A: If a nursing neonate has a 5:1 suck/swallow ratio, this indicates non-nutritive suckling. The normal suck/swallow ratio is 2:1 or 1:1, which indicates that an adequate volume of milk is being obtained. If the suck/swallow ratio is 5:1 or greater, the neonate is probably getting very little or no milk and may become exhausted from trying to suckle, and the milk supply will decrease because of inadequate stimulation of the breast. The woman may need assistance from a breastfeeding specialist.

110. C: If a woman asks about bottle feeding human milk so the infant's father can experience feeding the infant, she should be advised to wait for at least 4 weeks. The suckling effort the infant makes is different with a woman's nipple than with a rubber nipple, and starting bottle feeding too early may result in nipple confusion and make the child resistant to nursing. Some infants are more sensitive to nipple changes than others.

111. B: Until a neonate regains body weight, the neonate should be nursed at least every 3 hours. If the neonate is sleeping, the mother should awaken the neonate because small infants can easily become dehydrated. Additionally, if the child wants to nurse more often, the neonate should be allowed to do so. Neonates usually nurse every 1 to 3 hours, so pacifiers should not be used to extend the time between feedings. Each session of nursing usually takes 20 to 40 minutes, so the mother gets very little rest in the first few weeks.

112. A: A normal percentage of weight loss for a neonate in the first few days of life is 5%. A weight loss of greater than 7% is cause for concern and may mean that the infant is not nursing adequately. As the mother's milk production increases, the neonates weight should stabilize and then begin to increase at the rate of about 0.5 to 1.0 ounce (15 to 30 g) daily for the next few months.

113. B: When expressing milk from the breast, a woman should start by grasping the breast with a C hold with the fingers about 2 to 3 centimeters from the areola and should move about the breast in a clockwise manner. If the hand stays in a fixed position, not all of the milk ducts will empty. Once the breast is grasped, the woman pushes back and then squeezes while moving the hand forward (milking motion).

114. A: Women may experience exacerbation of autoimmune disorders, such as lupus erythematosus, after labor and delivery because the woman's immune system is no longer suppressed. So that the mother's body does not reject the fetus as "foreign," the immune system remains suppressed during pregnancy. Because of this suppression, women with autoimmune disorders often experience reduction of symptoms or remission during pregnancy.

115. C: If, on the first post-partum day, the woman's fundus is firm and lochia appears normal but the woman complains of perineal discomfort and BP falls to 88/50 and pulse increases to 112, the nurse should suspect a hematoma. Hematomas occur with bleeding into the connective tissues and may occur in the vulvar, vaginal, and retroperitoneal areas. In the vulvar region, the discoloration and bulging are noticeable, but vaginal and retroperitoneal hematomas are hidden and harder to detect.

116. C: If a neonate's cardiac status appeared normal at birth but 48 hours later the neonate experiences a precipitous drop in circulation to the lower body, the likely congenital heart defect is coarctation of the aorta, which is a stricture of the aorta, proximal to the ductus arteriosus intersection. As the heart tries to pump the blood past the stricture, the blood pressure to the head and upper extremities increases decreasing blood pressure and circulation to the lower body and extremities. Symptoms may not occur until the ductus arteriosus closes, causing sudden loss of blood supply to the lower body.

117. A: Following delivery, if the fundus feels contracted and in the right position but free flow of bright red blood is evident vaginally, this is likely due to vaginal or cervical lacerations. Lochia is usually a darker red and dribbles more slowly. Anytime bleeding occurs with a contracted uterus, this is a warning sign that the patient should be examined for lacerations because the patient may experience significant loss of blood if the laceration is undetected and untreated.

118. C: The hormone that stimulates the alveoli to produce milk is prolactin. As the infant suckles, this stimulates the breast and causes the pituitary gland to release increased oxytocin, which in turn causes the muscles around the alveoli to contract and send the milk into the main lactiferous (milk) ducts (the "let down" reflex). If the breasts do not receive adequate and frequent stimulation, the level of prolactin begins to fall and eventually milk production stops.

119. B: If a woman reports that her neonate cries frantically when hungry, this likely means that the woman is missing signs of hunger because crying is usually a late sign. Signs of hunger include the infant making licking or sucking motions, rooting, and head bobbing. The infant may also hold the hands in fists or bring the hands to the mouth. If the woman strokes the infant's lips or cheek, the infant will turn the head and try to suck.

120. B: Following an unmedicated delivery, a neonate should ideally begin breastfeeding during the first 1 to 2 hours. During this time period, the neonate is usually most alert. The smell of the amniotic fluid remaining on the baby and the mother's smell are similar, and this smell helps to guide the infant to the breast and facilitate nursing. Therefore, the neonate should be offered the breast before the first bath.

121. A: A woman who develops postpartal DVT should be carefully monitored for signs of pulmonary embolus because small clots can easily dislodge and travel to the lungs. Signs and symptoms include dyspnea, tachycardia, pallor, cough, falling oxygen saturation level, and anxiety. Any woman with onset of these symptoms should immediately have head elevated to relieve dyspnea and be administered oxygen per facemask at 8 to 10 L/min and the physician notified.

122. C: Stages of milk production:

- Stage 1: Occurs during late pregnancy. Increased progesterone and estrogen levels to bring about changes in the breasts that prepare them for lactation.
- Stage 2: Occurs postpartum. Both progesterone and estrogen levels fall and prolactin levels increase in order to promote milk production.
- Stage 3: Occurs with weaning. Prolactin levels fall as the breasts have decreased stimulation.

123. B: In order to prevent post-dural puncture (spinal) headache, the woman should lie flat for several hours. When spinal anesthesia is administered, a small amount of cerebrospinal fluid may leak out, and if the fluid level in the brain is low, this can cause a headache, especially if the head is elevated, until the volume builds up again. Adequate hydration is also important, and caffeinated beverages may provide temporary relief.

124. A: During the *claiming* part of parent-neonate attachment, the parent usually first compares the child to other family members by looking for family traits and noticing how the neonate is similar: "She has her father's eyes." This is usually followed by the parent noticing differences: "His hair is darker than his brothers'." Last, the parent begins to notice those things that make the neonate unique: "Look at those long fingers!"

125. C: After delivery, a woman is likely to exhibit signs and symptoms of hypovolemic shock with blood loss greater than 1500 mL. The blood volume typically increases by about 1500 mL during pregnancy, so the woman usually tolerates considerable blood loss. Once the extra 1500 mL of blood is lost, every 500 mL of additional blood loss usually results in a 3% drop in hematocrit. Hypovolemic shock results in hypotension, tachycardia, pallor, cool skin (from vasoconstriction), anxiety, and confusion.

126. C: The phase of maternal role transition during which the woman begins to feel like a mother is letting go. Phases:

- Taking in (0-48 hours): Needs assistance of others and is focused on her personal needs, but may want to talk about labor and delivery and may exhibit excitement.
- Taking hold (2-10 days or weeks): Eager to learn and to take care of neonate but needs support and approval of others to gain confidence.
- Letting go: Gives up fantasies of "perfect baby," begins to see herself as a mother and part of a family, and resumes role with partner.

127. B: If a neonate's chest circumference is 34 cm, the head circumference would normally be about 36 cm. Normal measures:

Weight	2500-4000 g (average about 3400). Physiologic weight loss is 5-10% for full term and 15T for preterm.
Length	45-55 cm (average 50 cm).
Head circumference	32-38 cm (usually 2 cm greater than chest circumference)
Chest circumference	30-36 cm
Blood pressure	56-77/33-50 mm Hg
Pulse	120-120 bpm awake; 100 bpm asleep; 180 bmp crying
Respiration	30-60 per minute

128. A: An indication that the woman may not be bonding with her neonate is when the mother exhibits disgust when the infant urinates and refuses to change the diaper. Other indications include showing a lack of concern if the neonate cries; failing to try to talk to, touch, or interact with the neonate; ignoring the neonate completely; or expressing disappointment with the neonate's appearance or gender.

129. B: Paternal transition to parenting includes three stages:

- Commitment: The father accepts the responsibilities of parenthood and begins to make plans.
- Attachment: The father bonds with the infant through touch and interaction, such as singing to the neonate or holding and helping to care for the neonate.
- Preparation: The father adjusts his life to accommodate the needs of the infant.

130. B: If a woman admitted in labor plans to relinquish her infant for adoption, the nurse should acknowledge the adoption plans: "I understand the adoptive parents have been notified that you are in labor." Broaching the subject in a supportive manner allows the mother to express feelings about the adoption if she chooses to do so. It's unlikely that little else is on the woman's mind, so pretending otherwise only isolates the woman and her feelings.

131. C: To prevent contamination, reconstituted formula (or any opened formula) for bottle feeding should not be stored in the refrigerator for more than 24 hours. It's best to prepare one bottle at a time for use although women often prepare multiple bottles for use, such as during the night or while the woman is away from the infant and others are feeding the child, and liquid formula containers may hold enough to fill multiple bottles.

132. A: To facilitate bonding between the woman and her neonate if the woman chooses to bottle feed, the nurse should encourage the woman to maintain eye contact with the neonate during feedings. Maintaining skin-to-skin contact while feeding also helps to promote bonding. Holding the infant with the head higher than the body helps to prevent the child from aspirating and decreases risk of subsequent ear infections.

133. B: The neonate of a diabetic mother whose blood glucose levels were elevated above 145 mg/dL during labor is likely to experience hypoglycemia (<45 mg/dL) and hypocalcemia (<8 mg/dL). Hypoglycemia occurs because the mother's elevated glucose levels during pregnancy cause hyperplasia of insulin producing cells and increased insulin production. Hypocalcemia is common with neonates of diabetic mothers although the reason is not clear.

134. C: The primary risk factor for metritis (uterine infection) is Caesarean birth. The risk of infection is approximately 25 times higher with Caesarean birth than vaginal birth, a concern with the increased numbers of Caesarean births. For this reason, most women are administered single-dose antibiotic prophylaxis after delivery. Colonization of bacteria in the genital tract increases the risk of infection. Incidence tends to be highest in those of lower economic status although infection can occur in any woman.

135. B: A woman with gestational diabetes is at risk of delivering a neonate with macrosomia (birthweight > 4500 g). The maternal elevated glucose results in excess production of insulin in the fetus, and this causes excessive growth. These infants often exhibit extra fat deposits in the trunk and shoulder, and this increases the risk of shoulder dystocia. Macrosomia also increases the risk of Caesarean birth because of the size of the neonate.

136. A: If a woman with a history of bipolar disease develops marked hyperactivity about two weeks after delivery with signs of postpartum psychosis, including confusion and anger toward the infant, the first intervention should be to ensure the safety of the infant. The infant needs to be removed from the mother's care because of the risk of infanticide with postpartum psychosis. In some cases, especially if no other family member can care for the infant, child protective services may need to be notified.

137. C: If a neonate is born with gastroschisis (stomach and intestines herniating through an opening in the abdominal wall) the exposed organs should be immediately covered with moist gauze dressings and wrapped in plastic (around the neonate's body) to secure and prevent further fluid loss and hypothermia. The infant must be maintained in supine position to prevent intestinal ischemia. Surgery is usually done within 2 to 4 hours of delivery.

138. B: Following delivery, the best preventive measure to reduce the risk of developing deep vein thrombosis (DVT) is early ambulation. Whether Caesarean or vaginal birth, the woman should be assisted to ambulate within a few hours of delivery. Early ambulation also encourages urination and stimulates bowel motility, reducing the risk of constipation. The woman should be advised to avoid crossing the legs because doing so may decrease peripheral blood flow.

139. A: A first-line treatment for gestational hypertensive disorders is nifedipine although hydralazine or labetalol may also be used. However, they are administered intravenously while nifedipine is administered orally. Adverse reactions include dizziness, headache, flushing, and palpitations. The woman should be advised to avoid grapefruit. Use of nifedipine to control blood pressure must be balanced against potential fetal risk. Diuretics are generally avoided during pregnancy because of the risk of compromised placental perfusion.

140. C: A woman should be encouraged to room-in with her neonate during hospitalization in order to facilitate bonding. However, the woman should be assured that she can call for assistance with infant care at any time and that nurses will monitor both the mother and the neonate frequently. If the woman prefers to place her infant in the nursery for part of the time, the woman should also be supported in this choice.

141. C: On the day of delivery, a diabetic woman who has been receiving insulin for type 1 diabetes will probably require a lower dosage of insulin (and sometimes no insulin). The glucose level often drops precipitously after delivery, so the woman may require treatment for hypoglycemia. Regular insulin should be administered rather than longer acting insulin until glucose levels stabilize.

142. A: If a neonate has a hematocrit of 67%, this likely indicates polycythemia. Polycythemia (hematocrit >65%) develops in utero in response to oxygen deprivation. The fetus produces additional red blood cells as a compensatory measure. Polycythemia may also occur in neonates who are small or large for gestational age if the cord is milked after delivery. Polycythemia increases the viscosity of the blood. An exchange transfusion may be done to reduce the hematocrit to prevent neurological deficits.

143. B: If a Haitian woman states that she does not want to name her baby girl, the nurse should assume that delayed naming is a cultural norm. In fact, Haitians usually wait until after the first month to give their neonates a name. Naming holds special importance in many cultures, and names may be chosen to reflect religion, such as names chosen from the Bible or the Koran. Some Africans believe that the name may affect the child's fate. In some cultures, such as traditional Chinese, the father decides on the name.

144. B: Postpartum blues typically begins a day or two after delivery, peaks at 5 days, and subsides by about 10 days. Postpartum blues is characterized by emotional lability during which the woman may have mood swings and feel depressed and anxious. The cause is not clear but is likely some combination of physical factors (hormonal and body changes), psychological factors (anxiety, fear of caring for the child), social factors (loss of support), and/or cultural factors (unhappiness with gender of child, cultural expectations).

145. A: X-linked disorders affect primarily male offspring. The female carries two X chromosomes—one from the father and one from the mother. Because one chromosome is normal, this chromosome can compensate for the defective chromosome. However, if the male offspring receives a defective X chromosome, the Y chromosome cannot compensate, and the male will exhibit the disorder.

146. C: If a woman expresses concern that her 3-year-old child does not seem to love the neonate, the nurse should advise the woman that young children develop affection over time. It is normal for a young child to feel some degree of jealousy when an infant is brought into the home, and since the infant interacts minimally in the first few weeks, the young child may show little interest, but this should change over time if parents remain attentive and supportive.

147. B: A woman who is nursing her neonate usually needs to increase fluid intake by about 1000 mL per day to compensate for the 23 to 27 ounces of milk produced each day for the neonate. She should also increase calories by about 500 per day. However, this may vary depending on the woman's usual caloric intake and weight. If a woman is overweight and trying to lose weight, the woman should avoid reducing calories for at least the first 6 weeks until milk production is well established.

148. C: An antidepressant that is generally considered reasonably safe to continue during pregnancy for women with a history of severe depression is citalopram (Celexa®) although some studies indicate it may slightly increase the risk of persistent pulmonary hypertension in the neonate. Other SSRIs that are often continued during pregnancy are sertraline and fluoxetine. The risks should be balanced against the risk of exacerbation of depression. Paroxetine (Paxil®) has been linked to heart defects, and MAO inhibitors, such as tranylcypromine (Parnate®), should be avoided during pregnancy.

149. B: A neonate exposed to or infected with herpes simplex is treated with acyclovir. The risk of transmission of maternal infection to the neonate is about 50% with primary infection and 1 to 2% with secondary outbreaks. Infected neonates usually exhibit symptoms by 10 to 12 days, including skin, eye, and mucous membrane blistering. HSV may spread to internal organs, including the brain. Women with active lesions should have Caesarean birth within 4 hours of membranes rupturing.

150. A: Conditions associated with oligohydramnios (<500 mL) include urinary tract anomalies. After week 20 of gestation, most amniotic fluid is produced by fetal urine, so if urine production is inadequate, the volume decreases. Oligohydramnios can lead to pressure deformities (such as club foot), pulmonary hypoplasia, and compression of the umbilical cord. Chromosomal abnormalities (trisomy 21, 18, and 13) and obstructional lesions of the GI tract are associated with polyhydramnios (>500 mL).

151 C. Laboratory findings associated with disseminated intravascular coagulation include:

- Prolonged prothrombin and partial prothrombin times.
- Decreased platelet counts and fragmented RBCs.
- Decreased fibrinogen.

DIC is a secondary disorder of pregnancy, triggered by various conditions, including placental abruption, hypovolemic shock, eclampsia, post-partal hemorrhage, and sepsis. Treatment includes replacement blood products, anticoagulants, cryoprecipitate, coagulation inhibitors, and coagulation factors.

152. B: When assisting a patient to take a sitz bath to relieve swelling and discomfort of hemorrhoids, the nurse should assure that the water temperature does not exceed 105° F (41° C). Patients should continue a sitz bath for approximately 20 minutes. Patients who will continue sitz baths at home should be taught that, at this temperature, the water feels comfortably warm when tested on the wrist but not hot.

153. A: If the normal speaking voice is 50 to 60 decibels, the noise levels in the nursery and NICU should be maintained at 45 decibels or lower because excessive noise can be very stressful to neonates, resulting in overstimulation. Women should be advised to avoid exposing their neonates to loud noises, such as radios and TVs at high volume. If the neonate becomes stressed, the neonate's oxygen requirements increase, and the neonate may experience increased episodes of apnea and bradycardia.

154. B: With kangaroo care, the neonate in minimal (or no) clothing is placed between the mother's bare breasts to provide warmth and skin-to-skin contact. This can be done immediately after birth, but provides benefits to both mother and infant if continued, especially for preterm neonates. Neonatal benefits include better regulation of vital signs, calming, decreased periods of apnea, increase in weight gain, fewer nosocomial infections, and enhanced bonding.

155. C: If a neonate has a patent ductus arteriosus, the usual initial treatment is indomethacin. If given within 10 days of birth, the medication closes about 80% of defects. Patent ductus arteriosus (PDA) occurs when the ductus arteriosus that connects the pulmonary artery and aorta fails to close after birth. This results in left to right shunting of blood from the aorta back to the pulmonary artery, increasing the blood flow to the lungs and causing an increase in pulmonary hypertension that can result in damage to the lung tissue.

156. B: In the neonate, the nurse should immediately report any periods of apnea that last more than 20 seconds. Periodic breathing with periods of apnea lasting for 5 to 15 seconds is common in the neonate, but prolonged apnea is abnormal and may indicate respiratory distress. The neonate should be carefully examined for changes in skin color and depressed heart rate during episodes. Stimulating the infant may trigger respirations. Other indications of respiratory distress include grunting respirations and sternal and intercostal retraction.

157. A: The wet neonate's temperature falls rapidly after birth if not promptly dried and warmed because of evaporation when the wet skin is exposed to air currents. Temperature drops rapidly (skin temperature falls 0.3 °C/minute) after birth with exposure to ambient room temperature but should stabilize within 8-12 hours. Temperature is often measured by axillary method (for 3 minutes) and ranges from 36.3-37.0 °C. To avoid a temperature drop, the neonate should be examined under a warmer.

158. C: Following birth, damage to the neonate's upper brachial plexus (C5 to C7) is likely to result in Erb's palsy, which affects both the upper arm and the forearm. Movement is diminished or absent with the arm extended at the side and the forearm prone. Brachial plexus injury is associated with macrosomia, breech presentation, and shoulder dystocia. In most cases, recovery occurs within 3 to 6 months, but some infants may require surgical repair although prognosis is poor for surgical intervention. Pseudoparalysis (lack of movement because of fracture) may be misdiagnosed as brachial plexus injury.

159. A: The purpose of administering vitamin K to a neonate it to facilitate clotting. Neonates lack vitamin K at birth, and are, therefore, at risk of developing clots until vitamin K begins to be synthesized in the intestines when the neonate begins to feed. The neonate is administered an injection of vitamin K1 (AquaMEPHYTON) in a single dose of 0.5 to 1.0 mg to prevent episodes of bleeding in the first week of life.

160. A: Parents should be taught to place a neonate on the back when the neonate is sleeping and unattended at all times to decrease the risk of sudden infant death syndrome (SIDS). Ideally, the baby should sleep in the same room with a parent for the first year, but in a separate crib on a firm mattress with a fitted sheet but no blankets, toys, of other bedding. The slats of the crib must be no more than 6 cm apart to prevent the neonate from getting the head caught between the slats.

161. A: Starting immediately after hospital discharge, the neonate should have "tummy time" 2 to 3 times daily for 3 to 5 minutes each time. During this time, the neonate should be constantly attended. Tummy time helps to prevent flat areas of the head and helps to strengthen the neck and shoulder muscles as the child lifts the head. The frequency and duration of tummy time should increase as the neonate gets older.

162. B: The normal position for the neonate's ears is with the insertion point of the top of the ear parallel to the outer canthus of the eye. The ears should be proportionate to the head size, soft and pliable, and cartilage should be firm by term. Low set ears are associated with a number of different congenital disorders, including trisomy 13 (Patau syndrome), trisomy 18 (Edwards syndrome), and intellectual disabilities.

163. A: When placing a newborn in a safety car seat, the seat should be rear facing and reclined 30 to 45 degrees (about half-way back) as this prevents the neonate's head from falling forward in a crash and blocking the airway. If the seat is reclined too far, the infant may slide backward (toward the front of the car) during a crash, injuring the head. A safety car bed may be necessary for premature infants.

164. C: If a neonate must undergo a medical procedure, sucrose analgesia (SweetEase™) should be given to the infant 2 minutes before the procedure begins. A pacifier is dipped in sucrose analgesia (24% solution) and given to the neonate to suck. The pacifier can be redipped every 2 minutes up to 4 times. Sucrose solution may be used in addition to other analgesia to provide comfort. Contraindications include less than 32 weeks of gestation, hyperglycemia, feeding problems, severe illness, opioid sedation, paralysis, and NPO status (unless okayed by physician).

165. C: Score of 10. Silverman-Anderson Index:

Characteristic	0	1	2
Chest/abdomen	Rise together with inspiration.	Abdomen rises but upper chest lags or sinks.	See-saw movement
Intercostals	No retraction	Minimal retraction	Pronounced retraction
Xiphoid process	No retraction	Minimal retraction	Pronounced retraction
Nasal flaring	None	Minimal	Pronounced
Grunt (expiratory)	None	Grunt heard with auscultation.	Audible grunt

166. B: The newborn hearing test that measures the integrity of the middle and inner ear and the outer hair cells of the cochlea is the otoacoustic emissions test. Otoacoustic emissions (OAE) are sounds generated by the cochlea, the inner ear structure. The audiologist conducts the OAE test by inserting a probe into the infant's external auditory canal, and stimulating the cochlea with several clicking noises. The audiologist uses a microphone to measure the evoked OAE sent off by the cochlea.

167. A: The eye prophylaxis for neonates that is generally the drug of choice is erythromycin to reduce the risk that the neonate will develop neonatal ophthalmia because of maternal infection with *Neisseria gonorrhoeae.* Erythromycin is effective against both gonococcal and chlamydial infections and is less irritating than silver nitrate. If the mother has had prenatal care and received a negative screening for sexually transmitted disease, the prophylaxis, although required by most states, can probably be refused with little risk to the neonate.

168. C: If air becomes trapped in the alveoli because of meconium aspiration during labor and delivery, the neonate is at risk for pneumothorax. Thick meconium staining of the amniotic fluid poses considerable risk that the fetus will aspirate and develop obstructions. During inspiration, the bronchioles dilate to accommodate air, and this usually allows air to enter the lungs, but the bronchioles contract on expiration, and this can result in air trapping. If the alveoli become too distended, they may rupture, resulting in the pneumothorax.

169. B: ABO incompatibility can occur if the mother is O and the fetus is B or A. In this case, the mother carries no antigens for A or B but has anti-A and anti-B antibodies. If the antibodies cross the placenta and enter the fetal circulation, they can cause fetal hemolysis. ABO incompatibility causes less severe problems than Rh incompatibility, but ABO incompatibility can cause problems during the first pregnancy because the anti-A and anti-b antibodies are already present.

170. C: If a neonate with Down syndrome has skin that appears mottled at times (pale in some areas and flushed in others), especially if the neonate is exposed to cool air, the most likely cause is cutis marmorata. With this disorder, the blood vessels contract and dilate at the same time. This condition is benign and resolves over time. Neonates with Down syndrome are prone to having cutis marmorata, so the parents should be advised about the condition to allay their fears.

171. A: In order for a child to be born with cystic fibrosis, an autosomal recessive disorder, both parents must carry the defective gene. When both parents carry the defective gene (carriers), then the risk that the fetus in each pregnancy will have the disease is 25% and the risk that the child will be a carrier is 50%. With most genetic disorders (but not all), carriers have no symptoms and must be detected through genetic testing.

172. C: If a neonate is born to an HIV infected mother, the neonate should begin antiretroviral medications with 6 to 12 hours. The neonate is tested (ELISA and rapid tests) within 24 hours of birth to determine if the neonate is positive with confirmatory testing carried out by DNA PCR. The neonate should take medications for the first 6 weeks, and the mother should avoid breastfeeding as there is a risk of 0.7% transmission for each month of breastfeeding.

173. C: In order to prevent intracranial hemorrhage, a neonate with thrombocytopenia requires a platelet count of at least 30,000. Thrombocytopenia in the neonate is rare but may be caused by increased rate of destruction or decreased production. Thrombocytopenia is common with neonatal infections, which increase the rate of platelet destruction. The need for platelet transfusion varies according to the condition of the neonate with stable neonates requiring transfusion at counts <25,000 and unstable <50,000.

174. B: If a neonate's mother was addicted to methamphetamine use during her pregnancy, the neonate in withdrawal will likely exhibit high-pitched crying, hyperreflexia, excessive lethargy and sleeping with abnormal sleep patterns, poor feeding, frantic fist sucking, fever, and tremors. Neonates of amphetamine-addicted mothers are usually small for gestational age and may have a small head circumference because of the vasoconstrictive effects on placental circulation and nutrition to the fetus.

175. A: Neonates who are bottle fed need to be burped every 2 to 3 ounces. Breastfed neonates should be burped after nursing on each breast. Bottle fed neonates swallow more air than breastfed neonates and need to be burped more frequently. Indications that the neonate is uncomfortable because of gas in the stomach include grimacing, squirming, regurgitating, and crying. The neonate may be burped while held on the shoulder or in sitting position.

How to Overcome Test Anxiety

Just the thought of taking a test is enough to make most people a little nervous. A test is an important event that can have a long-term impact on your future, so it's important to take it seriously and it's natural to feel anxious about performing well. But just because anxiety is normal, that doesn't mean that it's helpful in test taking, or that you should simply accept it as part of your life. Anxiety can have a variety of effects. These effects can be mild, like making you feel slightly nervous, or severe, like blocking your ability to focus or remember even a simple detail.

If you experience test anxiety—whether severe or mild—it's important to know how to beat it. To discover this, first you need to understand what causes test anxiety.

Causes of Test Anxiety

While we often think of anxiety as an uncontrollable emotional state, it can actually be caused by simple, practical things. One of the most common causes of test anxiety is that a person does not feel adequately prepared for their test. This feeling can be the result of many different issues such as poor study habits or lack of organization, but the most common culprit is time management. Starting to study too late, failing to organize your study time to cover all of the material, or being distracted while you study will mean that you're not well prepared for the test. This may lead to cramming the night before, which will cause you to be physically and mentally exhausted for the test. Poor time management also contributes to feelings of stress, fear, and hopelessness as you realize you are not well prepared but don't know what to do about it.

Other times, test anxiety is not related to your preparation for the test but comes from unresolved fear. This may be a past failure on a test, or poor performance on tests in general. It may come from comparing yourself to others who seem to be performing better or from the stress of living up to expectations. Anxiety may be driven by fears of the future—how failure on this test would affect your educational and career goals. These fears are often completely irrational, but they can still negatively impact your test performance.

Review Video: 3 Reasons You Have Test Anxiety
Visit mometrix.com/academy and enter code: 428468

Elements of Test Anxiety

As mentioned earlier, test anxiety is considered to be an emotional state, but it has physical and mental components as well. Sometimes you may not even realize that you are suffering from test anxiety until you notice the physical symptoms. These can include trembling hands, rapid heartbeat, sweating, nausea, and tense muscles. Extreme anxiety may lead to fainting or vomiting. Obviously, any of these symptoms can have a negative impact on testing. It is important to recognize them as soon as they begin to occur so that you can address the problem before it damages your performance.

Review Video: 3 Ways to Tell You Have Test Anxiety
Visit mometrix.com/academy and enter code: 927847

The mental components of test anxiety include trouble focusing and inability to remember learned information. During a test, your mind is on high alert, which can help you recall information and stay focused for an extended period of time. However, anxiety interferes with your mind's natural processes, causing you to blank out, even on the questions you know well. The strain of testing during anxiety makes it difficult to stay focused, especially on a test that may take several hours. Extreme anxiety can take a huge mental toll, making it difficult not only to recall test information but even to understand the test questions or pull your thoughts together.

Review Video: How Test Anxiety Affects Memory
Visit mometrix.com/academy and enter code: 609003

Effects of Test Anxiety

Test anxiety is like a disease—if left untreated, it will get progressively worse. Anxiety leads to poor performance, and this reinforces the feelings of fear and failure, which in turn lead to poor performances on subsequent tests. It can grow from a mild nervousness to a crippling condition. If allowed to progress, test anxiety can have a big impact on your schooling, and consequently on your future.

Test anxiety can spread to other parts of your life. Anxiety on tests can become anxiety in any stressful situation, and blanking on a test can turn into panicking in a job situation. But fortunately, you don't have to let anxiety rule your testing and determine your grades. There are a number of relatively simple steps you can take to move past anxiety and function normally on a test and in the rest of life.

Review Video: How Test Anxiety Impacts Your Grades
Visit mometrix.com/academy and enter code: 939819

Physical Steps for Beating Test Anxiety

While test anxiety is a serious problem, the good news is that it can be overcome. It doesn't have to control your ability to think and remember information. While it may take time, you can begin taking steps today to beat anxiety.

Just as your first hint that you may be struggling with anxiety comes from the physical symptoms, the first step to treating it is also physical. Rest is crucial for having a clear, strong mind. If you are tired, it is much easier to give in to anxiety. But if you establish good sleep habits, your body and mind will be ready to perform optimally, without the strain of exhaustion. Additionally, sleeping well helps you to retain information better, so you're more likely to recall the answers when you see the test questions.

Getting good sleep means more than going to bed on time. It's important to allow your brain time to relax. Take study breaks from time to time so it doesn't get overworked, and don't study right before bed. Take time to rest your mind before trying to rest your body, or you may find it difficult to fall asleep.

Review Video: The Importance of Sleep for Your Brain
Visit mometrix.com/academy and enter code: 319338

Along with sleep, other aspects of physical health are important in preparing for a test. Good nutrition is vital for good brain function. Sugary foods and drinks may give a burst of energy but this burst is followed by a crash, both physically and emotionally. Instead, fuel your body with protein and vitamin-rich foods.

Also, drink plenty of water. Dehydration can lead to headaches and exhaustion, especially if your brain is already under stress from the rigors of the test. Particularly if your test is a long one, drink water during the breaks. And if possible, take an energy-boosting snack to eat between sections.

Review Video: How Diet Can Affect your Mood
Visit mometrix.com/academy and enter code: 624317

Along with sleep and diet, a third important part of physical health is exercise. Maintaining a steady workout schedule is helpful, but even taking 5-minute study breaks to walk can help get your blood pumping faster and clear your head. Exercise also releases endorphins, which contribute to a positive feeling and can help combat test anxiety.

When you nurture your physical health, you are also contributing to your mental health. If your body is healthy, your mind is much more likely to be healthy as well. So take time to rest, nourish your body with healthy food and water, and get moving as much as possible. Taking these physical steps will make you stronger and more able to take the mental steps necessary to overcome test anxiety.

Review Video: How to Stay Healthy and Prevent Test Anxiety
Visit mometrix.com/academy and enter code: 877894

Mental Steps for Beating Test Anxiety

Working on the mental side of test anxiety can be more challenging, but as with the physical side, there are clear steps you can take to overcome it. As mentioned earlier, test anxiety often stems from lack of preparation, so the obvious solution is to prepare for the test. Effective studying may be the most important weapon you have for beating test anxiety, but you can and should employ several other mental tools to combat fear.

First, boost your confidence by reminding yourself of past success—tests or projects that you aced. If you're putting as much effort into preparing for this test as you did for those, there's no reason you should expect to fail here. Work hard to prepare; then trust your preparation.

Second, surround yourself with encouraging people. It can be helpful to find a study group, but be sure that the people you're around will encourage a positive attitude. If you spend time with others who are anxious or cynical, this will only contribute to your own anxiety. Look for others who are motivated to study hard from a desire to succeed, not from a fear of failure.

Third, reward yourself. A test is physically and mentally tiring, even without anxiety, and it can be helpful to have something to look forward to. Plan an activity following the test, regardless of the outcome, such as going to a movie or getting ice cream.

When you are taking the test, if you find yourself beginning to feel anxious, remind yourself that you know the material. Visualize successfully completing the test. Then take a few deep, relaxing breaths and return to it. Work through the questions carefully but with confidence, knowing that you are capable of succeeding.

Developing a healthy mental approach to test taking will also aid in other areas of life. Test anxiety affects more than just the actual test—it can be damaging to your mental health and even contribute to depression. It's important to beat test anxiety before it becomes a problem for more than testing.

Review Video: Test Anxiety and Depression
Visit mometrix.com/academy and enter code: 904704

Study Strategy

Being prepared for the test is necessary to combat anxiety, but what does being prepared look like? You may study for hours on end and still not feel prepared. What you need is a strategy for test prep. The next few pages outline our recommended steps to help you plan out and conquer the challenge of preparation.

Step 1: Scope Out the Test

Learn everything you can about the format (multiple choice, essay, etc.) and what will be on the test. Gather any study materials, course outlines, or sample exams that may be available. Not only will this help you to prepare, but knowing what to expect can help to alleviate test anxiety.

Step 2: Map Out the Material

Look through the textbook or study guide and make note of how many chapters or sections it has. Then divide these over the time you have. For example, if a book has 15 chapters and you have five days to study, you need to cover three chapters each day. Even better, if you have the time, leave an extra day at the end for overall review after you have gone through the material in depth.

If time is limited, you may need to prioritize the material. Look through it and make note of which sections you think you already have a good grasp on, and which need review. While you are studying, skim quickly through the familiar sections and take more time on the challenging parts. Write out your plan so you don't get lost as you go. Having a written plan also helps you feel more in control of the study, so anxiety is less likely to arise from feeling overwhelmed at the amount to cover.

Step 3: Gather Your Tools

Decide what study method works best for you. Do you prefer to highlight in the book as you study and then go back over the highlighted portions? Or do you type out notes of the important information? Or is it helpful to make flashcards that you can carry with you? Assemble the pens, index cards, highlighters, post-it notes, and any other materials you may need so you won't be distracted by getting up to find things while you study.

If you're having a hard time retaining the information or organizing your notes, experiment with different methods. For example, try color-coding by subject with colored pens, highlighters, or post-it notes. If you learn better by hearing, try recording yourself reading your notes so you can listen while in the car, working out, or simply sitting at your desk. Ask a friend to quiz you from your flashcards, or try teaching someone the material to solidify it in your mind.

Step 4: Create Your Environment

It's important to avoid distractions while you study. This includes both the obvious distractions like visitors and the subtle distractions like an uncomfortable chair (or a too-comfortable couch that makes you want to fall asleep). Set up the best study environment possible: good lighting and a comfortable work area. If background music helps you focus, you may want to turn it on, but otherwise keep the room quiet. If you are using a computer to take notes, be sure you don't have any other windows open, especially applications like social media, games, or anything else that could distract you. Silence your phone and turn off notifications. Be sure to keep water close by so you stay hydrated while you study (but avoid unhealthy drinks and snacks).

Also, take into account the best time of day to study. Are you freshest first thing in the morning? Try to set aside some time then to work through the material. Is your mind clearer in the afternoon or evening? Schedule your study session then. Another method is to study at the same time of day that you will take the test, so that your brain gets used to working on the material at that time and will be ready to focus at test time.

Step 5: Study!

Once you have done all the study preparation, it's time to settle into the actual studying. Sit down, take a few moments to settle your mind so you can focus, and begin to follow your study plan. Don't give in to distractions or let yourself procrastinate. This is your time to prepare so you'll be ready to fearlessly approach the test. Make the most of the time and stay focused.

Of course, you don't want to burn out. If you study too long you may find that you're not retaining the information very well. Take regular study breaks. For example, taking five minutes out of every hour to walk briskly, breathing deeply and swinging your arms, can help your mind stay fresh.

As you get to the end of each chapter or section, it's a good idea to do a quick review. Remind yourself of what you learned and work on any difficult parts. When you feel that you've mastered the material, move on to the next part. At the end of your study session, briefly skim through your notes again.

But while review is helpful, cramming last minute is NOT. If at all possible, work ahead so that you won't need to fit all your study into the last day. Cramming overloads your brain with more information than it can process and retain, and your tired mind may struggle to recall even previously learned information when it is overwhelmed with last-minute study. Also, the urgent nature of cramming and the stress placed on your brain contribute to anxiety. You'll be more likely to go to the test feeling unprepared and having trouble thinking clearly.

So don't cram, and don't stay up late before the test, even just to review your notes at a leisurely pace. Your brain needs rest more than it needs to go over the information again. In fact, plan to finish your studies by noon or early afternoon the day before the test. Give your brain the rest of the day to relax or focus on other things, and get a good night's sleep. Then you will be fresh for the test and better able to recall what you've studied.

Step 6: Take a practice test

Many courses offer sample tests, either online or in the study materials. This is an excellent resource to check whether you have mastered the material, as well as to prepare for the test format and environment.

Check the test format ahead of time: the number of questions, the type (multiple choice, free response, etc.), and the time limit. Then create a plan for working through them. For example, if you have 30 minutes to take a 60-question test, your limit is 30 seconds per question. Spend less time on the questions you know well so that you can take more time on the difficult ones.

If you have time to take several practice tests, take the first one open book, with no time limit. Work through the questions at your own pace and make sure you fully understand them. Gradually work up to taking a test under test conditions: sit at a desk with all study materials put away and set a timer. Pace yourself to make sure you finish the test with time to spare and go back to check your answers if you have time.

After each test, check your answers. On the questions you missed, be sure you understand why you missed them. Did you misread the question (tests can use tricky wording)? Did you forget the information? Or was it something you hadn't learned? Go back and study any shaky areas that the practice tests reveal.

Taking these tests not only helps with your grade, but also aids in combating test anxiety. If you're already used to the test conditions, you're less likely to worry about it, and working through tests until you're scoring well gives you a confidence boost. Go through the practice tests until you feel comfortable, and then you can go into the test knowing that you're ready for it.

Test Tips

On test day, you should be confident, knowing that you've prepared well and are ready to answer the questions. But aside from preparation, there are several test day strategies you can employ to maximize your performance.

First, as stated before, get a good night's sleep the night before the test (and for several nights before that, if possible). Go into the test with a fresh, alert mind rather than staying up late to study.

Try not to change too much about your normal routine on the day of the test. It's important to eat a nutritious breakfast, but if you normally don't eat breakfast at all, consider eating just a protein bar. If you're a coffee drinker, go ahead and have your normal coffee. Just make sure you time it so that the caffeine doesn't wear off right in the middle of your test. Avoid sugary beverages, and drink enough water to stay hydrated but not so much that you need a restroom break 10 minutes into the test. If your test isn't first thing in the morning, consider going for a walk or doing a light workout before the test to get your blood flowing.

Allow yourself enough time to get ready, and leave for the test with plenty of time to spare so you won't have the anxiety of scrambling to arrive in time. Another reason to be early is to select a good seat. It's helpful to sit away from doors and windows, which can be distracting. Find a good seat, get out your supplies, and settle your mind before the test begins.

When the test begins, start by going over the instructions carefully, even if you already know what to expect. Make sure you avoid any careless mistakes by following the directions.

Then begin working through the questions, pacing yourself as you've practiced. If you're not sure on an answer, don't spend too much time on it, and don't let it shake your confidence. Either skip it and come back later, or eliminate as many wrong answers as possible and guess among the remaining ones. Don't dwell on these questions as you continue—put them out of your mind and focus on what lies ahead.

Be sure to read all of the answer choices, even if you're sure the first one is the right answer. Sometimes you'll find a better one if you keep reading. But don't second-guess yourself if you do immediately know the answer. Your gut instinct is usually right. Don't let test anxiety rob you of the information you know.

If you have time at the end of the test (and if the test format allows), go back and review your answers. Be cautious about changing any, since your first instinct tends to be correct, but make sure you didn't misread any of the questions or accidentally mark the wrong answer choice. Look over any you skipped and make an educated guess.

At the end, leave the test feeling confident. You've done your best, so don't waste time worrying about your performance or wishing you could change anything. Instead, celebrate the successful completion of this test. And finally, use this test to learn how to deal with anxiety even better next time.

Review Video: 5 Tips to Beat Test Anxiety
Visit mometrix.com/academy and enter code: 570656

Important Qualification

Not all anxiety is created equal. If your test anxiety is causing major issues in your life beyond the classroom or testing center, or if you are experiencing troubling physical symptoms related to your anxiety, it may be a sign of a serious physiological or psychological condition. If this sounds like your situation, we strongly encourage you to seek professional help.

Thank You

We at Mometrix would like to extend our heartfelt thanks to you, our friend and patron, for allowing us to play a part in your journey. It is a privilege to serve people from all walks of life who are unified in their commitment to building the best future they can for themselves.

The preparation you devote to these important testing milestones may be the most valuable educational opportunity you have for making a real difference in your life. We encourage you to put your heart into it—that feeling of succeeding, overcoming, and yes, conquering will be well worth the hours you've invested.

We want to hear your story, your struggles and your successes, and if you see any opportunities for us to improve our materials so we can help others even more effectively in the future, please share that with us as well. **The team at Mometrix would be absolutely thrilled to hear from you!** So please, send us an email (support@mometrix.com) and let's stay in touch.

If you'd like some additional help, check out these other resources we offer for your exam:
http://mometrixflashcards.com/MaternalNewborn

Additional Bonus Material

Due to our efforts to try to keep this book to a manageable length, we've created a link that will give you access to all of your additional bonus material.

Please visit
http://www.mometrix.com/bonus948/matnewnurse to access the information.